MW01132059

MADNESS

SRTD

STUDIES IN RELIGION, THEOLOGY, AND DISABILITY

SERIES EDITORS

Sarah J. Melcher
Xavier University (Cincinnati, Ohio)

and

Amos Yong
Fuller Theological Seminary (Pasadena, California)

MADNESS

American Protestant Responses
to Mental Illness

— Heather H. Vacek —

BAYLOR UNIVERSITY PRESS

Unless otherwise stated, Scripture quotations are from the New Revised Standard Version Bible, copyright 1989, Division of Christian Education of the National Council of the Churches of Christ in the United States of America. Used by permission. All rights reserved.

Cover Design by Kara Davison, Faceout Studio
Cover Image: "Contracture Provoquée," from Paul Regnard, *Sorcellerie Magnétisme, Morphinisme Délire des Grandeurs* (Paris: E. Plon, 1887).

Library of Congress Cataloging-in-Publication Data

Madness : American Protestant responses to mental illness / Heather H. Vacek.
  283 pages cm
  Includes bibliographical references and index.
  ISBN 978-1-4813-0057-5 (hardback : alk. paper)
1. Mental illness—Religious aspects—Christianity. 2. Protestantism—United States—History. I. Vacek, Heather H., 1969–
  BT732.4.M285 2015
  261.8'3220973—dc23

                              2014048047

For Gary, Luke, Mom, and Dad

and

all who navigate mental illness

Series Introduction

Studies in Religion, Theology, and Disability brings newly established and emerging scholars together to explore issues at the intersection of religion, theology, and disability. The series editors encourage theoretical engagement with secular disability studies while supporting the reexamination of established religious doctrine and practice. The series fosters research that takes account of the voices of people with disabilities and the voices of their family and friends.

The volumes in the series address issues and concerns of the global religious studies/theological studies academy. Authors come from a variety of religious traditions with diverse perspectives to reflect on the intersection of the study of religion/theology and the human experience of disability. This series is intentional about seeking out and publishing books that engage with disability in dialogue with Jewish, Christian, Buddhist, or other religious and philosophical perspectives.

Themes explored include religious life, ethics, doctrine, proclamation, liturgical practices, physical space, spirituality, or the interpretation of sacred texts through the lens of disability. Authors in the series are aware of conversation in the field of disability studies and bring that discussion to bear methodologically and theoretically in their analyses at the intersection of religion and disability.

Studies in Religion, Theology, and Disability reflects the following developments in the field: First, the emergence of disability studies as an interdisciplinary endeavor that has impacted theological studies, broadly defined. More and more scholars are deploying disability perspectives in their work, and this applies also to those working in the theological academy. Second, there is a growing need for critical reflection on disability in world religions. While books from a Christian standpoint have dominated the discussion at the interface of religion and disability so far, Jewish, Muslim, Buddhist, and Hindu scholars, among those from other religious traditions, have begun to resource their own religious traditions to rethink disability in the twenty-first century. Third, passage of the Americans with Disabilities Act in the U.S.A. has raised the consciousness of the general public about the importance of critical reflection on disability in religious communities. General and intelligent lay readers are looking for scholarly discussions of religion and disability as these bring together and address two of the most important existential aspects of human lives. Fourth, the work of activists in the disability rights movement has mandated fresh critical reflection by religious practitioners and theologians. Persons with disabilities remain the most disaffected group from religious organizations. Fifth, government representatives in several countries have prioritized the greater social inclusion of persons with disabilities. Disability policy often proceeds based on core cultural and worldview assumptions that are religiously informed. Work at the interface of religion and disability thus could have much broader purchase—that is, in social, economic, political, and legal domains.

Under the general topic of thoughtful reflection on the religious understanding of disability, Studies in Religion, Theology, and Disability includes shorter, crisply argued volumes that articulate a bold vision within a field; longer scholarly monographs, more fully developed and meticulously documented, with the same goal of engaging wider conversations; textbooks that provide a state of the discussion at this intersection and chart constructive ways forward; and select edited volumes that achieve one or more of the preceding goals.

Contents

Acknowledgments

I'm grateful for the many communities that have sustained and inspired me throughout this project. Lori Anne Bowen, Hannah McManus, Philip Shoe, and Kathryn Broyles offered friendship and support and, once upon a time, helped convince me that writing and teaching would be part of my future. Rebekah Eklund, Liz DeGaynor, Kate Bowler, Mandy McMichael, Mindy Makant, Wen Reagan, Brendan Pietsch, Angela Tarango, Denise Thorpe, Melanie Dobson, Celia Wolff, SueJeanne Koh, and Jeff Conklin-Miller proved to be joyful and encouraging companions, as did the wider Duke Divinity Th.D. and American Religious History communities. Susan Dunlap and Tammy Williams helped deepen my theological convictions about suffering and prompted me to want to research and write in response.

The people of Raleigh Moravian Church formed a cheering section much too large to name individually. They sustained me by the provision of love, food, fellowship, friendship, and song. I am especially thankful for the grounding presence of Pam Fishel, Mary Evelyn Jackman, Diane Murphy, Steve Reavis, Fran Saylor, and Craig Troutman. The broader Moravian world also offered support, including students, fellow trustees, faculty, and staff at Moravian Theological Seminary. Kelly Moore's shared passion for the subject of this book helped anchor the project, and her gift of friendship offered a lifeline on more than one occasion.

Many of the historical and theological questions that prompted my research emerged during my time as a student and volunteer chaplain at John Umstead Hospital in Butner, North Carolina. There, Marion Thullbery provided the sort of intentional wisdom and guidance—paired with pastoral concern for patients and students—that allowed my questions to solidify.

The following individuals read drafts of this volume, and I'm thankful for their insight. Amy Laura Hall nurtured my interest in theology and ethics of disability and mental illness and helped me ask bold, brave questions. Mary McClintock Fulkerson and Bonnie Miller-McLemore modeled the sort of scholarship and teaching that engages the church, the world, and the academy that I hope to produce. I am grateful to Mark Chaves for his careful reading and tough questions. Allen Verhey's gracious theological treatment of tough topics shaped my thinking. Together, these are scholars whose own work I benefited from encountering and whose questions, critique, and support I am glad to have received.

I've cherished the insight and companionship of fellow grantees at the Louisville Institute in Louisville, Kentucky, and of treasured colleagues in Crawfordsville, Indiana, during my time as a member of the 2013–2014 Teaching and Learning Workshop for Pre-Tenure Theological School Faculty at the Wabash Center for Teaching and Learning in Theology and Religion. My colleagues at Pittsburgh Theological Seminary have formed yet another rich community of scholarship and friendship. My writing-group companions—Leanna Fuller, Angela Hancock, Roger Owens, Jannie Swart, and Lisa Thompson—cheered me on during the final months of editing. Kathy Anderson's expert assistance made life at PTS easier in countless ways. Trent Hancock's help with the index was invaluable.

I might not be a historian without the initial nudge and the mentorship of Grant Wacker, and I'm grateful for his invitation and welcome to the guild. Grant affirmed the importance of this project from its earliest stages. The best gift I could offer Grant in return (beyond avoiding split infinitives and steering clear of other grammatical foibles) would be to produce well-researched, meaningful, and accessible history. I hope this volume offers a good start. First Grant, and later Carey Newman at Baylor University Press, challenged me to make the book better than I knew it could be. Carey's tutelage was helpful in shaping the manuscript into a final product. I'm indebted to both Grant and Carey.

My family receives my deepest thanks. From my parents, Ralph and Louise Hartung, I inherited a curiosity about the world, a love of learning, and the discipline and encouragement to tackle big projects. I am grateful to my husband, Gary, and my son, Luke, for their constant presence and love during the years this project took shape. While this is my book, it was our life together that made it possible, and for that, I am tremendously grateful.

Heather H. Vacek
July 2014

Introduction

Christianity and Mental Illness

In the early twenty-first century, every year one in four adults in the United States suffered from a diagnosable mental illness, and severe mental illnesses afflicted 6 percent of the population. Children suffered too—20 percent of teenagers lived with a serious mental disorder in a given year.[1] Mental maladies struck individuals of all ages, races, religions, incomes, educational levels, and upbringings. Despite the prevalence of mental illness, sufferers often hid their distress or were shunned when diagnoses or symptoms became public.

While treatments were available, not everyone sought help, and some died. In 2007, for example, nearly thirty-five thousand Americans took their own lives, making suicide the tenth leading cause of death. While tens of thousands lost their lives, even more came close—twelve reports of intentional self-harm occurred for every death.[2] More than 90 percent of those committing suicide experienced depression, other mental disorders, substance abuse, or some combination thereof. Yet, even after centuries of medical attention, public conversation about mental illness proved limited, and causes remained as mysterious as cures. Despite their widespread presence, those ailments continued to spark misunderstanding and fear. Sufferers faced stigmatization, and as a result, individuals and families often kept illness quiet and suffered in isolation, compounding the pain.

Christian responses proved no exception to the pattern of concealment and inattention. Mental illnesses in congregations often remained out of sight, whether purposely hidden or silently ignored. That "sufferers, their families, and the community [were] more likely to interpret [mental illnesses] in moral and religious terms" than they would with physical ailments shaped decisions to keep illness hidden.[3] The use of secular, instead of spiritual, treatments for mental distress prompted questions and concerns among believers. Even homeless Americans—who constituted the nation's largest population of mentally ill individuals—received mostly physical care from Christian churches.[4] Believers readily fed and clothed homeless men and women but did so largely without attention to their mental health.

The Christian tradition always included concern for health and healing. The biblical narrative recounted that Jesus Christ restored sight to the blind, enabled the lame to walk, and drove demons out of the possessed. His disciples carried on this work, and for thousands of years healing and wholeness for body, mind, and spirit were embedded in Christian belief and practice. Christianity promised physical and spiritual help in the face of distress, and followers of Christ focused not only on their own health but also on caring for others.[5] Given a deeply ingrained focus on healing, inattention to mental illness proved ironic.

Curious about connections between faith and health, late twentieth-century researchers probed connections between religion and mental distress. Studies suggested that religious belief and participation contributed to mental health.[6] Yet, as Kathryn Greene-McCreight—a clergywoman, theologian, and sufferer—noted, studies like these often made the sick feel worse. Faced with the perception that Christians should feel happy and full of joy, the afflicted often felt "guilty on top of being depressed, because they [understood] their depression, their lack of thankfulness, their desperation, to be a betrayal of God."[7] Participation in a church community might offer relief or bring condemnation, and ambivalence marked the reception sufferers encountered in religious communities.

Christian avoidance of mental distress proved ironic and, at times, grievous. In the late 1960s, for example, an ordained Presbyterian elder divulged his experiences with the church and his wife's mental illness but did so pseudonymously. "Jim Bryan," his wife, and their three children belonged to six congregations as they moved around the country. His wife's repeated hospitalizations with bouts of severe depression made life difficult in each church. When illness struck, word of the cause of her hospitalization spread, and Jim encountered what he named the "Nervous Glance" followed by "Pained Silence" from other parishioners. "The news of mental illness—depression, nervous breakdown, or psychosis of any kind," he recalled, swept "through the grapevine overnight."

"Faithful churchgoers," Jim observed with a dose of sarcasm, "who, I'm sure always take the log out of their own eyes before looking for specks in the eyes of their brothers, tend to close both eyes tightly and pretend that mental illness just doesn't exist." Jim reported that in some congregations, "four or five hospitalizations because of mental illness have gone unreported in church literature, unmentioned from church pulpits, and unprayed for during worship services." In contrast, he observed, "you quickly qualify for each of these if you happen to be injured in an automobile accident." As his family suffered, they usually failed to receive support or acknowledgment from fellow congregants. Even their minister struggled to offer more than a hesitant, "Jim . . . how are things?"

Stigma and fear, Jim realized, prompted silence and avoidance. They also inhibited the care the family desired. In the face of mental illness, Jim lamented that not just the congregations they joined but also the larger church had "failed in her educational and healing ministry." Some Christians, he noticed, were "still under the unfortunate illusion, a remnant of the Dark Ages, that mental illness is the sign of divine judgment for past sin." Other illnesses escaped similar theological diagnosis.[8]

Human suffering concerned American Christians, but not all shapes of distress earned the same response. Beginning in the colonial era, Protestants professed to care for the well-being of bodies, minds, and souls, but those living with mental illnesses often received minimal attention. Developing over three centuries, two distinct forces combined to inhibit Protestants' ability to fulfill their stated mission of caring for the whole person. Most significantly, shifting professionalization sequestered clerical (and lay Christian) authority in the private, spiritual sphere, leaving healing—physical and mental—as the responsibility of secular medical professionals. In addition, the social stigma surrounding mental illness deepened, making Protestants reluctant to engage sufferers lest they be tainted by association. Stigma emerged both from rising confidence in humankind's ability to solve problems and the persistence of theological notions that linked mental maladies with sin. Stigma linked mental maladies with weakness and deviance in ways that prompted avoidance. Those who suffered seemed at fault for their illness. Attentive to professionalization and stigma, this book traces the history of Protestant reactions to mental illness in America over three centuries. Though Christian inattention to mental illness formed the general pattern, five exceptions to the rule of benign neglect exemplify Protestant involvement and form the basis for theological reflection about ongoing Christian practice.[9]

Over three centuries, Americans defined diseases of the mind in many ways and did so from practical, spiritual, and medical perspectives. Distraction. Possession. Madness. Melancholy. Insanity. Mental illness. Often, terms that in one era were descriptive (such as insanity) turned pejorative in the next. By the nineteenth century, medical labels had joined—and often supplanted—descriptive and spiritual assessments. The most customary descriptions in each period indicated presumptions about the causes of illness and the professional groups that claimed authority to define and treat mental distress. "Possession," for example, popular before the rise of scientific medicine, reflected religious assessments of demonic forces at work in individuals. "Dementia praecox" or the more modern "schizophrenia" displayed definition by a medical establishment.[10] I deploy a variety of names for the experience of human suffering addressed in this volume. The labels reflect culturally specific experiences of mental ailments and include the following: madness, malady, insanity, distress, disorder, dysfunction, and illness. Whenever possible, I use the terminology that was normative in the period under study. I consider all of those ailments as "mental maladies," a term used as an umbrella categorization with spiritual, organic, medical, and sometimes moral components. "Malady" reflects the experience of those that suffered— they first suffered with symptoms such as depression, mania, visions, or anxiety. Only later did professionals classify those symptoms as disorder or illness.[11]

In America, care for the mentally ill changed dramatically from colonial times through the twentieth century, and not always for the better. The sick and their families, municipalities, medical professionals, clergy, and fellow citizens interacted to shape the provision of care, and responses evolved as the world around them changed. Chapters 1–5 offer a history of Protestant reactions to mental illness in the years between 1700 and 1980. Those chapters focus on five paradigmatic Protestants who professed interest in mental health: Cotton Mather, Benjamin Rush, Dorothea Dix, Anton Boisen, and Karl Menninger. Amidst widespread neglect of mental illness by Christians, those figures demonstrate both the range and the progression of attentive Protestant responses in a rapidly shifting medical, social, and religious landscape.

In chapter 1, the Puritan clergyman Cotton Mather's (1663–1728) story offers a case study of early pastoral authority on health and healing and presents theological assessments of illness during the colonial era. In chapter 2, the work of Benjamin Rush (1746–1813), a trained physician with Calvinist roots, highlights the initial professionalization of medicine in newly independent America and displays attempts to define and systematize the diagnosis and treatment of mental maladies as medical concerns. Those chapters show the slow, although incomplete, transfer of authority from clergy to medical professionals.

In spite of that shift, Protestants continued to fight for a caregiving role. Following the creation of the first American institutions offering dedicated care for the mentally ill, the public advocacy of the Unitarian Dorothea Dix (1802–1887) during the nineteenth century showed Christian outrage over inhumane treatment of the insane, particularly the indigent insane. By the turn of the twentieth century, Anton Boisen (1876–1965), a Presbyterian clergyman and seminary professor who spent time institutionalized as the result of mental illness, presented a plea to churches to train clergy to offer better care for those living with mental maladies. That move marked Protestant attempts to reclaim authority lost to medical professionals. The advocacy of Dix and Boisen appear in chapters 3 and 4.

After World War I, Karl Menninger (1893–1990)—the most revered American psychiatrist of the twentieth century, and a lifelong Presbyterian—appeared as the central figure at the intersection of medicine, the church, and mental illness. The Kansas physician's medical practice and public presence spanned nearly seventy years. For the betterment of the world, Menninger drew together scientific knowledge, deep compassion, his Calvinist sense of vocation, and a dose of Christian realism. Tireless, he offered an active Christian witness in the face of mental maladies. Few other twentieth-century Protestants, though, achieved Menninger's level of involvement. His life and work form the focus of chapter 5.[12]

Despite their differences, Mather, Rush, Dix, Boisen, and Menninger each responded to mental affliction with a sense of moral obligation and Christian duty, and all, implicitly or explicitly, claimed theological authority as they defined and addressed suffering. They also appealed to a mix of medical, scientific, moral, and clerical authority, depending on their professions and experiences. As those five Protestants reacted, they assumed that their assessments and solutions should apply to all individuals and in all cases; they considered their claims normative.

The historical chapters profile theological and practical assessments and place the work of five believers in a larger context that included prevailing understandings of madness, the state of medicine, commonly prescribed treatments for mental illness, the availability of institutional care, and social factors that shaped understandings of mental maladies. While the church lost its place as the primary authority in diagnosing the nature of suffering caused by insanity, some Christians refused to abdicate the provision of care for mental maladies to secular sources.

During the country's progression from a colonial outpost in the late 1600s to a world power in the 1950s—a period otherwise marked by tremendous ecclesial growth and institution building—the church, and particularly clergy, struggled to compete with outside authorities for the provision of care for mental illness. As urbanization, advances in science, the professionalization of medicine, population growth, the creation of institutions for the insane, and Enlightenment optimism about the possibility of a cure converged, Protestant clergy lost their position as sole providers of care and lone experts in the definition of mental ailments. Despite those changes, individual Christians, lay and ordained alike, continued to stake a claim to the solution.

Having outlined shifting lines of professional authority and traced how social stigma inhibited Protestant responses to mental distress, the concluding chapter offers a theological assessment in light of historical practice. It investigates Christian hospitality as an antidote to stymied reactions in hope of countering stigma and clearing the way for more faithful and attentive care for the suffering stemming from mental maladies. In total, this volume explores the past in order to shed light on the present; it engages history to strengthen theology and ongoing practice.[13]

The exploration of Protestants and mental illness demonstrates what appeared—and failed to appear—on congregational agendas. It also offers insight into how Christians engaged suffering, particularly seemingly intractable suffering. Within congregations, sufferers and their families struggled to voice their concerns about mental illness. Many simply remained silent and failed to receive the ministrations of the church. This volume explores why their journeys proved so difficult.

1

Making Theological Sense out of Suffering, Sin, and Sickness

Cotton Mather

> The Design of all this Essay, is to Lead the Reader unto HIM. . . .
> The Cure of a Sin-Sick SOUL, is that all Invalids ought to reckon
> their Grand Concern. . . . "Adverse health, the threat to and death of
> members of the body is considered rather terrible. But of all things
> which can happen to man, the worst is illness or loss of the mind. If
> we seek so diligently for medication for the sick body, why not with
> greater care work hard to find what cures and revives the mind?"
>
> —Cotton Mather, 1724[1]

In the winter of 1703, Cotton Mather lingered beside his wife's deathbed. Falling ill after a miscarriage, Abigail Phillips Mather had hovered near death for months. As spring approached, the smallpox epidemic that infected many Bostonians and afflicted Mather's children and neighbors settled into the already weakened body of his beloved wife. Navigating the epidemic as both a minister and the head of a household, Mather recalled the weight of providing care. "The little Creatures," he wrote of his sick children, "keep calling for me so often to pray with them, that I can scarce do it less than ten or a dozen times in a day; besides what I do with my Neighbors."[2] His children's suffering troubled the clergyman, and paying pastoral visits kept him busy. "But the most exquisite of my Trials," he confessed, "was the Condition of my lovely Consort." As his wife lay in the "Pangs of Death," the minister offered spiritual preparation for the transition to the world to come and comforted her with "lively Discourses upon the Glory of Heaven."[3] Concern for her soul shaped Mather's care, but so did marital devotion. "Two Hours before my lovely Consort expired," he recalled, "I kneeled by her Bed-Side,

and I took into my two Hands, a dear Hand, the dearest in the World. With
her then in my Hands, I solemnly and sincerely gave her up unto the Lord;
and in token of my real RESIGNATION, I gently putt her out of my Hands,
and laid away a most lovely Hand, resolving that I would never touch it any
more!"⁴ Illness and death were constants in Mather's life. Both physical and
mental ailments caused distress for those he cared for, and agonized wrestling with human suffering appeared throughout his diary. The musings
prompted by such episodes reveal another side of the colonial leader often
remembered as an inflexible and sanctimonious Puritan.⁵ They also offer
insight into Protestant views of illness in colonial America.

Cotton Mather (1663–1728) held a keen curiosity about the natural world
that, alongside deep Christian faith, shaped his interest in health and healing.
Thirteen of Mather's fifteen children preceded him in death; illness took the
lives of his first and second wives. His third wife suffered debilitating mental torment that often manifested in violent outbursts toward Mather.⁶ The
clergyman's inquisitiveness about sickness and healing arose not only from
observing illness in those he loved but also from his desire to rid himself of a
physical ailment—a stammer.⁷ His efforts grew, too, from a desire to make
sense of suffering and evil. Exploring sickness and investigating remedies
connected his faith to existential hardships. Primarily, though, as a devout
Puritan, he investigated health and disease to understand better God's good
creation. Mental illness proved part of that exploration.

Mather found the investigation of mental distress particularly important, and he attended to madness practically, scientifically, and theologically.
"If we seek so diligently for medication for the sick body," the clergyman
wondered, citing a Dutch physician, "why not with greater care work hard
to find what cures and revives the mind?"⁸ The melancholy of his parishioners, the "distraction" of fellow ministers, illness among his household staff,
and his third wife's outbursts all shaped the leading New Englander's perceptions of mental distress. Science proved a tool for deepening practical and
theological understandings. Rather than viewing faith and reason as separate
realms, Puritans like Mather saw both as gifts from a gracious God, gifts
to be deployed simultaneously.⁹ Within that unity of knowledge, Mather
worked hard to demonstrate scientific and theological connections. Deeper
comprehension of the natural world, he hoped, would bring closer communion with God's will, for himself and all New Englanders.¹⁰

The third-generation Puritan minister and theologian descended from
one of the most prominent families in colonial New England.¹¹ After graduating from Harvard College, Mather served Second Church (Old North)
in Boston, preaching weekly to the largest congregation in the colonies. In

June of 1690, at age twenty-seven, he was the youngest man elected a Fellow of Harvard College. A prolific writer, he published more than 450 works on a wide variety of subjects, including a history of the colonies, commentary on political developments, an exploration of witchcraft, a reconciliation of theology and science, and medical advice.[12] The sources for Mather's works proved as broad as his subjects, and in that written legacy, Mather drew from European and ancient intellectual traditions. In 1710, for example, the minister populated his brief *Essays to Do Good* with insight from Scripture, early Christian apologists, and theologians of the European Reformation.[13] He also reached beyond Christian sources for the volume, drawing on legal theory, the philosophy of Socrates, and the ancient Greek physician Hippocrates. With good reason, and like his Puritan forebearers, Mather claimed broad authority, and his opinions reached far. While his fellow colonists did not agree with him on all subjects, he serves as an authoritative colonial voice in a number of areas, including on matters of religion and health.

Mather's faith, ministry, and intellectual pursuits developed under the umbrella of American Puritan religious, intellectual, and social convictions. A theology anchored in the notion of covenant framed all aspects of Puritan life. God, colonial Calvinists asserted, covenanted to redeem humanity. Humans, in response to God's gracious act of salvation in Christ, covenanted to live in proper relationship with God and in mutual obligation to one another. For individual believers, this meant that true faith involved a daily obedience to the Law of God given in Scripture, and a continual effort to remedy sinfulness.[14] A sense of God's sovereignty and providence figured prominently in that covenantal framework. All aspects of life fell within bounds of the covenants, and believers viewed successes and failures as either divine blessings or punishment. Each appeared as just rewards for human actions. That Puritan theological backdrop prompted both Mather's inquiry and shaped his understanding of the suffering brought by illness.[15]

In the final years of his life, Mather compiled a medical journal, *The Angel of Bethesda*. Written in 1724 and published posthumously, the text ranked as the only comprehensive medical volume in the colonial period.[16] In it, he explored causes and cures for scores of ailments, including mental maladies. Always focused on the divine, the minister's medical account was interspersed with assertions of God's sovereignty and God's ability to heal. Mather viewed sickness and health in light of his Christian beliefs, and he entwined theological and medical observations. He laced theological writings with images of disease, and he mixed discussions of health with prayers. The prominent intellectual assumed that attending to one's own health and the welfare of others constituted part of a Christian life.

That a clergyman authored a medical volume shows the authoritative role religious leaders played in a wide range of arenas during the colonial era. Mather's work looms large in Puritan thought, an intellectual and religious tradition that shaped how Americans viewed the world around them in coming centuries, including issues of health and disease. More specifically, Mather's theological reflections about mental illness featured many of the presuppositions of later Protestant thought about illness. His work included assertions of the role of sin (original and individual) in sickness; it evinced a concern with the state of one's soul; and it also betrayed belief in supernatural causes of mental disease. Within a century and a half after Mather's lifetime, Americans defined madness as more a medical than a spiritual problem, but suspicions of supernatural influence persisted. The colonial-era minister attempted to claim mental disturbances as valid religious concerns.[17] Integrating medical and spiritual matters, his work displayed presumed connections between disturbances of the body, mind, and soul. Unlike later believers, Mather embraced scientific theory without forfeiting a sense of God's sovereignty. As a result, within the context of colonial health and healing, Mather's story offers a telling example of early American thought about sickness in general and mental illness in particular.

From the colonial era on, Americans attributed mental maladies to a combination of supernatural, moral, and medical causes. While the balance of those factors shifted over time, all three elements were present in Mather's assessment. When faced with mental distress, in the centuries after Mather's death, American Protestants debated the right relationship between the authority of science and medicine on one hand and religious and spiritual healing on the other. They explored theological and medical diagnoses, and assessed religious and medical cures. As they did so, prevailing social norms shaped their conclusions. Mather's thought introduces the basic components of an exploration that continued in the following centuries.

MADNESS AND MELANCHOLY:
A DISMAL SPECTACLE!

In February of 1724, Mather's diary marked the completion of *The Angel of Bethesda*. He prayed (with characteristic immodesty) that the volume might "prove one of the most useful Books that have been written in the World."[18] He drew the title of his comprehensive medical treatise from a New Testament passage about the healing power of Jesus Christ:

> Now in Jerusalem by the Sheep Gate there is a pool, called in Hebrew Bethesda, which has five porticoes. In these lay many invalids—blind, lame, and

paralyzed. One man was there who had been ill for thirty-eight years. When Jesus saw him lying there and knew that he had been there a long time, he said to him, "Do you want to be made well?" The sick man answered him, "Sir, I have no one to put me into the pool when the water is stirred up; and while I am making my way, someone else steps down ahead of me." Jesus said to him, "Stand up, take your mat and walk." At once the man was made well, and he took up his mat and began to walk. (John 5:2-9, NRSV)

Mather called his *The Angel of Bethesda* "an ESSAY upon the Common Maladies of Mankind," and, in it, he implored Christians to care for their teeth, bodies, and minds, all gifts from God. By combining scientific wisdom, theological reflection, and practical advice, the preacher hoped the volume would bring believers to the pool of healing.

Spanning more than sixty chapters, Mather's account described the symptoms of and offered remedies for a variety of ailments including vertigo, gout, intestinal worms, toothaches, and sore throats.[19] His advice spanned "lesser inconveniences" ("To Fasten the Teeth, Chew Mastick, often"; "For a Stinking Breath, Wash the Mouth often with a Decoction of *Myrrh* in Water"; "To take out the Marks of Gunpowder, Shott into the *Skin*, Take fresh *Cow-dung*, and having warmed it a Little, apply it as a thin Poultis, to the Part affected") as well as life-threatening conditions like smallpox and consumption (tuberculosis).[20] The volume drew from an extensive collection of contemporary and ancient medical literature, and a combination of folk and medical wisdom filled its pages. Most chapters noted treatments to relieve suffering, but a handful addressed prevention and the general maintenance of good health.[21]

Mather's attention to mental illness appeared in chapters on "Madness" and "Melancholy." The space allotted to those two afflictions demonstrated that he found mental disorders as worthy of attention as physical ailments. The minister's account described the symptoms of mania and melancholy briefly; it then speculated about causes and turned to recommended treatments. Missing in his presentation was any attempt to justify the reality of those conditions, indicating that defining madness and melancholy as illness evidently offered no challenge for his audience.[22]

In his brief characterization, Mather named madness a "DISMAL Spectacle!" He set it in contrast to human reason and compared the "calamity" of madness to "reason" and "enlightenment." The minister pointed to God as the gracious giver of those more rational powers and rued the presence of disordered thought and action. Madness, he observed, caused "Raging," "Shatter'd *Ideas* in the *Brain*," and "a Confused Manner."[23] Though he failed to explain the connection between cognitive and physical aspects of madness, his assessment made clear that he recognized both. Mental manifestations could inflict bodily effect, including "Extraordinary Strength in the Limbs, . . . Patience of Cold, and other Inconveniences."[24] Even without offering much descriptive detail, Mather made clear that madness affected sufferers deeply.

The clergyman offered a more thorough description of melancholy. With the "Distemper" of melancholy, he noted "the *System of our Spirits*, comes to be dulled, and sowred." He characterized sufferers as serious, sad, miserable, and thoughtful and observed that their behavior often appeared as "Nonsense" and "Folly" to those around them.[25] Mather found melancholy difficult to shed, despite appearing bizarre to others. "The *Fancies* and *Whimsies* of People over-run with *Melancholy*," Mather noted, "are so Many, and so Various, and so Ridiculous, that the very Recital of them, one would think, might somewhat serve as a little *Cure for Melancholy*."[26] Naming those peculiarities failed to bring cures, and, lamentably, melancholy itself seemed to exacerbate suffering. "These *Melancholicks*," he observed, "do sufficiently *Afflict themselves*, and are Enough their *own Tormentors*. As if this *present Evil World*, would *Really* afford Sad Things Enough, they create a World of *Imaginary Ones*, and by *Mediatating Terror*, they make themselves as Miserable, as they could be from the most *Real Miseries*."[27] Melancholy, like madness, brought deep distress.

Mather did not characterize mental and physical illnesses as fundamentally different sorts of ailments, but his description of madness and melancholy in *The Angel of Bethesda* did differ from his commentary on physical afflictions. He named the universal reach of mental distress. "What is the Whole World," he reflected, "but an Entire *Mad-house*?"[28] He also refused to draw a crisp distinction between humans afflicted with madness and melancholy and healthy ones. Instead, he observed that all suffered from mental distress, at least in some area of their lives.[29] "*Every Man is Mad* in some *One Point*," Mather asserted. "There is at least *One Point*, wherein *Reason* will do nothing with him."[30] Mental illness seemed unavoidable, and that even held true among those Mather loved.

While *The Angel of Bethesda* did not, Mather's diary included descriptions of mental illness within the clergyman's household. In 1703 he documented the departure, during the prior winter, of a servant who "had for so many Years been a Blessing" to his family but who was no longer able to work after the "Distraction" that followed her affliction with smallpox.[31] A decade later, Mather worried that had his first wife survived her fatal illness, news of the death of one of her brothers—and the disgraceful "idle, profane, drunken, and sottish" state of another—surely would have caused her to lapse into mental illness. Learning about those family calamities, he pre-dicted, would "without a Miracle, have brought . . . a Disorder of Mind upon her" and made her incapable of her usual role of supporting him.[32] Mather's diaries also described the erratic conduct of his third wife, Lydia Lee George Mather.[33] Lydia's unpredictable behavior included "prodigious Proxysms" and violent outrage that caused Mather "dreadful distress."[34] His wife's "rag-ing madness" and "miserable distraction" left the minister at a loss. After an outburst in 1724, Mather cried, *"Quid agam? Redemptor mi! Quid agam?"* ("What should I do? My Redeemer! What should I do?").[35] Mather was no stranger to the suffering and disruption caused by mental distress and knew that healing sometimes failed to appear.

COLONIAL MEDICINE AND CLERICAL AUTHORITY

Mather developed his treatise on sickness amidst a nascent American medical establishment. Illness and injury affected most colonial residents and seemed to strike indiscriminately. A 1713 measles epidemic, for example, took the lives of the minister's second wife, infant twins, and two-year-old daughter as well as a servant. Mather and six older children escaped death.[36] Few col-onists received formal medical care during outbreaks. Educated citizens had access to a variety of medical writings for advice, but limited access to medi-cal knowledge reduced the possibility of prevention and cure of both simple and complex illnesses. In addition, few formally trained physicians practiced in early America.

With high costs of travelling to Europe to obtain medical training, and few incentives for European physicians to journey across the Atlantic, apprenticed doctors provided most medical care in the colonies' first century.[37] Those practitioners were sometimes college graduates in other fields who worked with established doctors, but many were untrained, self-proclaimed "physicians." By 1720 only one Boston doctor had received formal medical training; all others learned their art via apprenticeship.[38]

Eventually a few men formally educated in topics related to medicine appeared in colonial America. During the eighteenth century, Harvard—though it taught mostly clergy—offered courses in "physic," the art of heal-ing disease.[39] Twelve of the first 149 graduates from Harvard apprenticed as physicians after graduation. Before the first medical schools opened, other schools, including Yale and the College of Philadelphia, taught courses in anatomy, chemistry, physics, and surgery.[40] Demand for medical training grew, although slowly.

With inconsistent training and no professional standards, the authority of physicians on medical matters remained unsteady in colonial times. In contrast, Mather's authority as a public intellectual allowed him to express ambivalence toward doctors, even men who had received training. Midway through *The Angel of Bethesda*, for example, the minister paused to detail "The Uncertainties of the PHYSICIANS."[41] His commentary fell just after his discussion of consumption, a common ailment with a high mortality rate. Mather noted that many depended on the advice of physicians for comfort and for their lives, but as evidence of the downside in seeking their help, he displayed a wide variety of contradictory counsel offered by medical men in the face of consumption. Doctors differed about the causes and the cures for the disease, and some, Mather shared, even died from the ailments they professed to treat. With good reason, the authority of clergy to speak about health and healing remained largely unchallenged.

Despite skepticism about professional help, Mather urged sufferers to seek the help of physicians, but only if they remembered that true healing came from Christ:

> *O Thou afflicted*, and under *Distemper*, Go to *Physicians*, in *Obedience* to God, who has Commanded the *Use of Means*. But place thy *Dependence* on God alone to Direct and Prosper them. And know, That they are all *Physicians of no Value* if He do not so. Consult with *Physicians*; But in a full Perswasion, That if God leave them to their own Counsels, thou shalt only *Suffer many Things from them*; They will do thee more *Hurt* than *Good*. Be Sensible, *Tis from God, and not from the Physician, that my Cure is to be looked for*.[42]

Only because they too were creations of God could the help of doctors yield good results.[43] Even with such caution, Mather's writings show a role for both spiritual and medical cures. Accounts of his ministry indicate that he offered care for the ill and made pastoral visits to the ailing. Yet, he also called on physicians for himself and family members when sick. His willingness to seek help displayed the understanding that medicine was a gift of God. The clergyman made it clear that God could work through physicians, but no guarantee existed.[44] Mather's reflections about medicine introduced dilemmas that Christians struggled with in later centuries. Was God at work in the secular medical world? How should Christians relate to secular help? How should the faith of physicians shape their medical practice? Mather answered such questions in light of a sovereign God who was present in all spheres of life.

As a clergyman who felt called to address the suffering that illness caused, Mather displayed broad expertise and claimed authority beyond care for the soul alone. While he did not formally practice medicine, many colonial clergymen served in both capacities, a practice Mather supported. The dual careers of clergy stemmed from understanding ministers as healers—of body and soul—but also resulted from the simple fact that their flocks needed their expertise. Given temporal suffering, Mather saw ministers as being in a unique position to help by dispensing both spiritual counsel and medical knowledge.

Although Mather never claimed to practice as a physician, he exerted medical authority during epidemics when he perceived indifference or conflict amongst the medical community. In 1713, for example, having lost family members to an outbreak of the measles, he weighed in and urged physicians to distribute treatment directions. Then, aware that medical professionals might criticize his effort, Mather published his own instructions in *A Letter, About a Good Management under the Distemper of the Measles, at this time Spreading in the Country. Here Published for the Benefit of the Poor, and such as may want the help of Able Physicians.* The minister felt compelled to help and deemed it necessary to share the results of his own study.[45]

Mather's 1713 publication failed to raise the ire of physicians, but his actions during a smallpox outbreak eight years later did. Having convinced himself of the value of inoculations against disease long before the arrival of the epidemic in Boston (by studying European medical literature), Mather advocated vaccinations for fellow citizens. He did so in the face of resistance from medical professionals in both the colonies and Europe. Though the high risk of disease and death from immunization deterred wide support, Mather persuaded one (nondegreed) physician, Dr. Zabdiel Boylston, to inoculate. Other doctors decried the intrusion of a minister into medical matters.[46]

Widespread opposition exploded on both medical and theological grounds. Not only was vaccination risky, many also claimed it interfered with God's providence.[47] For more than a generation, Puritan preachers had proclaimed that epidemics (along with damage from hailstorms, fires, and earthquakes) revealed God's judgment for the sins of the people.[48] In the face of death and illness, those jeremiads from the pulpit urged a spiritually lax citizenry to reclaim their faithfulness and to live as God's covenanted people. God would reward faithfulness just as God punished transgression. Inoculation sparked theological concerns because it seemed to prevent warranted divine punishment for human sinfulness. For those wary of vaccination on theological grounds, tending to sickness proved acceptable, but anticipating God's judgment and preventing illness did not. Perhaps surprisingly, Mather disagreed. Though certain of God's providence, his confidence in science as a gift of God molded his theological diagnosis.[49] Medical and theological concerns remained part of the same whole for Mather—inoculation was among God's provisions for humanity.

The clergyman vocalized his views, and the resulting disagreement within and between the medical and theological communities sparked heated public debate.[50] Tensions grew sharp enough that one opponent tossed a grenade through a window of Mather's home during the controversy, an event that convinced the minister that the actions of his opponents were orchestrated by the devil.[51] Eventually, other Boston clergy and physicians supported Mather and Boylston's efforts, in part because inoculation proved effective. The smallpox episode betokened an extension of clerical authority—in the name of the physical and spiritual welfare of the people—into the practice of medicine.[52] Incursions of this sort decreased with the rise of medical science and remained controversial, but colonial clergy, as general intellectuals with few peers that were as well educated, held the book knowledge to stake such claims. Mather extended his clerical authority into the medical realm but did so under the banner of superior medical knowledge and undergirded by spiritual concerns.

Given the scattered nature of colonial medicine, it is logical that, during the period, clergy retained authority in diagnosing illness and offering advice about care. As well-read—and, in many townships, the best-read—members of the community, they passed on remedies of which they were aware and, in the case of Mather, published their recommendations. In a world understood to be fully God's creation and domain, they did so with equal, if not superior, authority from those beginning, more formally, to practice medicine.[53]

After Mather's time, spheres of professional authority shifted, and clerical forays into medicine, like Mather's, may have precipitated some of the change. The minister's support of science in the face of medical and theological opposition, for example, had unintended consequences. Mather's approach to inoculation opened a doorway for the "undermining" of the widely held "conception of pestilence as a sign of God's wrath."[54] For Mather, recommending vaccination did not prevent him from understanding divine purpose in all illness. For others, however, that connection loosened, especially as medicine professionalized. Over the next century, illness was likely to be viewed as a medical problem that warranted secular medical treatment, not primarily a providential reality against which all God-given means should be deployed. Shifting perceptions would give physicians more authoritative voices than clergy in attending to medical matters.

In his day, Mather's broad authority remained intact, but as the colonial era ended, more formal medical training emerged and bolstered confidence in physicians. In November 1765, courses in medicine, taught by physicians trained in Europe, began at the Pennsylvania Hospital.[55] Six years later, the College of Philadelphia granted the advanced medical degree for the first time, to four men.[56] By the turn of the eighteenth century, Harvard had established its medical school, and medical schools also opened at Dartmouth, Queens (later Rutgers), and the University of Transylvania.[57] Despite the appearance of medical schools, however, instruction in medicine lacked standardization, and practitioners often disagreed about both diagnosis and treatment. Even with the presence of hospitals and physicians in the colonies, not everyone had access to, or chose to consult, a medical practitioner, and so lines of authority changed slowly. Colonists still gleaned medical knowledge from almanacs and newspapers, and turned to patent medicines (elixirs) and folk medicine and folk practitioners for assistance.[58] They also continued to turn to clergy like Mather for advice about physical and divine cures and causes.

THE GRAND CAUSE OF SICKNESS

Mather understood all things—life, death, illness, health, nature, and humanity—theologically, and that shaped his exploration of the purpose and causes of sickness. Rarely did his writing separate sickness and theological reflection. A 1700 sermon, for example, showed his seamless mixing of theological and medical imagery. Describing one who had sinned, Mather observed, "He has the Palsey of an unsteady Mind; He has the Feavour of Unchasity . . . He has the Cancer of envy; He has the Tympany of Pride."[59] In his discussion of the usefulness of sickness for prompting self-reflection, he offered the following analogy: "I pray, Lett our *Sickness* itself, be such an *Emetic*, as to make us *Vomit* up our *Sin*, with a penitent *Confession* of it."[60]

Mather viewed the experience of illness as wasted if not used for its spiritual benefit. "Our Sickness is utterly lost upon us," he claimed, "if it render not a CHRIST more *precious* unto us than ever."[61] Sickness served to draw believers closer to God and more attentive to God's will. Even in the case of illness in children, Mather hoped that "the Uncomfortable Circumstance of my Child" would turn parents toward the Creator. "*My God will humble me*," he hoped, "for the Share which I have in the Sin of our *First Parents*. May my Repentance for our *Original Sin*, be brought unto its *Perfect Work*, by the View of what *My Child* . . . is now suffering from it."[62] Mather found sacred purpose in all natural phenomena.

Because colonial Puritans like Mather saw both illness and health as purposeful within God's covenant, understanding the connection between sin and illness proved central in Mather's curiosity about sickness and healing. As a result, he began his medical volume with theological reflections about the source of illness. Mather's first chapter, "Some Remarks on The Grand CAUSE of Sickness," reflected on the origin of evil. In that discussion, he anchored the cause of all human ailments, whether physical or mental, in a theology that presumed lasting impacts of personal and original sin. Acknowledging the difficulty of the topic, Mather noted, "*Whence Evil Comes*, has been as *Vexing* a *problem* as ever was in the World."[63] The clergyman, however, found a clear solution to the longstanding problem: the evil of sickness and disease stemmed from sin. "Bear in Mind," he counseled, "That *Sin* was that which first brought *Sickness* upon a *Sinful World*, and which yett continues to *Sicken* the World, with a World of Diseases."[64]

Mather saw sin as the cause of sickness in two ways. First, "the *Sin* of our *First Parents*, was the *First Parent* of all our *Sickness*."[65] Affirming original sin, Mather cited Genesis: Adam and Eve's choice to eat—not from the tree of life, but from the tree of knowledge—damned the world to suffer the "wretchedness" of sin. Illness in innocent infants provided proof of original sin as a cause of sickness. In a later chapter devoted to "Infantile-Diseases," Mather lamented, "Oh! The Grievous Effects of *Sin*! This wretched *Infant* has not arrived upon years of sense Enough, to *Sin after the Similitude of the Transgression committed by Adam*. Nevertheless, the *Transgression of Adam* . . . has involved this Infant in the Guilt of it."[66] In one way or another, all human ailments resulted from the lasting effects of original sin.

Alongside original sin, Mather argued that sickness resulted from individual transgression. "Remember, That the *Sin* of every individual Man," he observed, "does not but *Repeat* and *Renew* the *Cause* of *Sickness* unto him."[67] While the precise source of mental ailments might remain unknown, he argued individual sins against God did bring madness, even when physical causes also existed. Sometimes, through their own "willful repudiations" of God's covenant, individuals brought sickness upon themselves.[68] Again, Mather found support of his assertion in Scripture, quoting Psalm 107:17: "*Fools, because of their Transgression, and because of their Iniquities are Afflicted*, with Sickness."[69] The minister assumed that those working against God could be afflicted in response. He described, for example, "a critic of the clergy who after speaking in church was quickly and justifiably punished with madness."[70] Mather also assumed personal heavenly rebuke when he observed sickness in those he loved. Always searching the state of his own soul, he viewed his wife Lydia's insanity and violent paroxysms as a divinely ordained test of his patience and an invitation to pray more earnestly.[71] Illness, then, could be punishment, or at least chastisement for individual sin. Mather refrained, though, from naming which illnesses stemmed from original sin and which stemmed from individual sin. Nonetheless, the minister spent more time in *The Angel of Bethesda* discussing the relationship of sin to mental distress than he did in chapters on other ailments. Mather offered no reason for that expanded reflection.

While he urged Christians to attend to personal sins, Mather offered no condemnation of those afflicted with mental illness. The same was not true for those afflicted with venereal diseases. He dismissed those sufferers as wretched sinners in his chapter "Kibroth Hattaavh, or Clean Thoughts, on, The Foul Disease."[72] The minister found the topic so distasteful, such a "Nasty Discourse," that he refrained from suggesting remedies. He assumed those who suffered deserved to continue in their distress: "As for any Remedies under this *Foul Disease*,—You are so Offensive to me, I'll do nothing for you. You shall pay for your Cure."[73] Apparently, some remained deservedly beyond the help of medical ministrations, but not those living with mental maladies.

Mather was sure that sin lay behind illness and confident that sickness prompted believers to turn toward God for healing. The role of *"Sickness,"* he argued in *The Angel of Bethesda*, was "to awaken our Concern, first, for the *pardon* of the Maladies in our *Souls*."[74] Regardless of its specific cause, Mather viewed illness as a chance for introspection, an opportunity to identify and root out one's own sin. He offered that counsel to his parishioners and dispensed it for himself. In the fall of 1711, for example, having spent time visiting sick neighbors, Mather fell ill with the same "uneasy Malady; The Flux with Vomiting." He understood the interruption from illness as God's call "to look inward" and be "thankful for His merciful Saving of [me]." Sickness provided an opportunity to consider "Maladies in [my] own soul."[75] Both physical and mental ailments provided a prompt for the believer to turn toward Christ, to confess sin, and to seek assurance of salvation.[76] For Puritans like Mather, assurance of God's gracious salvation existed alongside perpetual uncertainty about the state of one's own soul. They knew, though, that they could pave the way for God's saving work. Colonial Calvinists understood conversion to be an ongoing process, and so attending to the spiritual role of illness in that process proved logical and purposeful.[77]

THE ROLE OF THE SUPERNATURAL

Despite speculation about its origins, causes of mental illness remained elusive in colonial America. Mather's commentary assumed mental disorders were connected to the supernatural realm, whether spurred by sin, demonic possession, divine punishment, or a struggle of faith. The ascription of otherworldly influence persisted partly because biological explanations remained unknown.[78] For Puritans like Mather that understood the world to be God's dominion, wonders—rainbows, storms, earthquakes, deadly fires, and

physical abnormalities—were manifestations of God's sovereignty.[79] Not all
apparitions were attributed to divine causes, though, and belief in witchcraft
and the devil also shaped understandings of the forces at work in the world.

Dissent and nonconformity garnered attention in colonial society, particularly when strangely behaving individuals threatened the desired decorum.
Whether presumed to stem from witchcraft, mental illness, or willful disobe-
dience, nonnormative beliefs and behaviors often brought opposition, expulsion, and even death. The Salem witch trials of 1692–1693 demonstrated the
hysteria that could erupt when society suspected the presence of willful deviance.[80] Despite often being linked with the frenzy surrounding the Salem
trials, Mather experienced severe illness during the years of the trials, and
records show his presence at the trials on only two occasions. The minister authored a document, signed by all Boston clergy, advising the government about the trials, but the treatise displayed ambivalence—it both urged
caution and recommended that legal proceedings continue.[81] The minister
refrained from presuming personal guilt in public accusations of witchcraft and even provided shelter and care for some of the accused.[82] Mather's
writings, though, made clear his belief in witchcraft. Unusual phenomena
like the aurora borealis and two-headed snakes formed evidence for him of
witchcraft's presence and power.[83] The clergyman's interest in witchcraft,
like his interest in medicine, stemmed from his intellectual curiosity about
the workings of God's world.

Demonic forces also played a role in Mather's interpretation of madness.
The clergyman assumed that the devil undermined God's intentions and
thereby attempted to destabilize proper social order. He observed that some
individuals, because of "the state of their humors," found themselves susceptible to possession by Satan or demons.[84] Spotting a direct connection, one of
Mather's sermons argued for "an unaccountable and unexpressable interest
of Satan often times in the Distemper of madness."[85] Specifically, the devil
could inflict madness upon those seeking to do God's work in the world.
Reflecting on the state of William Thompson, a minister suffering from
melancholy, Mather observed that Satan became "irritated by the evangelic
labours of this holy man" and "obtained the liberty to throw him into a Balneum Diaboli."[86] Attribution of demonic causes also appeared in *The Angel
of Bethesda* as Mather concluded some melancholy resulted from demonic
forces: "There is often a Degree of *Diabolical Possession* in *Melancholy*," he
asserted. He also noted, "*Maniacks* are sometimes more or less *Dæmoniacks*."[87]
Mather's writings display a varied diagnosis of insanity over the course of his
life, but throughout, biological, moral, and supernatural explanations blend.

Colonists distinguished between madness and witchcraft, and suspected that the latter arose from willful participation with evil. They also discerned a difference between being a witch and being bewitched—the former a matter of choice, the latter the result of possession.[88] Mather assumed that possession by the devil caused only the most extreme forms of madness, likely including the "furious and forward pangs" and "horrid rage" of his third wife.[89] In addition, thoughts of atheism or blasphemy evinced demonic possession, he asserted, and might spur suicidal thoughts. In his later writings, satanic connections to madness diminished. Similarly, they played only a background role, an underlying but remote suspicion, as later Protestants assessed the causes of mental illness.

ATTENDING TO THOSE IN NEED

Regardless of their origins, mental distress prompted individual and communal reaction. Before formal medical definitions and treatments of mental illness arose, colonists offered practical, institutional, and spiritual responses to the social and economic problems that appeared.[90]

American residents generally tolerated insane citizens, assuming madness could strike those of any social class or profession. With little social infrastructure, care of mentally ill neighbors fell most often to families and local communities. The dispersed, agrarian shape of early colonial life left "distracted" or "lunatick" persons less visible to society as a whole, even if troublesome to a few. The community's attention shifted to the mentally ill only when their presence proved threatening. At times, towns legally designated dependent individuals as the responsibility of the community. The concern was largely economic, and municipalities established guardianship laws to protect individual and communal interests.[91] The pauper insane garnered support more reluctantly, but they received assistance in almshouses or from other local families. Colonists viewed insanity as episodic rather than chronic, and proper attention allowed individuals to recover and return to full participation in family life.

In both colonial New England and colonial Virginia, mentally ill individuals whose own families could not, or would not, care for them boarded with others. Caretakers received compensation from either the family or the municipality. In the event that a citizen's illness threatened public safety, residents made other provisions, including the construction of small living structures to contain violent men and women. Because of limited resources and harsh living conditions for nearly all residents, however, citizens felt responsibility for only dependents from their own communities— towns worked to rid themselves of vagrants and others without local legal residence. Eventually, most cities opened almshouses for the care of a variety of dependent citizens, including widows, the poor, and the mentally ill. Beyond almshouses, few colonial facilities for the insane existed. In part, little infrastructure developed because population density remained low and ad hoc solutions remained effective.

Alongside the provision of care, society extended wide tolerance of mental illness to those in positions of leadership or authority. Two eighteenth-century congregations, for example, accommodated their clergymen despite bizarre behavior. In 1738 Joseph "Handkerchief" Moody, a minister from York, started wearing a handkerchief over his face, never again appearing without it in public.[92] The pastor's congregation tolerated his behavior for three years—even after he could no longer face his congregation and preached with his back turned. Another minister, Samuel Checkley, "suffered a series of personal losses in the 1750s and from that period on he was unable to speak without weeping."[93] He began delivering his sermons in gibberish, but his congregation refrained from firing him. Instead, they hired someone to help. Churches not only tolerated leaders with mental illnesses, they found them capable of continuing their duties despite affliction.

Formal, institutional care appeared only as the colonial era closed, decades after Mather's death. Hospitals for the insane had operated in Europe for centuries, but limited communal efforts to care for the mentally ill appeared in colonial America. The earliest institutional care appeared in general hospitals. The first facility, the Pennsylvania Hospital, admitted insane patients from its opening in 1752.[94] Of the 102 diagnoses given at the hospital between 1757 and 1758, 24 specified "lunacy."[95] The first hospital on American soil devoted to the care of the mentally ill opened in Williamsburg, Virginia, in the fall of 1773.[96] Early American institutions housed just a few patients; most sufferers continued to be cared for at home and in the local community, and those that were admitted to facilities often languished for years without cure.

The impetus to provide care arose from not only practical but also religious motivations. For Mather, attending to suffering in the world proved central to his conception of the Christian life. "Let no man pretend to the name of a Christian," he proclaimed, "who does not approve the proposal of a perpetual endeavour to do good in the world." "Much must be done," Mather urged, "that the miseries of the world may have suitable remedies provided for them; and that the wretched may be relieved and comforted.... In a word, the kingdom of God in the world calls for innumerable services from us."[97] Doing good in the world, Mather argued, formed an obligation for Christians, part of their covenant responsibility.

As society claimed general responsibility for citizens in need, Mather argued that Christian discipleship required caring for one's neighbors, even eccentric or troublesome ones. While persons afflicted with melancholy "often make themselves Insupportable *Burdens* to all about them," he asserted that those around "Malancholicks" must bear the other's suffering with patience, generosity, and humor.[98] The minister felt the weight of his own counsel: "There is a poor, distracted man in my Neighbourhood," the minister noted in a 1713 diary entry, "for whom and for whose Family, I must contrive to do what Kindness I can."[99] God's covenant with the people called for them to care for one another.

Mather named prayer as the initial response to madness: Those that did not suffer directly should first offer individual prayers of thanks for "the use of *Reason*, wherewith" the individual is "*Enlightened*." "How Thankful to [their] Gracious God" healthy individuals should be, "for the Powers of Reason, in the free Exercise thereof, Conferred upon [them], and Continued unto" them. Then, on behalf of those suffering, he recommended "Supplications for the Rescue of the *Mad*," asking for God's pity on those whom God created.[100] For susceptible men and women, prayer could also keep madness at bay. Individual petitions drew sufferers closer to God: "We are never brought unto a *Right Mind*, but in and by a Thorough *Conversion* unto God."[101] With physical ailments, Mather made clear that God answered prayers for cures. In 1711, for example, the minister suffered from severe headaches. He first sought relief in physical cures including "Unguents, and Plaisters, and Cataplasms, and Epispaspics. . . . But all to no purpose." Eventually, he resorted to prayer. After confessing his sinfulness, he begged God for "the Removal of [his] Malady" and found immediate relief.[102] Claims of instantaneous healing appeared less frequently in Mather's discussion of mental maladies, but in 1693 he noted the effectiveness of the congregation's prayers in bringing healing to "a Young Woman, horribly *possessed* with Devils."[103] Other corporate religious responses also appeared in the colonies. Personal journals from the period, for example, showed that Puritan leaders, including Mather and the Massachusetts judge Samuel Sewall, held days of prayer and fasting for "distracted neighbors."[104] Organized public action revealed a sense of communal responsibility and a solution rooted in Christian practice. Prayer proved an individual and a corporate duty that was both religious and civic. It oriented all suffering, including mental distress, within God's providential workings and could prompt divine healing.

Beyond prayer, in *The Angel of Bethesda*, Mather commended a variety of material treatments for madness and melancholy, and most of those cures reflected the prevailing theory of disease. The colonial understanding of disease—physical or mental—was more than a thousand years old and assumed illness stemmed from an imbalance in the four major fluids or humors of the human body: cold, dry, hot, and moist.[105] Health was a matter of equilibrium among those humors, and imbalance, or disease, called for restoring the body to proper order through bleeding, purging, sweating, dietary remedies, and herbs.[106]

For madness, Mather recommended ingested treatments, beginning with a carefully monitored diet: "Both the *Meats* and the *Drinks* of the *Mad, should be very cooling.*" Herbal remedies supplemented a proper diet and included St. John's wort and the flowers of pimpernel. Mather suggested opiates, one of few available medicines, for relief from the suffering caused by madness. He also presented a number of topical remedies: "Living *Swallows*, cut in two, and laid reeking hot unto the shaved Head, have been præscribed, as a Cure for *Madness.*" Finally, he shared additional physical treatments including bleeding and purging: "*Bleeding* often Repeated, has done Something to Extinguish the Fury of the *Animal Spirits,*" and "*Madmen* have sometimes been perfectly Cured by *Saavation.*"[107] In caring for madness, the use of these and other age-old physical treatments persisted for more than a century after the colonial era.

Similarly, Mather compiled a range of topical, ingested, and behavioral recommendations for melancholy. Some might be cured by wearing a bag of saffron over their hearts or find temporary relief by drinking a pint or more of cold water. Outdoor exercise such as horseback riding, especially with pleasant company, won approval, as did ingestion of "syrup of steel" and "Quincy's Elixir Hypocondriacum," a tincture of quinine. A more startling recommendation called for leeches applied to "hæmorrhoidal Veins." Of this treatment, Mather reported, "Tis incredible, how Lightsome and Easy they have grown upon it, and for many Months free from the *Melancholy* that had besotted them."[108] Even assuming the supernatural origins of illness and the effectiveness of prayer, colonists pursued physical treatments to provide relief from suffering.

Mather presumed clergy played a direct role in spiritual aspects of the treatment of mental disturbances. Sin interrupted the relationship between humans and God, and ministers held sole authority in discerning the state of the soul. Pastoral care focusing on spiritual development moved the individual toward closer relationship with the divine. Discerning the right pastoral response required an assessment of the source of melancholy. For melancholy stemming from "Spiritual Troubles," clergymen must exercise "Exquisite Care . . . to carry the *Troubled Sinner* through a *Process of Repentance*; And after a due Confession of his Guilt, and Impotency, and Unworthiness, *Lead him to the Rock*: Show Him a Glorious CHRIST, *Able to Save unto the Utter-most*, and *Willing to Cast out none that come to Him*."[109] Given the Puritan emphasis on discernment of the state of one's soul, clergy held a central role in ushering people through trials of doubt to awakening in God. But, perhaps stemming from his own experience, Mather warned ministers to be wary of the time consumed by talking with those suffering from melancholy. After several hours with sufferers, with no improvement occurring, he saw the work of Satan in keeping clergy from "their more *Useful Studies*." He advised ministers to make God's help clear but warned that spending too much time would be fruitless. "Bestow some *Suitable Book* upon them," Mather offered, but then "so take your Leave."[110] While authoritative guides about health and healing, clergy placed ultimate responsibility for recovery on God.

In contrast to the comfort offered to those whose melancholy resulted from spiritual distress, Mather warned that temporal distress caused by human action (or inaction) should be met with forceful counsel: "Rebuke the *Pining*, *Moaning*, *Languid*, and *Slothful* Sort of Christians, and let them know, that they must be rowsed out of their *Inactivity*, and abound more in *Direct* Acts, than in *Reflex* ones." Even in those cases, though, such activity should aim toward "a Soul Turning and Living unto God."[111] Mather's comments hint at a sense of personal laziness as a suspected root of distress, a condition that right thinking and right action would remedy.

As a clergyman, Mather felt responsibility to attend to the health of his flock. Given his understanding of the sovereignty of God and the weight of human sin, he found no reason to separate the physical, mental, and spiritual health of his parishioners.

SUFFERINGS FOR GOD

In the fall of his twenty-second year, Mather noted that he "had newly been thinking, *how all my Sufferings, might be rendered, after a sort, Sufferings for God*." He declared that he would "acknowledge the Hand of God, in all that befell" him. Rather than being "discouraged" when faced with trials, he decided to find "Reward" and "praise Him for it." That declaration in early adulthood was one Mather held to tightly throughout his life. A sense of God's sovereignty in all things formed the central conviction of the clergy-man's Calvinist theology. Good health might signal the Creator's approval, but suffering too provided evidence of being held (even if scolded) in the providential hand of God. Mather's writing never questioned God's motives in sending suffering. Rather, the minister simply turned to discern God's message amidst distress.

Few months passed in Mather's forty-three years of diary keeping without mention of illness. The minister was mindful of God's providence but also of the divine's ability to heal. He searched for the role he should play in bringing healing to bodies, minds, and souls. As one who partook of the secular wisdom of his age, Cotton Mather dispensed medical knowledge in medical terms. The pastor also shared theological wisdom about divine causes of and treatments for disease, insight he hoped would alleviate suffering. While distinct, those two roles formed part of the same task for Mather. A desire to understand God's creation more deeply, to draw nearer to the Creator, shaped his interest in medicine, as did his hope to care for God's people.

Mather's pragmatic and theological reflections on illness offer the sorts of assessments that later Protestants would both embrace and reject. While he devoted most attention in *The Angel of Bethesda* and other works to physical ailments, his inclusion of a quotation from a Dutch physician betrays his evaluation of the place of mental maladies:

> Adverse health, the threat to and death of members of the body is considered rather terrible. But of all things which can happen to man, the worst is illness or loss of the mind.[112]

Mather—by gathering available medical wisdom, reflecting theologically, and providing practical counsel—hoped to serve like the biblical angel at the pool in Bethesda in bringing healing to those around him, especially those afflicted with mental distress. Others, while discerning a divine call, would pursue different paths.

2

Christian Vocation and the Shape
of the Secular Profession

Benjamin Rush

> In reviewing the slender and inadequate means that have been employed
> for ameliorating the condition of mad people, we are led further to lament
> the slower progress of humanity in its efforts to relieve them, than any
> other class of the afflicted children of men. For many centuries they have
> been treated like criminals, or shunned like beasts of prey; or, if visited
> it has been only for the purposes of inhuman curiosity and amusement.
> Even the ties of consanguinity have been dissolved by the walls of a mad
> house, and sons and brothers have sometimes languished or sauntered
> away their lives within them, without once hearing the accents of a
> kindred voice. Happily these times of cruelty to this class of our fellow
> creatures and insensibility to their sufferings are now passing away.
>
> —Benjamin Rush, 1813[1]

In June of 1792, the Revolutionary-era physician Benjamin Rush recorded a
meeting with William Glendinning in his journal. The doctor noted that the
itinerant Methodist clergyman "had been insane" and "in a state of despair"
for four and a half years. Bodily pain, mental anguish, excessive sleep, and
a loss of interest in food and other people accompanied the minister's melancholy. A decade earlier, Glendinning had survived a suicide attempt.[2]
Rush reported that other sufferers did not. In 1804 he described the fate of a
Mrs. McCurrach, who "threw herself into the Skuilkill and perished." She
"had been melancholy for some months," Rush shared, "and had a few weeks
[earlier] been saved from death which she attempted to bring on herself by
taking 1 oz. liquid laudanum."[3] While the overdose failed to bring death, her
jump into a Pennsylvania river did. Curious about suffering in God's good

creation, Benjamin Rush (1746–1813) catalogued instances of mental disturbance throughout his journal. By practicing medicine, he hoped to remedy
physical and mental distress. The leading physician provided personal care
and fought for structural solutions to alleviate suffering. As he did so, his
repeated appeals for mentally ill Americans to receive humane treatment
demonstrated that many did not.[4]

Rush was born near Philadelphia two decades after Cotton Mather's
death. Like Mather, Rush proved well read in religion, science, and medicine. Unlike his New England predecessor, who served as a clergyman that
dispensed medical advice, Rush, a statesman and reformer, labored primarily as a physician. Though not a man of the cloth, the Presbyterian doctor's
Christian faith directed his wide-ranging endeavors, including his efforts to
improve the treatment of mental illness. While guided by faith, both men
deployed the scientific logic of their day to address suffering. The influence
of eighteenth-century Enlightenment empiricism on Rush's thought, however, prompted the transformation of madness from a religious to a scientific
phenomenon.[5]

In the years surrounding the American Revolution, Rush distinguished
himself as a prominent and outspoken member of society. His friends
included presidents Thomas Jefferson and John Adams, founding father
Benjamin Franklin, and the controversial patriot Thomas Paine.[6] In addition to corresponding with those men throughout his life (and working to
reconcile the feuding Jefferson and Adams in the early nineteenth century),
as a patriot, he served the country alongside them. Beginning in 1775, he
participated as a delegate to the Continental Congress and signed the Declaration of Independence the following year. Appointed as surgeon general of
the army during the Revolutionary War, he later quit, frustrated that politics
prevented necessary reforms in the medical care of troops. In 1797 President
Adams appointed him treasurer of the U.S. Mint, a position he held until his
death. Rush's reaction to public service proved mixed, and he later recalled
the time he spent in the service of his country with "pleasure and pain." The
doctor relished "acting for the benefit of the whole world, and of future ages,
by assisting in the formation of new means of political order and general
happiness," but he lamented the division sown by party politics.[7]

Rush provoked divergent reactions among his peers. Contemporaries
called him "wise, and again foolish; generous, and egotistic; a genius and an
intellectual fumbler."[8] The doctor was a forthright man with strong opinions,
and his enemies proved as famous as his friends. Among his adversaries, he
counted President George Washington and many fellow physicians. Nonetheless, he earned the respect of his colleagues, even those whose political or

medical opinions differed. Following Rush's death, John Adams reflected, "As a man of Science, Letters, Taste, Sense, Philosophy, Patriotism, Religion, Morality, Merit, Usefulness, taken altogether Rush [had] not left his equal in America, nor that I know in the world." After years of friendship and detailed correspondence, Adams lamented that he would miss that "main Prop" in his life.[9]

Despite broad political participation, Rush's principal work involved practicing, teaching, and reforming medicine. He attended to thousands of sick Americans and trained many of the period's physicians. The doctor practiced medicine at a transitional point in U.S. medical and social history, a period that brought the creation of a new country, the professionalization of medicine, and the creation of the first American medical institutions. Rush served at the nation's first hospital and taught at one of the earliest medical schools. In the final two decades of his life, he relinquished public pursuits and devoted himself to his patients, family, friends, and writing projects. Although Rush did not enter medicine to attend only to mental illnesses, they formed a focus of his public advocacy and framed his lasting medical legacy. Later advances in medicine negated many of his presumptions, but Rush's categorization of mental illnesses and proposals for treatment remained the standard for nearly a century and earned the doctor recognition as the father of American psychology.

In the narrative of American Protestantism and mental illness during the years of the early republic, the interaction of Rush's medical work with his religious convictions makes him a paradigmatic figure. The doctor's religious convictions shaped his vocational attention to mental maladies, but in the secular realm. While colonists like Cotton Mather claimed authority and expertise in both theology and medicine, changes in the early years of the newly formed country prevented almost all later clergy from being recognized as dually proficient. The professionalization of medicine during Rush's era unseated clergy as the foremost intellectual experts on matters of health and healing, and that change diminished church authority over physical and mental disease. As a leading voice among the era's physicians, Rush declared that medical men, not clergy, were the best arbiters of sanity. His work paved the way for a shift in treatment for distressed minds from the religious to the medical establishment.

Alongside the professional reorientation of clergy and physicians, Rush's work displays a change in assumptions about the role of sin in mental illness. The Puritan Mather had pinned the origins of mental distress, ultimately, in original and personal sin. Rush, instead, concentrated on physical and biological causes for all ailments. As the first American to systematize biological explanations, he treated mental illness as an organic malfunction. Rush practiced and wrote motivated by his Christian faith, but he dealt with mental distress as a disease to be treated, not as sin in need of spiritual care. The doctor sought physical, and not religious, cures, and other Americans followed his lead as biological theories replaced longstanding explanations rooted in the supernatural.

Like Mather, however, Rush's religious training and intellectual curiosity informed his medical pursuits. Both the physician's disciplined Calvinist inculcation and his hopeful Universalist leanings shaped his dedication to sick Americans. While in a different way from Cotton Mather, the Revolutionary-era physician's work demonstrated that his Christian beliefs fashioned his vocational choice and public involvement. Rush's career demonstrates one choice American believers made in response to their faith: they trained as physicians and sought to provide help in the face of suffering.

RUSH'S RELIGIOUS WORLD

Christianity infused Rush's world. In addition to remarks about illness, religious notes and reflections peppered his *Commonplace Book*. A keen observer, the doctor commented on the religious convictions of others, sermons he had heard, the launch of new congregations, and his own spiritual practice. He celebrated the strength he found in Christian faith and questioned the Deism of his peers. If measured by church attendance, Rush may have proved the most pious physician in Philadelphia.[10] Because of his religious upbringing, however, the doctor's faith extended far beyond sanctuary walls.

In July 1751, when Rush was just six, his father died, leaving his mother to ensure his religious and secular education.[11] After her husband's death, Susanna Rush and her children worshiped at Philadelphia's Second Presbyterian Church under the leadership of Rev. Gilbert Tennent, a key proponent of the First Great Awakening.[12] Out of respect for her late husband's religious heritage, Susanna also instructed her son in the traditions of the Episcopal Church.[13] In addition to his mother's tutelage, much of his early education fell to his uncle, Rev. Dr. Samuel Finley, who trained under New Side William Tennent, Gilbert's father.[14] Finley, the Tennents, and other New Side Presbyterians supported the religious revivals that swept through the colonies in the early eighteenth century and emphasized a renewed personal piety, a piety imparted to their young charges.

At age eight, Rush began attending Finley's West Nottingham Academy in Maryland. New Side Presbyterians founded the boarding school as a feeder to the newly formed College of New Jersey (later Princeton University). Years afterward, Rush recalled his uncle's tutelage as "highly calvinistical." His uncle's Calvinism, though, differed from the seventeenth-century Puritanism of Cotton Mather and his family members. Convictions of God's sovereignty and providence held firm but were now supplemented with a high regard for individual religious experience. As a result, beyond lessons in doctrine, Rush's uncle Finley prepared his students to connect their faith and their vocations. He exhorted Rush and others to resist corruptions of the world, to avoid indulgence, and to pursue lives that were both meaningful and useful to society.[15] Those lessons exerted lasting impact, even as the doctor's own religious convictions evolved beyond Presbyterianism.

As an adult, Rush's religious practice remained untethered to any particular tradition, and he found bits of religious truth in many groups. The doctor was convinced that most Protestants adopted "too partial notions of God, and his attributes," and thus extolled "one attribute at the expense of the rest."[16] His openness allowed Rush to speculate about the value of a plurality of traditions. "It would seem," he reflected, "as if one of the designs of Providence in permitting the existence of so many Sects of Christians was that each Sect might be a depository of some great truth of the Gospel, and that it might by that means be better preserved."[17] While maintaining theological preferences, Rush found value in multiple expressions of Christianity.[18] A wide view of Christian truth meant that he approached suffering and his role in ameliorating it with insight from a variety of theological frameworks.

Rush's religious convictions mirrored broader shifts in Protestant thought and practice resulting from the infusion of Enlightenment thought. As part of that eighteenth-century intellectual revolution, American thinkers embraced experiential knowledge rather than divine revelation as the "surest foundation of all reality."[19] The most direct source of the epistemological shift was intellectual development in Scotland, brought to the colonies through the migration of ideas and people. While American believers rejected more radical and skeptical elements of Enlightenment thought, a faith infused with the Common Sense Realism of the Scottish Enlightenment placed unprecedented authority in human free will and experience and lauded the use of pragmatic reason.[20]

To be sure, Christians had made use of logic for centuries. Cotton Mather deployed reason to understand the world, but the Puritan clergyman held fast to the conviction that God revealed all truth. Mather's approach matched the posture named in the medieval period as *"credo ut intelligam"* (I believe so that I may understand) or *"fides quaerens intelligam"* (faith seeking understanding).[21] God served as the starting point and the telos for Mather's intellectual inquiries.[22] Alternately, Rush, and those shaped by Enlightenment thought, assumed humans gained knowledge through the senses and began analysis of all matters from the starting point of individual human experience. Even in their religious lives, Enlightenment-era American Protestants trusted their own experience as empirical evidence for belief. Human inquiry served as the primary authority in making sense of the world and faith.

Though some early Americans shifted their confidence entirely to reason detached from divine influence, Rush was among those who both adopted Enlightenment principles and preserved elements of traditional Protestant belief. Rush maintained belief in both revelation and experiential reason, but because Enlightenment thought embraced an understanding of humans as inherently good, it undermined traditional Calvinist convictions about original sin, limited atonement, and predestination. Those doctrines seemed unlikely in light of optimism about human nature and abilities.[23] Rush questioned some age-old doctrines, but he did not fully reject the traditional faith. Many of his contemporaries embraced the detached God and mechanistic world of Deism, but not the Philadelphia physician. Undergirding all of the doctor's thought was the presumption of God, an active, necessary, and perfect being that could exercise final judgment.[24]

Over time, Rush's theological allegiance shifted from his familial roots. In adulthood, for example, amidst the climate of Enlightenment innovation, he studied conflicts over salvation theory between Calvinists (who maintained confidence in precise views of predestination) and others who favored the "Universality of the atonement." That reading, he reflected, "prepared [his] mind to admit the doctrine of Universal salvation."[25] Persuaded, in part, by Rev. John William Fletcher's *Appeal to Matter of Fact and Common Sense*, Rush adopted a more inclusive approach, one that assumed the salvation of all, not just those who had been "prenatally" predestined by God.[26] As he moved beyond some of his Calvinist inculcation, Rush held tightly to other convictions from his Reformed theological training. The doctor embraced hope in universal salvation but also allowed that "actively and negatively wicked" persons were consigned to hell.[27] Notwithstanding his Universalist leanings (and a preference for a God that saved), Rush never abandoned belief in consequences for sin including "future punishment, and of long, long duration," nor did he formally align himself with the emerging Universalist movement.[28] Rush sampled the diverse theological landscape but proved to be neither an orthodox Presbyterian nor a stereotypical Universalist. The Pennsylvania patriot understood himself as a committed Christian, one who confidently navigated multiple theological and intellectual frameworks.

Change in Rush's religious convictions likely shaped his understanding of human suffering. If God made salvation available to all, for example, disease did not serve, necessarily, as a sign of a human sin and distance from the

divine. Instead, infirmity was simply a reality of human life in need of amelioration, and healing should be provided by physicians, not clergy. Unlike
their Puritan predecessors, believers like Rush found supernatural intervention less plausible than naturalistic explanations for nearly all phenomena.
Paired with rising confidence in the ability of humans to solve all problems,
including physical and mental suffering, the rise of empiricism meant that
scientific analysis of the origins of disease supplanted religious ones.[29]

Political theory shaped by Enlightenment thought also played a role in
the evolution of Rush's theological convictions. After the American Revolution, and "based on the incontrovertible thesis that all men are equal," the
pious political leader found he could no longer embrace the predestining
God of Calvinism in light of the newly formed American republic, a country
where citizens had created their own future, at least politically. Nor, given
the political and scientific progress around him, did he believe that humans
were as evil or God as full of wrath as Calvin claimed.[30] Despite changes in
his thought, a biblically rooted faith continued to shape Rush's life. "The
Gospel of Jesus Christ," he advised his children, "prescribes the wisest rules
for conduct in every situation of life."[31] Rush may have rejected the strict
Calvinism of his forebearers, but not its call for personal discipline.

Rush also reserved a role for divine providence, especially in his own
life. In 1760, after graduating with a B.A. from the College of New Jersey,
and following a six-year medical apprenticeship in the colonies, Rush trained
for a career in medicine in Edinburgh, Scotland, earning his M.D. in 1768.[32]
Initially, he planned to pursue a career in the law. His mind changed, though,
after undertaking a period of prayer and fasting recommended by his uncle
Finley. "Providence overruled my intentions," the young man reflected,
"[and] I now rejoice that I followed Dr. Finley's advice. I have seen the hand
of heaven clearly in it."[33] His uncle's influence also showed in a letter Rush
wrote to a friend before leaving for Europe. He mused that he hoped to be
of "use to society when [he returned]."[34] Confidence about his place in God's
story was evident in his later comparison of himself to the prophet Jeremiah
and his conviction that God spared him from a near fatal illness in 1778.[35] For
Rush, divine providence dictated both his path and his purpose. Reflecting
on his own life, Rush noted, "Humble and unworthy instruments are often
employed in promoting the physical as well as moral happiness of mankind
in order to confound the splendor of those external circumstances which
attract and fix the esteem of the world." Certain of God's call, he understood
his role as a faithful servant rather than as a prophet.[36]

The physician's faith not only influenced his vocational pursuit but also
sustained him amidst the hardships and occasional criticisms that arose as

he provided medical care in eighteenth-century Philadelphia. Rush was always confident in his approach to medicine, but his methods sometimes met opposition. He declared, though, that "the comforts and support with which Christianity abounds to those who suffer persecution in the cause of truth and humanity" enabled him to continue serving patients even when "defamation and ingratitude" arose from critics.[37]

Rush's religiously rooted desire to serve the world shaped his participation in medicine and in a wide range of reform efforts. A sense of the need for public morality grounded in religious principles spurred, for example, forays into education. Rush campaigned for free public schools and the education of girls and women. In 1783 he helped found Dickinson College, as an alternative to Princeton, for Pennsylvanians.[38] The educated leader also opposed slavery, considering human bondage a "violation of the laws of nature and Christianity."[39] In 1773 he published *An Address to the Inhabitants of the British Settlements in America upon Slave-Keeping* and "endeavored to show the iniquity of the slave trade."[40] A year later, he helped found the Pennsylvania Society for Promoting the Abolition of Slavery and the Relief of Free Negroes Unlawfully Held in Bondage. Rush supported the formation of African American congregations in Philadelphia, including Richard Allen's Bethel African Methodist Episcopal Church.[41] In addition, he pled for temperance in both the army and society, and he argued for the benefits of limiting alcohol usage both for individuals and for the social body.[42]

As a physician, Rush had convictions about Christian charity that prompted him to make care available for citizens in need. In 1780 he participated in the founding of the Philadelphia Humane Society, a group that sought to educate citizens about health and hygiene. In 1786 he led the creation of Philadelphia's Dispensary for the Poor. The following year, with Deist-leaning Benjamin Franklin, he created the Philadelphia Society for Alleviating the Miseries of Public Prisons. He also worked for prison reform and the abolition of the death penalty in Pennsylvania. Beyond formal organizational involvement, Rush donated food, including watermelons and turkey, to Philadelphia jails in hopes that prisoners "should consider that God, by disposing the heart of one of his fellow creatures to show them an act of kindness, is still their Father and Friend."[43] The causes he championed displayed Rush's belief in the goodness of a loving Creator and his hope to make his endeavors of use to society and his life purposeful.[44] Notwithstanding Rush's diverse list of reform activities, medicine formed his primary mode of service.

REVOLUTIONARY-ERA MEDICINE:
PROFESSIONALIZATION, PRACTICE, AND FAITH

Medicine in American began to professionalize during the years Rush practiced. Amidst the formalization of medical theory and practice, Rush could have taken a purely secular approach as a physician. Faith continued to influence the doctor's orientation toward medical service, even as scientific medicine began to replace older, more ad hoc theories. Rush proved unable, or perhaps unwilling, to ignore his religious convictions.

The professionalization of medicine brought systemization to theory and practice. Propelled by Enlightenment optimism and empiricism, new hospitals were constructed, medical schools were incorporated, and physicians published the country's first medical journals.[45] Nevertheless, change progressed slowly. Apprenticeship continued, with two-thirds of practicing New England physicians in 1840 trained not in medical schools but by the older tutorial method.[46] Despite signs of professionalization, a lack of oversight, control, and shared standards persisted. Amidst that climate, Rush and a handful of other physicians that trained in Europe stepped in to refashion medicine in the United States.

In July 1769, following his medical studies and an internship in London, Rush launched his medical practice in the colonies. Working mostly in Philadelphia, he treated thousands in the course of his career, including many indigent citizens unable to pay. The doctor accepted barter in return for care and provided services for those who could pay nothing. A string of epidemics in the final decades of the eighteenth century—scarlet fever, croup, influenza, measles, smallpox, and cholera—kept him busy as he cared for the city's poor. To be sure, Rush attended to more aristocratic patients, but he admitted that he lacked the "principal means which [typically] introduce a physician into" that "business," including "the patronage of a great man," "the influence of extensive and powerful family connections," and "the influence of a religious sect or political party." Rush could not expect automatic patronage, a fitting reality given that sympathy toward the poor and the distressed directed his public work.[47]

The physician considered his service to impoverished Philadelphians part of his Christian responsibility. Resonating with the parable of the Good Samaritan, he repeated to himself the words "Take Care of him, and I will repay thee" "a thousand times" after leaving the sickrooms of the poor. He trusted in God's promises as he served his fellow citizens—promises of healing for the sick and strength for the servant. "To His goodness in accepting my services to His poor children," he ruminated, "I ascribe the innumerable blessing of my life; nay more, my life itself." Rush assumed divine blessing took the place of monetary rewards. The doctor reported that "including the business [he] did without charging for it, and bad and absolved debts," he had "not been paid for more than one fifth of the labor of [his] life." [48] Indeed, Rush described his first years of practice as a time of "constant labor and self-denial." "My shop," he noted, "was crowded with the poor in the morning and at meal times, and nearly every street and alley in the city was visited by me every day."[49] Though his service brought personal difficulty, Rush did not attempt to move beyond his base of needy patients.

Because patient need—and not social standing or religious affiliation— dictated Rush's clientele, the doctor worked feverishly and sometimes willingly put himself in harm's way. He confessed to risking infection from his patients and that at times he became infested with viruses and vermin after visits.[50] In 1780 an outbreak of "break bone fever" even brought Rush near death.[51] While recovering, the weary physician dreamed about the value of his service to needy citizens:

> I dreamed that a poor woman came to me . . . and begged me to visit her husband. I told her hastily, that I was worn out in attending poor people, and requested her to apply to another Doctor. "O! Sir (said she, lifting up her hands) you don't know how much you owe to your poor patients. It was decreed that you should die by the fever which lately attacked you, but the prayers of your poor patients ascended to heaven in your behalf, and your life is prolonged only upon their account."[52]

While confessing to be "little disposed to superstition," Rush reported that he awoke in tears. The vision left a lasting impression: "It enreased [*sic*] my disposition to attend the poor and never, when I could not serve them, to treat them in an uncivil manner." Shortly after the dream, and to ease the burden of attending to the growing needs of the city's poor, Rush hired his first assistant.[53]

Alongside his medical practice, Rush was well known as a teacher of medicine. Initially, he took on apprentices, boarding them in a neighbor's barn, providing training, and offering advice as they established their own clientele.[54] In August 1769 the College of Philadelphia elected him professor of chemistry, and he taught while maintaining his private practice.[55] In 1787 he helped found the College of Physicians of Philadelphia. Two years later, the medical school at the College of Philadelphia appointed him professor of theory and practice of medicine. There, Rush trained (directly or indirectly) a large majority of physicians in the newly independent country.[56] He proved centrally positioned to participate in the leading medical conversations and controversies of his day.

Unlike many of his contemporaries, beyond simply dispensing treatments, Rush emphasized preventative medicine and public health practices. He argued, "Obviating diseases is the business of physic [medicine] as well as . . . curing them," and he told his students it "required as much skill to prevent diseases as to cure them."[57] His efforts improved health measures in the city of Philadelphia and in the nation's army. Before other physicians did so, Rush recommended a bland diet comprised mostly of vegetables alongside "active" exercises including walking, running, dancing, fencing, swimming, and talking as preventative measures.[58] While a surgeon general, his 1777 treatise, "To the Officers in the Army of the United States: Directions for Preserving the Health of Soldiers," pioneered military hygiene. He suggested banishing linen shirts (which were too likely to retain perspiration), keeping hair short and well groomed, and limiting rum consumption.[59] Without such changes, he feared more soldiers would die from poor sanitary conditions than from combat. He assumed that the well-being of all aspects of society required healthy citizens.

Beyond advocating prevention, Rush attended to acute illness. Some of his medical techniques, however, provoked controversy among his peers (and condemnation by later medical professionals). Rush was one of the first Americans to challenge the older system of medicine that rooted the source of disease in the balance of the body's fluids. He advocated, instead, a theory advanced by his Edinburgh teacher, William Cullen, pointing to disturbances in the nervous or vascular system as the cause of disease.[60] Venesection, or bloodletting, formed a logical response to disease assumed to lie in the circulatory system. Rush's widespread practice of bloodletting and his use of calomel (mercury) to purge the body, particularly during the 1793 yellow fever epidemic, however, earned him critics. His passion for "heroic medicine" also diminished the once strong stream of referrals he received from other Philadelphia physicians.[61]

Nevertheless, widespread illness assured a steady client base. The yellow fever epidemics of the 1790s proved particularly deadly. In 1793, before a cold snap killed the then unknown cause of the outbreak—mosquitoes—more than 10 percent of the population of Philadelphia died.[62] In September of that year, Rush estimated one hundred citizens died daily.[63] During the epidemic, he was the first to proclaim that public hygiene efforts could stem the disease's spread.[64] When yellow fever returned, in addition to treating patients, he proposed draining Philadelphia's marshes and gutters of their "noxious miasma."[65] Though city leaders failed to heed his advice, by Rush's count, deaths from the yellow fever epidemic would have been 50 percent higher without the heroic treatments he prescribed. Critics disputed his claim, and supporters praised his efforts. Regardless, he saw divine help in the "success which attended the remedies it pleased God" to lead him to introduce "into general practice."[66] Rush continued to attend to patients amidst opposition and even when he contracted illnesses. The doctor remained dedicated to healing others—to upholding the ancient Hippocratic oath and his Christian responsibility to alleviate suffering. Motivated by his Protestant faith, and shaped by the intellectual revolution of the Enlightenment, Rush approached diagnosis and treatment simultaneously as a medical professional and a committed believer.

MENTAL MALADIES: EVERYDAY OBSERVATIONS

The doctor's faith shaped his impetus to care, his approach to treatment, and the fulfillment he found in restoring patients to health. Rush attended to citizens in need of both physical and mental ministrations, but for the Philadelphia physician, healing madness brought greater satisfaction than ameliorating physical distress. "There is a great pleasure," he wrote near the end of his life, "in combating with success a violent bodily disease, but what is this pleasure compared with that of restoring a fellow creature from anguish and folly of madness, and of reviving within him the knowledge of himself, his family, his friends and his God!"[67] Rush approached the search for cures confident that an orderly, divinely created natural world would yield answers when studied. The doctor proclaimed that to think otherwise was "to call in question the goodness of the Supreme Being, and to believe that he acts without unity and system in all his works."[68] Rush relied on the help of a loving Creator to bring cures for physical and mental ailments.

Concern, curiosity, and divine call prompted the doctor to record instances of mental distress throughout his decades of practice. In January 1798, for example, he recounted the death of a friend, Rev. Jacob Duché. Among other ailments, Duché was "much disordered in the evening of his life, with a tendency to palsy, and with Hysteria." Rush noted the man "sometimes laughed and cried alternately all day." Despite his friend's affliction, Rush remembered him as "truly amiable, pious, and just."[69] In Rush's view, mental illness seems not to have changed Duché's essential character, only his behavior. As Rush chronicled instances of mental disease, he noted that family members sometimes sought legal action to control ailing relatives. He relayed that, in court, the family of John Vanderen, a local miller, used the man's proposal to "bring the waters of the Wissahiccon Creek to Philadelphia by means of pipes" as evidence of his insanity. Despite speaking "shrewdly and wittily in his own defense" at the 1790 trial, Vanderen found himself committed to the Pennsylvania Hospital for the remainder of his life as a result of his actions.[70]

Rush also documented men and women that took their own lives. The doctor rarely drew a direct connection between suicide and insanity but assumed the presence of some sort of mental disorder in many cases. For example, in notes for a "Lecture on the Medical Jurisprudence of the Mind," Rush concluded, "Suicide is madness."[71] During an economic crisis in 1792, he mentioned the suicide of a Frenchman resulting from unsuccessful economic investment.[72] Two years later, he "paid a visit of condolence" to a Mrs. Capper, "whose husband shot himself . . . from a dread of meeting his creditors." That entry included his attempt to soothe the widow's concerns about the state of her husband's soul. Displaying his theological leanings, Rush "endeavored to comfort her from consideration of universal repentance after pardon of death."[73] Suicide, in Rush's view, did not prove to be an unpardonable sin. In August 1800 he marked twenty-four suicides in New York since the spring, "3 of whom were servant girls, one in consequence of being rebuked by her mistress."[74] Three years later, he prepared a list of medical questions for Meriwether Lewis to gather responses to on his exploration of the west with William Clark. As Rush thought about the Native American people Lewis would encounter, he wondered, "Is suicide common among them?" and whether "Ever from love?"[75] Finally, Rush noted his debate with the Frenchman Comte de Volney about suicide and whether it proved "justifiable where a sense of evil predominated over a sense of good" (Volney's view) or whether it "[arose] from derangement" (Rush's assertion).[76] Although speculation about causes did not accompany his portrayal of most cases of insanity, Rush noted causes in most of his reports about those who took their own lives. Madness that drove citizens to end their lives warranted deeper explanation.

On February 3, 1810, Rush recorded a more personal connection to mental illness. "This day," he wrote, "my son John Rush arrived from New Orleans in a state of deep melancholy brought on by killing a brother officer in the Navy." "Neither the embraces nor tears of his parents, brothers, or sister," Rush remembered, "could prevail upon him to speak to them. His grief and uncombed hair and long beard added to the distress produced by the disease of his mind."[77] The younger Rush never recovered from the shock of killing his close friend, Lieutenant Benjamin Taylor, in a duel. With the exception of one brief return to his parents' home, John spent the next twenty-seven years in a cell on the wards his father knew well in the Pennsylvania Hospital. Rush mentioned his son's illness in letters to Thomas Jefferson, but the family never made the young man's condition public.[78] Rush called for the removal of stigma associated with mental maladies but also supported privacy for those who suffered. It remains unclear whether Rush and his family sought to protect their son or themselves—or both—from public shame. In the final years of his life, his son's affliction personalized Rush's compassion for those suffering from mental maladies and deepened his desire to find treatments.

CHANGING VIEWS OF MADNESS

In 1812, a year before his death, Rush published *Medical Inquiries and Observations upon the Diseases of the Mind*, outlining the symptoms, causes, and treatments of mental illness. Seeking to improve care for those who ailed, Rush systematized his observations about mental disorder, and that effort began the country's transition to a medicalized understanding of madness.[79] He hoped—by categorizing the biological causes of mental illness—that "those diseases [could] be brought under the dominion of medicine" and be cured.[80] Like Cotton Mather, the experienced physician attended to mental diseases to bring healing. Mather, though, had grounded his considerations of causes of emotional distress in sin. Rush, instead, deployed Enlightenment empiricism and focused on biological details. In doing so, he sought to "convince the world that mental disease was to be equated with organic disease," illness that could be prevented and treated just like physical ailments.[81]

Biological definitions of mental disease, like those offered by Rush, prompted a reassessment of other conceptions. Most significantly, medical views of madness challenged human sinfulness as the sole source of disease. Rush acknowledged the reconsideration of causes when he contended that many "anti-social" behaviors considered sinful, actions including "suicide, impulse to murder, habitual lying, drunkenness, and compulsive stealing, might [instead be biologically rooted] emotional disorders."[82] Personal culpability for ailments remained a possibility for Rush, but the rise of scientific medicine provided the primary rationale. By the end of the eighteenth century, explanations of mental illness based in human biology and personal ethics prevailed over religious definitions grounded in original and personal sin, at least among many physicians.[83]

Rush's observations and systemization took place amidst broader changes in understandings of mental illness, and a number of intellectual developments influenced those shifts. As the doctor's confidence in biological definitions displayed, Enlightenment thought favored naturalistic rather than supernatural explanations for many phenomena, including human behavior and sickness.[84] Certainty in the ability to explain natural occurrences was paired with belief that study and experimentation would uncover solutions. The act of categorization itself demonstrated trust that through description and organization, human effort would yield remedies for the problem of madness. When Rush and other medical men harnessed scientific wisdom to explain illness, they downplayed or dismissed presumptions of direct, divine involvement in causing sickness.

American thinkers like Rush also took up European speculation about the role of the passions in causing madness in a way that shifted the focus of causality from sin to personal ethics.[85] In a framework that assumed a "strong connection between mind and body," excess passions "were thought to be the conduit through which the mind operated on the body to cause illness" and "abnormal mental functioning."[86] Medical writers noted that excess passions—including "envy, pride, jealousy, love, hate, grief, wealth, and power"—could prompt emotional or physical disease.[87] The focus on a connection between emotions and bodily health countered claims, influenced by longstanding Christian assumptions, that "soul and body [were] of different natures" (one immortal, the other material) and had "limited possibilities of interaction."[88] The newer position collapsed concerns about mind and body and placed both under the purview of biological medicine. Mental illness became a problem of a diseased physical mind rather than a troubled, immaterial soul.[89]

Medical school dissertations offer one of the main sources of insight into the development of medical theory from the Revolutionary era. As late eighteenth-century medical students wrote about the role of excess passions in insanity, they pointed to a "failure of self-control" in prompting illness.[90] When "moral irregularities and excessive passions" brought on madness, Americans assumed that human intervention—their own actions or the help of physicians—might cure, or at least ameliorate, mental disorder. When illness lingered despite treatment, physicians suspected not deficiencies of their own efforts but rather an inability of patients to control their passions and behaviors.[91] Patient failure, and not physician limitations or divine design, perpetuated illness. Similar shifts toward individual responsibility appeared in other aspects of American life. The revivals of the First and Second Great Awakenings, for example, offered individuals more responsibility for their own salvation; self-interest increasingly characterized economic relationships; and "the Enlightenment itself offered the possibility of human control over hitherto unthinkable frontiers."[92] Ushered in by Enlightenment developments, the rise of scientific medicine brought the possibility of new cures, but it also shifted some blame for persistent mental ailments to those who suffered.

While physicians gained confidence in their ability to diagnose and treat mental illnesses, absolute certainty remained elusive, and a variety of theories (medical and spiritual) tended to coexist. Notwithstanding Rush's primary focus on biological factors, the doctor was comfortable maintaining some belief in the supernatural alongside scientific inquiry. He posited an indirect role for sin in sickness, declaring that "the powers of the human mind" were "thrown out of their order by the fall of man."[93] Original sin might play a role in precipitating mental disorder, but Rush refrained from explicitly rooting illness in sin and from pointing to spiritual cures for sickness. In the Puritan era, Cotton Mather understood that sin—whether original or personal—lay behind mental disease. When Rush and his medical contemporaries did address the role of sin in illness, they proved less likely to suspect mental illness as the result of the will of God or the design of the devil.[94] Atop reliance on biological explanations, that change left personal morality, rather than divine punishment or even original sin, as a more frequently suspected cause.

Despite belief in the possibility of divine intervention, Rush remained sure scientific insight would prove that "all diseases [were] curable," given time to discover cures. Often he blended faith and practical action in his medical practice. In a letter to his wife, the doctor confessed, "While I depend upon divine protection and feel that at present I live, move, and have my being in a more especial manner in God alone, I do not neglect to use every precaution that experience has discovered to prevent [becoming ill]."[95] The doctor professed belief in "intellectual as well as physical miracles" but relied on the former to bring cures.[96] While such opinions helped debunk sin as the cause of many mental conditions, transitions in public viewpoints came slowly.

Lacking broad access to scientific studies about mental ailments, most laypersons lagged medical professionals in their adoption of biological causes as primary explanations. Some proved comfortable ruminating about origins of mental distress but refrained from declaring causes definitively. The diaries of Methodist clergymen in America, for example, speculated "that a loss of mental balance" could be either spiritual or physiological in nature.[97] In 1796, as the Methodist itinerant James Meacham traveled his preaching circuit, he encountered a woman "who once was happy in God, & as [he was] told was once of the most sensible Woman of her age." Acknowledging that the woman was now "quite out of her reason," Meacham (unlike physicians eager to declare organic origins of disease) refrained from diagnosing either spiritual or biological causes at fault. Instead, he asked, "Who can account for these things? Is it possible that Satan can have power to [chain] the right reason of a Human Soul, up in the dark caverns of distraction? Or is [it] a constitutional disorder?"[98] While lacking certainty, Meacham proved comfortable allowing both natural and supernatural origins of mental distress. By the twentieth century, for most Americans, medical advances that challenged notions of supernatural causation displaced sin as the presumed primary underlying cause of mental maladies. But, in the century following Rush's work, without the ability to pinpoint exact causes of, or cures for, mental illness (even with continued medical advances), laypersons and professionals alike looked both to medicine and to morality to explain mental maladies.

Changes in understandings of the causes of mental illnesses shifted lines of authority in attending to insane Americans. With growing, if uneven, confidence in the ability of science to bring cures, medical care usurped religious authority like that provided by Cotton Mather, a transition Rush supported. Rush believed physicians needed to "assert their prerogative" and "rescue mental science" from "the usurpation of schoolmen and divines."[99] Physicians, not clergyman, he proclaimed, were the "best judges of sanity."[100] A 1767 sermon demonstrated that some clergy shared that view. Preaching after a suicide, Rev. Samuel Phillips urged his parishioners to seek medical attention at "the first sign of distraction": " 'Don't say as many do, that no Physician can relieve us because our Trouble is altogether a Trouble in Mind, and Body not at all affected.' " This attitude, he argued, was " 'wrong' because 'Trouble of mind' often starts with 'Trouble in the body.' " The sermon emphasized somatic aspects of madness and stressed the importance of a physician's intervention to interrupt the course of illness. Indeed, Phillips claimed that religious ministrations were appropriate only when care from a doctor failed to help.[101] In 1785, after two failed suicide attempts, the Methodist clergyman William Glendinning's friends took him, not to a fellow minister for counseling, but to a doctor for medical treatment.[102] To be sure, suffering souls continued to turn to clergy in times of mental anguish, but Phillips' recommendations and the actions of Glendinning's friends demonstrated that even ministers found medical alternatives preferable.

DEFINITIONS OF DISEASE

Independent of the presumed origins of mental illness, late eighteenth-century physicians continued to deploy the same basic categories of insanity used by Cotton Mather—melancholia, mania, madness—although more as degrees of illness than as separate conditions. While he was the Revolutionary-era leader in categorizing mental disease, Rush was not the only American physician to write about insanity. The Philadelphia doctor recommended a definition of insanity in a 1794 medical dissertation by another practitioner, Edward Cutbush. Rush affirmed the work's conviction that "a false perception of truth; with conversation and actions contrary to right reason, established maxim, and order" characterized mental illness.[103]

Akin to his view of physical illness, Rush concluded that the symptoms, causes, and successful treatments of mental illness pointed to madness originating in the blood vessels of the brain. Before justifying his theory that problems with the vascular system caused madness, he detailed earlier medical theories of mental distress he hoped to overturn. He rejected dysfunctions of the liver, spleen, intestines, and nerves as causes of insanity. While asserting that dysfunction of the blood vessels formed the primary source of madness, Rush also presented "remote and exciting causes of intellectual derangement." Those contributing causes might be physical and included the following: falls and other direct impacts to the brain, isolation, odors, famine, excessive "use of ardent spirits," "inordinate sexual desires and gratifications," blood transfusions, great pain, "extremely hot and cold weather," intestinal worms, and irritation from foreign objects, such as a small bullet, lodged somewhere in the body.[104] Beyond physical causes, he highlighted factors that taxed cognitive functions and caused madness. They included the intense study of many subjects (including trying to fix the exact date of biblical prophesies and the disappointment that occurs after the predicted date passed), switching the mind too rapidly from one subject to another, "inordinate schemes of ambition or avarice," extravagant joy, excessive anger, terror, disappointed love, fear, grief, public and private defamation, and absence from one's native country. No one was immune to mental illness, and Rush offered an example of a "clergyman in Maryland [who] became insane in consequence of having permitted some typographical errors to escape in a sermon which he published upon the death of general Washington."[105] Altogether, Rush's observations informed his conviction that physical and experiential factors, not supernatural forces, caused mental maladies.

In addition to outlining causes of madness, Rush documented attributes and conditions that predisposed individuals to suffer. He observed a hereditary disposition to mental maladies. He listed dark hair color, great wit, the acquisition of sudden fortunes, and, in Christian countries, "infidelity and atheism" as predisposing conditions. Noting that "maniacs seldom live to be old," Rush named those between ages twenty and fifty as most likely to suffer. Single people suffered more than the married, the rich more than the poor, those living in colder climates more than those living in warmer ones, and those with creative occupations (poets, painters, sculptors, musicians) more than those with logic-oriented professions (chemists, naturalists, mathematicians, and natural philosophers).[106] Rush found women more likely to suffer than men, although each gender experienced events that predisposed them to mental illness.[107] Women had a greater predisposition "imparted to their bodies by menstruation, pregnancy, parturition [giving birth], and to their minds, by living so much alone in their families."[108] Rush found men more likely to experience madness stemming from the experiences of war or from excessive drink and identified men as more likely to commit suicide.[109]

While clear that supernatural forces did not cause mental illness, Rush argued that mental distress could manifest with religious expression. Certain kinds of mental disease, he observed, appeared

> most frequently in the enthusiasts in religion, in whom it discovers itself in a variety of ways; particularly; 1) In a belief that they are the peculiar favourites of heaven, and exclusively possessed of just opinions of the divine will as revealed in the Scriptures. 2) That they see and converse with angels, and departed spirits of their relations and friends. 3) That they are favoured with visions and the revelation of future events. And, 4) That they are exalted into beings of the highest order.[110]

As evidence, Rush remarked that he had "seen two instances of persons who believed themselves to be the Messiah" and had "heard of each of the sacred names and offices of the Father, Son, and Holy Ghost having been assumed at the same time by three persons under the influence of this partial form of derangement in a hospital in Mexico."[111] With those observations, Rush noted that—while in the past such persons were fined, put in prison, or even put to death—medical science now saw their actions as illness rather than impiety.

Despite a long list of causes and predisposing conditions, Rush contended that madness might simply appear, even in good, moral, otherwise healthy individuals:

> To the history that has been given of the correspondence between the ravings and conduct of mad people and their natural tempers and dispositions, there are several exceptions. These are, all those cases in which persons of exemplary piety and purity of character, utter profane, or impious, or indelicate language, and behave in other respects contrary to their moral habits. The apparent vices of such deranged people may be compared to the offensive substances that are sometimes thrown upon the surface of the globe by an earthquake, mixed with the splendid fossils formerly mentioned, which substances had no existence in nature, but were formed by a new arrangement in the particles of matter in consequence of the violent commotions in the bowels of the earth.[112]

Rush and his peers admitted that medical science could explain some, but not all, occurrences of mental disease. Cases like the seven-year insanity of a virtuous, young church member prompted physicians like Daniel Sanders to fall back on supernatural explanations. The Vermont doctor declared illnesses like the young woman's to be among the "mysteries of Providence."[113] Regardless of their presumed origins, mental illnesses warranted a response.

CORPORATE AND INSTITUTIONAL RESPONSES

Following Rush's lead, most physicians came to treat mental illness primarily as a medical concern rather than a social, economic, or spiritual problem. As a result, the assumed proper locus of care began to shift from the home and community to medical institutions.[114] Mental and physical maladies, as they had in the earlier colonial era, continued to draw public attention. The responses they prompted, though, grew more coordinated as the colonies matured.

In 1751, with assistance from Rush and Benjamin Franklin, a group of Philadelphia Quakers petitioned the Pennsylvania Assembly, seeking financial support for the colony's first hospital. Philadelphia was the largest city in the colonies, and Quakers had stepped aside from political participation after their pacifist beliefs came in conflict with the need to defend the colony's western border. As part of their turn to philanthropic work, they hoped to launch a medical facility.[115] While intending the hospital to treat both the physically and the mentally ill, the petition to the assembly began with a plea about care for the mentally disturbed:

> That with the number of people the Number of lunaticks, or Persons distempered in Mind, and deprived of their rational faculties, hath greatly increased in this Province.
>
> That some of them, going at large, are a terrour to their neighbors, who are daily apprehensive of the violences they may commit; and others are continually wasting their substance, to the great injury of themselves and families, wickedly taking advantage of their unhappy condition, and drawing them into unreasonable bargains . . .
>
> That few or none of them are so sensible of their condition as to submit voluntarily to the treatment their respective cases require, and therefore continue in the same deplorable state during their lives; whereas it has been found, by the experience of many years, that above two thirds of the mad people received into Bethlehem Hospital, and there treated properly, have been perfectly cured.[116]

An appeal for care of the insane in the largest colonial city made sense. Growing population densities in cities made madness more visible, more difficult to contain in almshouses and family homes, and thus more problematic. Hospitalization offered safety for the public and care for the insane.

The proposal for a new hospital succeeded, but the institution failed to guarantee helpful treatment. The facility admitted insane patients from its opening in 1752, but sufferers received largely custodial, and sometimes violent, care until Rush joined the staff in 1783. Prior to Rush's direct administration, patients endured "hot and cold showers alternately," had "their scalps . . . shaved and blistered," and were "bled to syncope and purged until only mucus came from their intestines." They "were chained by ankle or waist to the wall of the cell," and because "mad people were not supposed to appreciate temperature differences . . . cells were not heated."[117]

Harsh treatment persisted for decades and seemed logical to caregivers. The Enlightenment heralded human reason and equated a loss of reason with a loss of humanity. Despite medical advancements, Americans viewed the mad as less than human. Even Rush contended, "A man deprived of his reason partakes" in "the nature of . . . animals."[118] Nonetheless, the poor treatment of that patient population, and the lack of cures, disturbed the doctor and prompted his deeper explorations of mental distress. His work was part of a wider movement for reforming care, one shaped both by humanitarian impulses rooted in the Enlightenment and by Christian convictions about love of neighbor.[119] Though religion no longer played the primary role in defining madness, it influenced treatment protocols, particularly in the development of specialized institutional care.

HUMANE TREATMENT METHODS

After the turn of the nineteenth century, American institutions incorporated treatment approaches that differed from ones practiced in the early years of the Pennsylvania Hospital. New ideas about "moral treatment" influenced the creation—and later the reform—of facilities for the insane throughout the nation. Several private institutions formed and emphasized the treatment protocol pioneered by French physician Philippe Pinel and mirrored in the work of English reformer William Tuke. Similarly, their new approaches sought to eliminate, or at least minimize, the abuses and harsh treatments found in facilities like London's Bethlehem Hospital. Though most of the new American facilities opened after Rush's death, they offered the sort of correctives he found necessary from his experiences at the Pennsylvania Hospital.[120]

Moral treatment named both a disposition toward care and a set of techniques. Working independently, and believing that insanity could be cured, Pinel's and Tuke's reforms included similar presumptions. They worked to orient treatment around kindness and careful attention to the emotional and physical needs of each patient and sought to impart hope and instill confidence in healing.[121] Pinel's *traitement moral* was known in England and America as "moral treatment," but his methods (and the French *moral*) had no explicit "moralistic content." It did not assume, for example, that moral faults caused mental illness. Instead, the new methods concentrated on behavioral aspects of insanity and attended to treatments more so than specific diagnoses.[122]

Personal experience and religious convictions motivated the creation of those new methods. The conditions at the asylum that Pinel took charge of in 1793 upset the French doctor (who at one point had considered the priesthood). In response, he removed physical restraints from patients, avoided "heroic" measures including bleeding and corporal punishment, and instead created a well-ordered environment to promote health. Presuming that "madness did not 'imply a total abolition of the mental faculties,'" he appealed "to the patient's reasoning abilities." Doing so required authoritative asylum leadership to "persuade patients to internalize the behavior and values of normal society." Pinel's approach, which required confinement in asylums, brought surprising improvements in patients and bolstered confidence that treatment should include psychological approaches.[123]

In 1796 William Tuke, a Quaker merchant, opened the York Retreat in England. Distressed by abuses in existing institutions (including the death of a Quaker woman who died six weeks after being admitted to an asylum), Tuke and the Quaker community established their own facility. Treatment took on much the same form as it did in Pinel's French institution. Based on Quaker virtues of gentleness and quietness, the York Retreat was created as "a place in which the unhappy might obtain refuge—a quiet haven in which the shattered bark might find a means of reparation or safety."[124] Tuke hoped to treat both mind and spirit. The staff at the York Retreat relied on the Quaker belief in the Inner Light that assumed that this divine spark was never fully extinguished in humans, even by disease. They hoped to help patients recover their sense of the divine in themselves. Life for patients at York included exercise, work, and recreation.[125] Governed by the Friends General Meeting, the hospital's rooms were well heated and ventilated, and the eleven-acre property included room to grow crops and raise cows. All but the most violent patients were free to travel throughout the facility and grounds.[126]

Moral management made its way to the United States most directly as the result of close relationships between Quakers on either side of the Atlantic. The Friends Asylum (originally, the Asylum for the Relief of Friends Deprived of Their Reason), established in 1813 in Philadelphia and opened in 1817, appeared as the first private hospital in the United States dedicated to the care of those with mental illness. Over the next decade, mental hospitals opened in Boston (McClean Hospital, 1821), New York (Bloomingdale Asylum, 1824), and Connecticut (Hartford Retreat Center, 1824). Each of those institutions followed the York Retreat model. Most facilities, however, paired moral treatment (including "occupational therapy, religious exercises, recreation, and the employment of mechanical restraint . . . only when absolutely necessary") with medical therapeutics.[127] And, despite the emergence of specialized treatment facilities, few medical journals before 1824 discussed mental disease, and so the majority of American physicians, even if they had access to the latest medical theory, likely knew little about moral treatment.[128]

RUSH'S TREATMENT PROTOCOL

Though Rush's work predated the appearance of those religiously based institutions, his treatment repertoire included a blend of moral treatment and medical care. He promoted humane treatment environments, and his work contributed to the shift in American care. To facilitate healing, Rush believed, "great regard should be had to cleanliness in the persons and apartments of mad people." To protect patients from being exposed to the public as showpieces, he asserted, "mad people should never be visited, nor even seen by their friends, and much less by strangers, without being accompanied by their physician." Isolation offered protection for the one who suffered, hindered the disease from being known to the community, and allowed doctors to control asylum environments.[129] Hoping to make treatment more agreeable to women, Rush argued that female patients should be housed separately from men and cared for by female attendants. Finally, when suicide proved a possibility, all precautions possible should be taken to prevent it.[130]

Unlike those who focused exclusively on behavioral treatments, Rush also recommended physical remedies. The doctor's physical treatments aimed at restoring healthy harmony to patients. With mental disorders understood to stem from an excess of passions or imbalance in bodily systems, physicians sought to restore balance and reason in patients.[131] Rush's arsenal included treatments used throughout the eighteenth century in America: bloodletting, purges, emetics, forced salivation by ingesting mercury, a reduced diet, stimulating drinks (such as Madeira wine), and baths (both warm and cold). In addition, in order to stimulate the blood, he commended "frictions" to the trunk of the body and physical exercise. Rush deployed existing medical treatment to treat emotional disorders, but he also invented two devices to treat mental illness. The first—a tranquilizer chair—strapped patients in, keeping them upright, in order to "save the head from the impetus of the blood as much as possible."[132] He also devised a "gyrator." The machine spun patients on a turntable, in hopes that centrifugal force would restore proper blood flow to the brain. Injuries resulting from both devices led to their abandonment, both by Rush (who preferred bloodletting) and by other practitioners.[133]

At times, Rush supplemented physical treatments with psychological ones, although his reliance on physical cures meant that he lagged European counterparts in turning more exclusively to psychological approaches.[134] Cotton Mather hoped that conversation with a clergyman would help sufferers root out sin and turn to God. Alternately, Rush urged insane patients to write their "thoughts and secrets on paper." He hoped that reviewing what they had written would shock sufferers into rejecting their disturbed thoughts.[135] Rush found value in talking with patients, but in a different way than his Puritan predecessor. Mather had noted that conversation between a clergyman and sufferers could alleviate madness. Rush assumed that patients benefitted from talking to their physicians instead of their spiritual leaders. Such attention, he argued, signaled that the physician took the disease seriously, even if he was bored by the details: "It will be necessary, therefore, for a physician to listen with attention to [the] tedious and uninteresting details of its symptoms and causes."[136] Mather and Rush recommended conversation with different objectives. Mather hoped to help individuals root out sin that lay at the core of their illness and to connect individuals to God for healing; Rush anticipated healing by validating the experience of illness.

Despite the primacy he gave to medical care, be it physical or psychological, Rush sometimes recommended the assistance of a clergyman. He advised that when individuals thought they were unpardonable (or assumed they had committed an unforgiveable sin) they should seek council from a clergyman. In addition, "if the disease be derived from a sense of guilt, it is generally connected with ignorance or erroneous opinions in religion," he argued, and "the former must be removed, by advising the visits of a sensible and enlightened clergyman."[137] For those suffering religious delusions, Rush recommended either a physician or a pastor to remind patients that God rarely delivered prior revelations to lone individuals or without witnesses. Religious assistance remained helpful, but only in a subset of cases.

Beyond physical treatment and conversation, Rush recommended nonphysical cures that echoed the psychological approaches of European moral treatment. He advocated keeping busy, industriousness, being social, and even reading novels (so that the mind was kept active, even if the body was not). He observed that "building, commerce, a public employment, an executorship to a will; above all agriculture have often cured this disease. The last, that is, agriculture, by agitating the passions by alternate hope, fear, and enjoyment, and by rendering bodily exercise or labour necessary, is calculated to produce the greatest benefit."[138] In addition, he encouraged "certain amusements" including checkers, cards, shooting, the theater, listening to children playing, listening to music, matrimony, memorizing or copying prose, and travel for the treatment and prevention of mental maladies. To combat mental disease, Rush deployed a wide range of treatment options, and perhaps out of necessity, given that no approach proved effective in all cases.

A PUBLIC ADVOCATE

Alongside attending to his own patients, documenting medical theory about mental ailments, and recommending treatments, Rush continued to seek funding to ensure better treatment for sufferers. Thanks to his influence, the Pennsylvania Hospital, which opened in 1752, included a ward for the insane. From 1783 until his death, he served as an attending physician at the facility, and in 1787 he undertook "exclusive care" of the "maniacal patients" and made careful observations of the pathology of mental illness, hoping to improve treatment.[139] Not content simply to provide good care, the doctor sought ways to expand healing efforts to more of the population. In March of 1792, prompted by a short publication by Rush, the lower house of the Pennsylvania Assembly allotted £15,000 to build a separate "madhouse" for the insane at the hospital.[140] In January of 1803, the doctor met with the hospital's managers and proposed that "a man of education" be appointed "to superintend the Lunatics, to walk with them, converse with them, &c., in order to awaken and regulate their minds."[141] The compassionate physician advocated for the best care possible for those suffering with mental illness, not simply confinement.

Rush found good health to be a combination of social, political, economic, and environmental factors and bristled at obstacles that prevented many from seeking treatment.[142] In a November 11, 1789, letter to the Board of Managers of the Pennsylvania Hospital, the sympathetic physician noted that without proper physical space to house patients, he could not provide adequate treatment for those suffering from mental maladies:

> Gentlemen: Under the conviction that the patients afflicted by Madness should be the first objects of the care of a physician of the Pennsylvania Hospital, I have attempted to relieve them, but I am sorry to add that my attempts which at first promised some Improvement were soon afterwards rendered Abortive by the Cells of the Hospital.
>
> These apartments are damp in Winter & too warm in Summer. They are moreover so constituted, as not to admit readily of a change of air; hence the smell of them is both offensive and unwholesome.

> Few patients have ever been confined in these Cells who have not been affected by a cold in two or three weeks after their confinement, and several have died of Consumption in consequence of this cold. . . .
>
> Should more wholesome apartments be provided for them, it is more than probable that many of them might be Relieved by the use of remedies which have lately been discovered to be effectual in their disorder.[143]

Nearly a decade later, he wrote again to the board of managers. He called for better physical care and recommended employment for patients.[144] Alongside direct appeals to the board of managers, Rush took his fight public, publishing a series of articles in the city newspapers and petitioning members of the state legislature for funds for a new wing for the insane in the Pennsylvania Hospital.[145]

Three years before his death, Rush wrote to the board of managers once more and outlined specific recommendations based on twenty-five years of experience. He proposed separating patients by gender and severity of disease, providing recreational activities, appropriate staffing, and comfortable accommodations, and limiting the number of visitors. Rush's commitment to society and his fellow humans meant that he cared about more than medical innovation. Society was bettered only if the conditions of those who suffered most improved. He knew that insufficient funding prevented the implementation of all of the requests he made to the hospital's board of managers, but he hoped that they would have adopted some that assured both the "comfort of the mad people" and the "reputation of the institution."[146]

As Rush systematized understandings of mental illness and pushed for revised treatments, he sensed the challenges ahead and pled for God's guidance. He opened *Medical Inquires* by connecting his work to God's providence and his call as a Christian:

> In entering upon the subject of the following Inquiries and Observations, I feel as if I were about to tread upon consecrated ground. I am aware of its difficulty and importance, and I thus humbly implore that BEING, whose government extends to the thoughts of all his creatures, so too direct mine, in this arduous undertaking, that nothing hurtful to my fellow citizens may fall from my pen, and that this work may be the means of lessening a portion of some of the greatest evils of human life.[147]

Reflecting on his medical proposals, the doctor pointed to God as their source: "It is not to him that willeth, nor to him that runneth, but to the overruling hand of Heaven alone that we are to look for the successful issue of human actions whether of body or mind."[148] Rush assumed that all in nature was God's creation, including the minds of physicians. He was also sure that individual health and societal health were linked. His pious upbringing and quest for faithfulness shaped his public work, whether medical or political. Pain, in Rush's eyes, including the suffering that stemmed from mental maladies, formed primarily a medical problem, but one that Christians had a responsibility to address through medical innovation and advocacy.

"HE AIMED WELL"

Rush's autobiography included portraits of the signers of the Declaration of Independence. There, he offered a pithy description of his own character: "He aimed well."[149] Rush, shaped by both Protestant and Enlightenment values, studied medicine to alleviate the distress of others. Although he met opposition, he helped many, and his contributions to medicine won wide recognition, evidenced by the "handsome ring" sent to him "from the Emperor of Russia."[150] As part of his work, Rush demonstrated a concern for public health and turned public and professional attention to mental illnesses as valid medical concerns. He shaped early institutional care for sick citizens and proved a model of Christian charity. The doctor believed hard work to combat suffering and injustice was the Christian responsibility the Divine Creator called and enabled him to accomplish.

Illness afflicted most colonial and Revolutionary-era Americans. Mental maladies invaded the lives of fewer citizens but appeared frequently enough to be deemed worthy of attention by church leaders, the medical community, and society. While the professionalization of medicine had begun, treatments for all types of illnesses remained far from modern or standardized. Only by the early nineteenth century did many Americans, especially physicians like Rush, shift to view sickness primarily through medical and not spiritual lenses. Though widespread lay adoption of that shift lagged elite acceptance, the role of the church in defining mental distress had changed forever. No longer could a voice like Cotton Mather's carry the authority it once had about the causes of and solutions for physical and mental suffering. Voices like Rush's demanded a hearing.

Still, Christians continued to feel called to alleviate suffering and felt compelled to find new ways to participate in tending to the distress of their fellow humans brought by mental maladies. Rush believed that a new day had begun and that "times of cruelty to this class of our fellow creatures and insensibility to their sufferings are now passing away."[151] While improvements appeared, and despite Rush's optimism and best efforts, suffering and inadequate care continued for those living with mental maladies. Other Christians noticed. In the coming century, as medical approaches to mental illness gained scientific complexity, and as institutionalization grew more standardized, believers like the reformer Dorothea Dix and the pastor Anton Boisen would forge new paths. They did so amidst growing suspicion that mental maladies that were unresponsive to treatments might signal moral deficiencies in those afflicted. Dix and Boisen, like Rush, however, remained undeterred in their efforts to bring change.

3

Advocating for the Helpless, Forgotten, and Insane

Dorothea Dix

> I come to present the strong claims of suffering humanity. I come to
> place before the Legislature of Massachusetts the condition of the miserable,
> the desolate, the outcast. I come as the advocate of helpless, forgotten,
> insane, and idiotic men and women; of beings sunk to a condition from
> which the most unconcerned would start with real horror; of beings
> wretched in our prisons, and more wretched in our almshouses.
>
> —Dorothea Dix, 1843[1]

Legend held that while walking down a Boston street in 1841, Dorothea
Dix overheard two men denouncing the squalid conditions at the Middlesex County jail in East Cambridge, Massachusetts, an institution that housed
criminals and the insane side by side. The conversation, one she might have
otherwise ignored or forgotten, struck a nerve. Dix had been feeling guilty
about her self-centeredness. Focusing on "improvement of her mind at the
expense of her heart," she had neglected not only her closest acquaintances
but also her fellow citizens. Other accounts reported that her exposure to
the plight of mentally ill Americans housed in prisons took place when the
Unitarian minister James T. G. Nichols begged her to take over his Sunday
school class with female inmates. Either way, the horrid conditions she found
while visiting the jail sparked the work that made her famous and fulfilled
her search for a God-given vocation.[2]

Dix (1802–1887) spoke of that encounter as her Damascus Road experience. It spurred her quest—as a calling from God—to remedy the plight
of America's insane. In the years that followed her visit to the Middlesex

County jail, she toured hundreds of prisons, almshouses, institutions, and private homes, gathering evidence about America's inadequate treatment of the mad. Aiming to improve and expand care for those living with mental disease, she shared her findings and spearheaded reform efforts throughout the United States. Benjamin Rush's attention to mental maladies took place in his study and in Pennsylvania sick rooms. Dix's crusade occurred on the public stage in state legislatures and in dilapidated almshouses and prisons. From 1843 to 1865, without formal training in medicine or institution building, her efforts helped launch and expand thirty hospitals for the insane. By taking up the cause of the nation's mentally ill, she found a place where the world's need, her passions, and her God-given abilities aligned.[3] In doing so, Dix blazed a new trail in Protestant advocacy.

In an Enlightenment-shaped world that granted medical men authority in treating disease, the Boston reformer refused to ignore suffering. As a result, Dix's nineteenth-century support for mentally ill Americans changed again the relationship between Protestants and mental illness. While Christians had always looked inward toward the state of their souls and outward toward faithful action in the world, in the nineteenth century, American Protestants grew more certain that the proper reach of their faith extended beyond their homes, congregations, and townships, to the new nation. That reach included its rapidly expanding social institutions. Beyond providing care for family members and neighbors, believers felt called to ensure help for all in need. Churchgoers made provisions for that work in a variety of ways. They formed benevolence societies with goals of abolishing slavery, curbing intemperate drinking, and distributing Bibles.[4] They took matters into their own hands and provided care for the ailing and destitute. Often, they enlisted governmental resources to aid their Christian mission to ameliorate suffering. Dix pioneered the final approach, relying not only on her own determined discipline but also on the sympathies of fellow believers to procure funding for mental institutions. Dix demonstrated that not all Protestants that attended to mental illness were physicians or clergymen. She responded to suffering by claiming authority from her identity as Christian, called to help fulfill God's mission in the world. Her example, visible to men and women around the nation, helped cement the conviction that faith demanded individual public action to alleviate suffering. The tenacious reformer operated with a new sort of authority, a moral authority rooted in her Protestant faith.[5]

Dix's career as a social activist did not begin until she was forty-one years old, and yet she appeared indefatigable in the four decades that followed. A woman with humble New England beginnings, she transformed into a renowned and respected advocate for the country's insane. She crisscrossed the nation inspecting public institutions. She dined and vacationed with intellectual and social elites. A Protestant, she garnered the attention of Pope Pius IX with her work. An American living before the enfranchisement of woman, she commanded notice from state and national politicians. As her public career blossomed, the Presbyterian minister Theodore L. Cuyler lauded Dix's "conquer[ing of] a half dozen legislatures."[6] A layperson, she was appointed by President Abraham Lincoln as the Superintendent of Women Nurses for the Union during the Civil War.[7] Before those feats, however, she endured decades of uncertainty, personal struggle, and relentless campaigning.

Dix's public advocacy took place during a time of immense religious, medical, and social optimism. A combination of Enlightenment hopefulness, giddiness over the successful new country, and confidence in the power of religion to effect change made a cure for all ills—medical or social—seem possible. Americans were convinced of their ability to solve problems, cure disease, and bring about social change. A sense of God's divine blessing of the new nation fueled that hope. A democratic spirit paired with energy from religious revivals infused Protestantism and emboldened individual Christians to make changes in the world around them. Although some of that optimism later proved misplaced—especially when it came to the ability to cure mental maladies—Dix's story exemplifies the power of a desire for social change rooted in religious mission and fueled by scientific and political optimism.[8]

Alongside the expanding reach of Protestant ambition, and continuing a process begun in the prior century, the professional and individual domains claiming authority over illness shifted again. The clergyman Cotton Mather understood physical and mental maladies as spiritual problems; attending to sin and the human relationship with a sovereign God formed a logical response but required pastoral guidance. The blend of faith and Enlightenment empiricism of physician Benjamin Rush brought mental illness solidly under medical jurisdiction. Other doctors adopted Rush's approach, and the transition co-opted clergy authority. By 1850 ministers were turning to asylum physicians for advice about the mental health of their parishioners, and Americans agreed that mental illnesses were best cared for in medical facilities, by medical professionals. To be sure, Protestant clergy continued to counsel the troubled, but their focus changed to helping parishioners navigate religious life amidst illness and the country's rapidly changing economic and social systems. By the Civil War, expertise in matters of mental illness diversified into three realms: some defined the problem, some directly provided treatment, and others helped ensure medical facilities were available to house those in need. Christians dabbled in all three areas in antebellum America but, following Dix's lead, firmly grabbed hold of the final role.

WELL PREPARED FOR AN UNCERTAIN FUTURE

Years before her work as a reformer, Dix's family provided a mixed set of lessons that shaped the fiercely independent character that enabled her mission. From her grandparents, the young woman received tutelage in philanthropy and wealth. Dix was the granddaughter of a self-made Bostonian—a doctor, merchant, and land speculator who married into money.[9] The riches her grandfather Elijah accumulated funded moral reforms including the construction of a school and prison in Worcester, Massachusetts. He also built a large home in Boston where Dorothea later lived. The elder Dix's professional pursuits and philanthropy ended abruptly after his unexpected death when Dorothea was seven.[10] Thanks to a modicum of inherited wealth and, later, her publishing income, as an adult, Dorothea, who never married, lived independently with adequate means. Her frugal lifestyle helped, as did memories of her earliest years.

Dix's father offered an example of capriciousness and struggle that Dorothea hoped to avoid. The black sheep of his family, Joseph Dix dropped out of Harvard, entered a marriage that his family disapproved of, moved to rural Maine, and remained perpetually destitute and frequently ill. In New England, he took up Methodism during the revivals of the Second Great Awakening and worked as an itinerant lay minister. His family of origin marked his religious conversion as a move into commonness. As elite Congregationalists, they viewed Methodism as "a crude, homespun evangelism" that appealed to society's downtrodden, not those of high social standing.[11] Joseph's only daughter shared the wider family's sense that Methodism lacked the controlled and respectable faith that she grew to admire in Congregationalism and its offshoot, Unitarianism.[12]

After her birth in Hampden, Maine, Dorothea's immediate family moved frequently. They lived in poverty, at times only steps from the almshouse. Unpredictable and suspected to be an alcoholic, Joseph proved prone to extreme "religious spells" as the family wandered through the New England frontier. Dix recoiled from her father's emotion-filled Methodism and detested being forced to help him bind religious tracts for sale. Joseph's explosive faith, though, imparted a deeply personal piety and a quest for personal perfection.

As an adolescent, Dorothea seized responsibility for her life. Her mother, Mary, after giving birth to Dix's two brothers ten years her junior, proved too ill to rear children. Early biographers painted a picture of a home devoid of love that included emotional, if not physical, mistreatment.[13] Whether or not such abuse occurred, Dix tried to wipe her parents from her memory and throughout adulthood referred to herself as an orphan.[14] At age twelve, Dorothea fled to Boston to live with her paternal grandmother, for whom she was named. Dorothy Lynde Dix's home offered an escape for Dorothea but also a cold, disciplined environment, and the two women sustained a tense relationship. In a letter to a friend, the younger Dix bemoaned that living with her grandmother required "moral and physical courage to face the Medusa!"[15] After a year under her grandmother's roof, she left Boston to help care for her brothers, who had been abandoned with an aunt in Worcester. Lacking financial resources, and unsure of her place in her grandmother's will, Dix opened her first school, hoping to care for her brothers and become self-sufficient.

The education that enabled Dix to teach came from a variety of sources. Her father provided training in the Bible and classics. After leaving home, she acquired a borrowing card for a Boston research library thanks to the help of her uncle, the librarian and scholar Thaddeus Mason Harris. The scores of books she checked out occupied her for three or four hours each night as she read and commented on literary classics, physical and natural sciences, and philosophy. Attendance at public lectures in Boston added insight into astronomy, mineralogy, and botany. Like Mather and Rush before her, Dix was interested in the natural world and science as a study of God's handiwork and providence.[16] Also like her Protestant predecessors, scientific progress failed to dislodge her sense of God's presence in the world.

Aware of her God-given, keen intellect, Dix struggled with how best to put it to use. Always purposeful, she hoped improving her education would not only provide income but also shed light on her place in God's providence.[17] The young teacher's education extended beyond book learning and lectures. Time living with relatives in Boston and Worcester had introduced Dix to upper-class social norms of behavior and dress. Both book learning and education in social norms became valuable tools as she later navigated the country investigating treatment of the insane.

Eventually, Dix returned to Boston with her brothers, becoming the head of her own household at age sixteen. She was well educated, but as a woman in the nineteenth century, she lacked access to a wide range of venues to deploy her knowledge. Teaching formed an acceptable outlet. Dix opened schools and worked at a pace that her friends deemed obsessive.[18] At her first school, in addition to imparting knowledge, she hoped to "rescue some of America's miserable children from vice and guilt, dependence on the Alms-house, and finally from what [she feared would] be their eternal misery."[19] Intellectual, social, and spiritual salvation were overlapping goals in the young woman's teaching. Dix proved a strict, demanding, and inflexible instructor.[20] Students described her as "stern," "overbearing and dictatorial."[21] The determined teacher wanted to instill a disciplined morality in her students, an attribute her own decades of public work later displayed.[22] While never fully content with her teaching career, she spoke of her time in the classroom as "the cause and work, for which and to which Providence has adopted . . . me." She became one of Boston's "most prominent young schoolmistresses," but, while teaching formed a satisfying pursuit, it was not her permanent vocation.[23]

Related to her teaching, Dix earned wide recognition as an author of children's books. The first, *Conversations on Common Things; or, Guide to Knowledge: With Questions* (1824), she published at age twenty-two. To compile that reader, which was intended for use with lower-level schoolchildren, she corresponded with a number of prominent scientists and scholars, asking questions and seeking new knowledge. The text became a financial success, going through sixty editions before the Civil War.[24] Over the next decade, Dix published four more books, largely in the form of devotional guides for families and children. Together, publishing and operating schools provided a means for the focused New Englander to further her own education and to exert authority. As a writer and a teacher, both acceptable occupations for a woman in Jacksonian America, Dix was able to use her intellectual gifts in the public realm.[25] Her work not only received praise from Boston's leading citizens but also made her a public figure and provided needed income.[26]

Dix's education, income, and access to prominent Bostonians marked her as an elite member of American society, but she preferred to think of herself as an outsider. While preparing material for a never-published memoir, she reflected, "The whole of my years, from ten years till the present, differ essentially from the experience and pursuits of those around me."[27] In many ways, she was right. Dix garnered public accolades but maintained just a handful of close friendships, and a sterile emotional distance marked most of her relationships. Because she never married, she failed to conform to a primary social norm for nineteenth-century women.[28] Often a loner, Dix corresponded and dined with the nation's most prominent women and political and religious men but spent much of her later life inside almshouses, prisons, and asylums gathering data. She preferred to travel alone, even through unfamiliar European countries.[29] She survived—and clung to a sense that she failed to fit in society—because of her confidence that her life had a divine purpose, if only she could discover it.[30]

Bright and hardworking, Dix had her grandfather's philanthropic legacy and strong intellectual grounding, but neither the security of unlimited inherited wealth nor the satisfying assurance of a lifelong vocation. Even with some success providing education for children, she was dissatisfied, her future remained uncertain, and the work that cemented her place in American history remained decades away.

A WORLD IN TRANSITION

Not only was Dix's early life marked by frequent change but from 1800 to 1850 the world around her also underwent dramatic social, economic, religious, and medical transformations. Those shifts shaped reactions to the nation's dependent citizens, including the poor, prisoners, and the mentally ill.

Demographic transitions anchored social change. In the post-Revolutionary era, Americans migrated from rural areas to cities, and an influx of immigrants from Europe helped fuel urban growth. In 1790 only six cities boasted populations more than 8,000; by 1850, eighty-five did. No American cities included more than 50,000 residents in 1790; by 1860 New York City alone housed half a million residents. Four more cities held 100,000 to 250,000 citizens, and twenty more cities contained populations between 25,000 and 100,000.[31] Alongside those shifts, the country transitioned from a largely rural agricultural economy to urban mercantile and factory capitalism.[32] Though much of the country's population remained in rural areas, growth in cities yielded higher levels of poverty, and population concentration made squalid conditions and behaviors deemed deviant, such as mental maladies, visible to more Americans.

As citizens moved and modes of production evolved, daily activity that once revolved around families and household industries now centered on the workplace and social institutions. Society grew increasingly segmented, with "firm boundaries" emerging between "the domestic and the economic," between men, who spent their days in the public, economic sphere, and women, who spent their days at home.[33] As a result, family life privatized, and public (and quasi-public) institutions, including schools and hospitals, appeared to address educational and welfare needs once provided by individual households.[34]

A distinction also grew between capitalists and laborers, with the latter increasingly valued for their productivity and contributions to the market economy. Despite the egalitarian rhetoric pervasive since the American Revolution, social life remained stratified, and more so than in the prior century, Americans deemed one another good members of society based on their economic productivity. Those unable or unwilling to work, including the poor and the mentally ill, emerged as socially problematic citizens. An increasingly rich merchant class that sought continued productivity helped fund the early development of educational and welfare institutions.

Religious change also reshaped antebellum America and paved the way for spiritually motivated activism like Dix's. In 1776, despite denominational distinctions in belief and practice, a broad evangelical consensus undergirded much of Protestant life. By 1850, though, the American Protestantism in which Dix was firmly entrenched was experiencing upheaval. As charismatic leaders rose to shape new traditions, Protestantism diversified. New sects and denominations took a variety of forms, from the frontier revivalism of Joseph Dix to the rationalist reaction to the perceived emotional excess of awakenings by Boston's elite Congregationalists and Unitarians. Joseph's daughter stood at the crossroads of those, sometimes contradictory, religious impulses.

The revivals of the Second Great Awakening unsettled traditional Protestant denominationalism and brought lasting theological change. Sharing emphases on new birth, conversion, and salvation with the revivals of the early eighteenth century, the movement spread farther geographically. The nineteenth-century awakenings also deemphasized the Calvinist notion of human depravity. Instead, clergy and believers influenced by theological Arminianism focused on a "loving and beneficent God," a moral universe, human possession of free will, and the perfectibility of humanity.[35] For those with Arminian affinities, optimism rather than pessimism increasingly animated religious thought. Just as Americans had successfully defined their political future, they now felt free to contribute to their own salvation and found themselves emboldened to bring that redemption to others. That hopefulness shaped the development of both social outreach and medical care.

Emerging just after the nation's successful declaration of independence, those theological changes were accompanied by a profoundly egalitarian spirit. Religious populism enabled many, including Dix, to define and embrace a personal faith and piety that shaped both their life choices and engagement in the world.[36] Clergy retained spiritual authority, but they now shared it with laity in novel ways. Ministers preached about salvation, but individual men and woman held responsibility for claiming their eternal destinies. Unlike the earlier Puritans, many Americans now felt sure of both their salvation and their virtue.

No longer needing clergy to validate their religious experiences, believers could trust their own instincts. Dix admired and professed loyalty to a number of clergymen, but they were figures of her choosing. She looked to them to help inform—but not dictate—how her faith should be enacted. In those men, she found inspiration, but she needed no permission to interpret how her faith shaped her actions. While she spoke and corresponded frequently with prominent clergymen, an egalitarian impulse allowed her to declare her religious mission and then to pursue it outside of church or denominational structures. When, at last, Dix found her calling, she proved sure of her vocation. Dix claimed religious authority for her vocation and implored others to live up to Christian ideals.[37] Emboldened by her faith, she acknowledged few limits to her ability to pursue her God-given mission in the world.

A SPIRITUAL HOME FOR A TROUBLED SOUL

A variety of religious influences molded Dix's piety and sense of her purpose in the world. In her childhood, her father worked to indoctrinate his daughter with his fiery faith. Under his roof, Joseph's evangelicalism required, for example, that she bear witness to her conversion by confessing her sins, trusting only in God's mercy, and working toward her own salvation. The pressure to testify about the details of her faith shaped her piety, but given her reserved nature, she found her father's emotional and volatile revival religion hard to bear and longed for alternatives.[38]

Others shared Dix's desire for a less enthusiastic, more rational religion. Indeed, some Americans declared the revivals of the Second Great Awakening excessive displays of emotionalism and hoped to maintain decorum and counter spectacle with reason. The democratic spirit that marked religion after the Second Great Awakening meant believers were free to advocate alternatives to revivalism, and objections shaped, in part, the liberal evangelical trajectory that first appeared in the Unitarianism of the first half of the nineteenth century.[39] It was amidst those liberal Protestants that Dix found her spiritual home.[40]

Unlike their more revivalist Protestant counterparts, early Unitarians appealed not only to Scripture but also to reason as a source of authority. William Ellery Channing, the minister of Federal Street Church in Boston, and eventually Dix's pastor and mentor, proved the most influential of the first generation of Unitarians. Channing and likeminded believers also ascribed authority to the "spirit of the age," an assumed collective sum of individual reason.[41] Claiming this threefold authority (Scripture, reason, and culture) imparted a particular focus to more liberal Protestantism. Religion, Channing asserted in an 1824 ordination sermon titled "The Demands of the Age on the Ministry," "must be dispensed by men who at least keep pace with the intellect of the age in which they live."[42] Clergy should still attend to theology, but "the bulk" of their attention should be turned outward toward intellectual and social concerns.[43]

Liberal Protestants declared their responsibility for identifying and reme-
diating social problems. The primary task, given what Channing and others
saw as "unprecedented demands" of modern life, was a call for engagement
beyond "the cell of the monk" and "the school of the verbal disputant," and
"into life and society."[44] Channing hoped to progress beyond doctrinal dis-
putes and attend to the "grossly defective" society with a realistic optimism.[45]
He advocated a view of Christianity that held "but one purpose, the perfection of human nature, the elevation of men into nobler beings."[46] Christians,
he argued, should look inward to perfect themselves and then move out into
the world to raise the station of others, a sentiment that resonated deeply
with Dix. According to Protestant liberals, human effort and innovation,
rather than the miraculous or divine intervention, helped shape the world
as God intended.

Dix's religious journey included several temporary stops before she found
a home in Channing's congregation, and each location added to the insight
and motivation for her later advocacy work. After leaving Maine for Boston
in her teens, Dix worshiped at Hollis Street Church with her grandmother
in the family's rented pew. Appearing in that Congregational setting seemed
to mark Dix as free of her frontier revivalist roots. Nonetheless, much of
her father's Methodist devotional influence continued. She prayed daily, read
Scripture, and sought God's will for her life.[47]

Dix also failed to shake a sense that her sin interrupted the needed drive
for perfection.[48] She viewed humans as "woefully fallen" and human nature
as "hot-blooded, reckless, venal, and predisposed to betray the soul to ever-
lasting shame."[49] At least she suspected that of herself. Dix's writings from
early adulthood displayed a preoccupation with her own sin. She noted that
a half-dozen "faults must be abandoned by [one] seeking prosperity: sleep,
drowsiness, fear, anger, laziness," and "loitering." She confessed to suffering from all six.[50] Despite human sinfulness, Dix was also sure God called
individuals to serve in specific ways. "We are not sent into this world merely
to enjoy the loveliness therein," she reflected. "No, we were sent here for
action—for constant action. The soul that seeks to do the will of God with a
pure heart fervently, does not yield to the lethargy of ease."[51] She remained
deeply uncertain of her calling in the world but convinced that God would
reveal it in time if she remained faithful.

While in Worcester caring for her brothers, Dix worshiped with members of her extended family at the Second Congregational Society. The
minister there, Rev. Dr. Aaron Bancroft, served as the first president of the
American Unitarian Association and "emphasized the harmony between
reason and religion," a message that resonated with the intellectual young

woman.[52] It was under Bancroft's influence that Dix first migrated toward Unitarianism's logical, embodied impulse. She traded an inward preoccupation with the possibility of salvation for an external focus on public service that ushered it in (in her life and the lives of others).[53] In Unitarianism, Dix found assurance that her God-given intellect, if properly and practically deployed, could contribute to her salvation through her work in the world.

After Dix returned to Boston, Rev. John Pierpont, minister of Hollis Street Church, helped continue her theological transition. Pierpont emphasized the social obligations of Christians and assumed that the church's ministry should extend beyond the wall of the congregation to all Bostonians.[54] That approach seemed correct to Dix, and her writing from that period displayed her focus on the suffering humanity of Jesus as a model for her own life. Increasingly, she understood Christ as a man of action and Christianity as a call to follow his caring example. A hymn from one of her children's books displayed that sentiment:

> That mutual wants and mutual care
> May bind us man to man.
> Go clothe the naked, feed the blind,
> Give the weary rest;
> For sorrow's children comfort find,
> And help for all distressed.[55]

Pierpont's teaching and ministry to the city's poor inspired Dix's schools in Boston. Rev. Joseph Tuckerman, pastor of the Congregational Church in Chelsea, provided a similar influence. In addition to sermons about Christian responsibility to care for the poor, his ministry included firsthand provision for the material needs of impoverished Bostonians. By helping Tuckerman collect shoes, clothing, and books for the city's impoverished children, Dix witnessed how an individual working in cooperation with institutions could prompt social reform, an awareness that undergirded her later reform efforts.[56]

Finally, at William Ellery Channing's Federal Street Church in Boston, Dix found what she called "a church of my own," and she aligned fully with the optimism and hopefulness of the Unitarian movement.[57] Like Tuckerman, Channing proclaimed that God's servants should minister in the world rather than remain isolated in churches. Channing himself was never active as a social reformer, but his conviction that Christians should attend to social problems deeply influenced Dix.[58] Unlike many of his contemporaries, though, Channing refused to see the world around him as actually undergoing beneficial progress. Improvement remained only a possibility. Instead, he saw "an age of sin and moral decline, 'obviously and grossly defective when measured by a Christian standard.'" Christians, in Channing's eyes, had a duty to "press vigorously 'into life and society'" to prompt change.[59] The elder Unitarian statesman's urging to work in the world, and his sense of ongoing human depravity, matched Dix's understanding of faith and society.[60] His slight of "heart-felt religion" and piety did not. Dix maintained that "a man certainly cannot be religious without good morals" but that "one can have good morals without the essence of religion, *viz*, vital piety."[61] While many found the revivalist and rational impulses of Protestantism antithetical, Dix refused to reject the lessons of her father's fervent piety in her transition to a more rational and active faith.

Protestant influence remained strong in American life in the antebellum years—it shaped Dix's work and made others receptive to her pleas. Despite modernizing impulses that might have watered down its cultural influence, religion offered hope for individual perfection and promise for success of the country's nascent institutions.[62] In 1829 President Andrew Jackson's first inaugural address reflected the early century religious and institutional hopefulness alongside an optimistic anthropology. "I hold," proclaimed Jackson,

> to the doctrine that man can be advanced; that man can be elevated; that man can be exalted in his character and condition. We are told on high authority, that he is made in the image of his God; that he is endowed with a certain amount of divinity. And I believe man can be elevated; man can become more and more endowed with divinity; and as he does, he becomes more Godlike in his character and capable of governing himself. Let us go on elevating our people, perfecting our institutions, until democracy shall reach such a point of perfection that we can exclaim with truth that the voice of the people is the voice of God.[63]

Conviction that change was good marked Dix's era. Some of the optimism of the Jacksonian era diminished in the aftermath of the Civil War, but before then, individual initiative and institutional growth—both fueled by changes in Protestantism—occupied center stage.

Despite growing theological and denominational differences, both liberal and more traditional Protestants sought to engage in the world around them. Nineteenth-century Protestants, whether they sided with revivalists or endorsed a more "rational" faith, kept a focus on individual salvation but paired it with a sense that this personal salvation bore social consequences, and Christians collaborated to bring change.[64] Under the leadership of those like Presbyterian minister Charles G. Finney, for example, "abolition leagues, temperance societies, [and] missionary programs" formed and worked actively for social improvement.[65]

Notwithstanding a growing sense of the proper role of faith in the larger world, Dix continued to search her own soul. She worried about the presence of evil and wrote that only a life "virtuously sacrificed for the benefit of others" allowed one to escape such peril.[66] In particular, frequent illness and growing exhaustion from her teaching, writing, and charity work gave her reason to reflect on the religious meaning of illness. Dix considered her ailments "spiritual tests" and, sometimes, "deserved punishment."[67] She feared succumbing to sloth amidst her illness and wrote to a friend that sickness proved evidence of "a hidden disposition . . . a secret desire to escape from labor."[68] While never explicit that she assumed the same about the sickness in others, it seems plausible, even if Dix reserved the harshest judgment for herself. Dix understood illness firsthand.

Christianity played a central role, not only in forming Dix's understanding of the world but also in shaping the national consciousness as the country experienced demographic and economic changes. Though many Protestants collaborated to enact their faith by seeking social improvement, other believers pursued their religious vocations alone. Given her preference for an individualistic faith, that Dix's religious mission took place beyond formal denominational structures seemed expected.[69]

As her faith prompted her to survey her world, ailing Americans drew Dix's attention. Amidst other cultural shifts, medical science continued to evolve during the antebellum era, including treatment for insane citizens. Dix's concern brought her in contact with both patients and an emerging group of physicians specializing in the care of insanity.

MEDICAL SPECIALIZATION

In the first half of the nineteenth century, serious illness remained a threat for most Americans. Medical care improved, but only sporadically. From 1790 to 1825, infectious diseases wreaked havoc, especially in port cities that received immigrants. Urbanization and immigration meant more citizens ailed, further reducing physician effectiveness. As in the prior century, yellow fever epidemics persisted. Malaria, smallpox, and bubonic plague abated, though, in part because of more widespread inoculation and the use of cinchona bark to counter malaria.[70] The origins of most diseases, however, physical or mental, remained as mysterious as effective cures.

Most antebellum physicians practiced as generalists, a reality necessitated by the need to treat a wide variety of patients without the help of hospitals in many locations. After 1830, however, the changes in theories of disease led to one of the early medical specializations, surgery. Paired with the emerging use of anesthesia, surgeons now attended to more than just broken bones.

The growing infrastructure of asylums led to the other early subfield of medical practitioners—alienists, specialists in the care of the mentally ill. It was with those physicians, who often served as asylum superintendents, that Dix formed her closest alliances. By doing so, she would not only further her own cause but also help build their public credibility.

Physicians continued to train in the United States, but leading antebellum doctors still sought schooling in Europe.[71] Many that practiced in the United States lacked formal education, and without many teaching hospitals, training through apprenticeship continued, especially in rural areas. Charlatans plied their trade, and medical sects including homeopathy, hydropathy, Grahamism, and Thomsonianism appeared and drew adherents.[72] Lacking reliable cures, patients gravitated to any treatment that brought relief.

The respect that physicians gained during Benjamin Rush's era waned in the early decades of the nineteenth century. With a great diversity of care available—and public feuds between physicians about whose techniques were best—public trust of medical professionals diminished.[73] Continued use of bloodletting and purging also failed to endear the ailing to doctors. Training practices like dissection caused public outrage and even riots in Philadelphia. In addition, by 1840 medical innovation seemed to be lagging other scientific development.[74] Physical and natural sciences drew more certain conclusions than did medicine. The workings of the human body remained mysterious. Compounding this, post–Declaration of Independence attacks on elitism made citizens fear the rising professional power of doctors.[75] Many advised cultivating personal hygiene in order to avoid the need to see a physician. As a result, America's physicians lost, for a period, some of the authority they had gained in the prior century. That lost authority migrated, not back to the ministers that held it in colonial days, but to common citizens that presumed the right and the ability to discern the therapy they needed and the best sources for that treatment.

Despite trouble with their public image, physicians remained optimistic about their abilities and effectiveness.[76] Formal professionalization of the practice of medicine had begun in the years following the American Revolution, but Jacksonian-era deregulation dismantled most of the nascent licensing standards.[77] In the absence of state or federal regulation, physicians joined in medical associations. In 1847 the American Medical Association formed and studied the state of medical education in the country, aiming to standardize training and further differentiate between regular (professional) and irregular practitioners.[78]

While professional disagreements continued, changes hinted at the coming standardization and modernization of medicine. The continued development of the physical sciences prompted physicians to abandon older theories of disease. Many now argued for medicine as science, instead of an art. Moving beyond the longstanding view of humorial causes and cures, physicians defined localized bodily origins of disease, and the assumption that disease stemmed from lesions in specific areas of the body changed treatments.[79] The use of bleeding and purging declined by 1850 and largely had disappeared from physicians' toolkits by 1870. Generalized treatments no longer made sense amidst a growing understanding of the specific origins of disease.[80]

Altogether, demographic, economic, religious, and medical changes made understandings of all illness—mental and physical—ripe for reconsideration and reform. Dix's part in that process, however, remained a few years away.

EUROPEAN RESPITE

Falling victim to serious illness, including an ailment such as her father's alcoholism, terrified Dix. She hoped that disciplined work and strong morals would ward off sickness, but her tireless teaching eventually produced the opposite effect. In March 1836 she experienced a physical and emotional breakdown. Dix brooded over congestion in her lungs, ongoing depression, thoughts of suicide, and lack of clarity about God's purpose for her life.[81]

Always analyzing, Dix searched for religious meanings of her suffering. Like Cotton Mather, she assumed connections between illness (physical and mental) and sin. Health, she thought, depended on observing divine laws; illness resulted from breaking them. Sickness alerted believers to their wrongdoing. "God never withholds the train of . . . results he has annexed to wrong conduct," she reflected, "and the pain that visits the involuntary transgression is often our first index to a broken law."[82] Whether or not her breakdown helped her empathize with others, the time she spent recovering provided insight into moral treatments for mental illness. She struggled, however, to navigate a path through her melancholy.

The introspective Dix felt sure that her condition was just punishment, a "chastisement" inflicted by God "for the soul's health."[83] Her friends, including Rev. Channing and Ralph Waldo Emerson, convinced her that a sea voyage and tour in Europe were necessary to cure her ills and paved the way for her stay, sending her with letters of introduction to their acquaintances overseas.[84] Noting compulsive work—and not laziness—as the root of her illness, a letter written by Channing explained that Dix "injured her health by her singular devotion to her work."[85]

One of Channing's European connections—the Liverpool resident William Rathbone III—and his family nursed Dix back to health. Rathbone (a Quaker with Unitarian sympathies, politician, and philanthropist) and his wife offered her compassionate care and intellectual company during the many months she remained in their home. Once refreshed, she remained in Liverpool, studying prevailing theories of disease and European approaches to public care.[86] While recovering, Dix observed social reform efforts in Europe, including work to overhaul the treatment of madness. She was inspired by the European quest to find new ways to determine who qualified for welfare programs, an effort resulting from investigations documenting poverty in the countryside. Through Rathbone, she met European social reformers including Samuel Tuke, the grandson of William Tuke, a pioneer of moral treatment for mental illness and now the proprietor of the York Retreat.[87] Dix visited the York Retreat and found a spirit of optimism about the possibility of curing mental illness through kind, gentle treatment. The approach resonated with her experience of receiving compassionate care at the Rathbone estate. Because of her exposure to European social reforms, her study of medicine, and the attentive care she received, Dix left Europe physically and mentally restored and with a renewed humanitarian drive and sense of purpose in life. Nascent American medical institutions posed a perfect target for her energies.

MEDICAL INSTITUTIONS FOR THE INSANE

Many colonial Americans had assumed that the work of an omnipotent God exceeded their understanding, and they accepted their fates—good and bad. By the nineteenth century, however, Enlightenment influence brought faith in human reason not only to understand but also to eliminate problems. Benjamin Rush, as a leading thinker of his era, expressed similar optimism, but assurance of human capabilities now proved stronger and more widespread. That confidence shaped views of mental illness. Americans like Dix assumed that illness, along with poverty, vice, ignorance, and insanity, were problems that human resourcefulness could remedy.[88] Public institutions seemed the effective place to start.

Hospital construction boomed in the nineteenth century. By the Civil War, 178 hospitals operated in the United States; one third of those were mental asylums.[89] Most often, the new institutions treated socially marginal individuals, including the insane, who no longer received care at home. General hospitals provided confinement more than diagnosis or treatment as they replaced care once administered in the infirmaries of almshouses.[90] Through the 1850s, those enterprises were "something Americans of the better sort did for their less fortunate countrymen; it was hardly a refuge [the well off] con-templated entering themselves."[91] Despite the good intentions of benefactors, by 1860 large city hospitals were overcrowded and often grossly unclean.[92]

The first institutions devoted to the care of the insane in America were private facilities with ties to Christian groups. The earliest, the Friends Asy-lum, opened in Frankford, Pennsylvania, in 1817.[93] Facilities like the Friends Asylum admitted just a handful of patients in their early years and eventu-ally restricted services to the wealthy, who could afford to pay for treatment. Until 1834, the Friends Asylum admitted only Quakers, and even many poorer Friends found themselves beyond assistance.[94] Superintendents at the first asylums believed that treatment was most effective when their charges were cared for surrounded by those from their own social class. That practice exacerbated the "growing exclusiveness" of care provided. Other mental hos-pitals served slightly more heterogeneous populations, but rising costs meant that the ability (or inability) of patients to pay for their care shaped admis-sions at each of the private facilities.

After 1824 the asylum landscape shifted.[95] The narrowness of the admis-sions process at the first hospitals, the limits to the availability of private philanthropy, and the high cost of protracted care for the incurably insane meant that early institutions failed to satisfy demand for treatment. At the same time, many physicians proved ready to adopt new practices. The approaches of William Tuke and Philippe Pinel earned broader awareness and influence among doctors and the social elite after their writings became widely available in America—Pinel's translation in 1806 and Tuke's *Descrip-tion of the Retreat* in 1813.[96] American physicians were optimistic that moral treatment would demonstrate the curability of mental maladies. Between 1825 and 1850, the treatment protocols advocated by Rush, Tuke, and Pinel moved beyond church-sponsored institutions. A new treatment arsenal that fed optimism about the ability to care for—and cure—mental maladies marked those twenty-five years.

During the same period, state-administered care for the insane emerged as the standard nationwide. Private hospitals failed to meet demand, but additional factors enabled the appearance of the first public asylums for the insane. The active social force of Protestantism accelerated change as Chris-tians put their faith to work in the world around them. In addition, and particularly in New England, a wealthy elite class found itself in competition with the newly rich and responded with philanthropic giving that combined with an availability of public funds. Finally, a "growing consensus" emerged that government had an obligation for the welfare of its citizens, an attitude that led to legislative approval of new institutions.[97]

Though nascent, church-run institutions failed to meet demand, accounts of burdensome community-based treatment also contributed to a desire for alternatives. An 1821 report by a committee investigating the insane in Connecticut, for example, lamented the horrible treatment of mad individuals and the burden they placed on their families. Of the relatives, the report noted:

> Their peace is interrupted, their cares are multiplied, their time is engrossed, and their fortunes reduced or entirely dissipated in attempting to restore to reason one unfortunate member. . . . The misery which they suffer is communicated to a large circle of friends and the whole neighborhood is indirectly disturbed by the malady of one.[98]

The report displayed the prevailing logic behind the change in focus from local family systems able and willing to attend to sufferers to a concern with the well-being of those providing care.[99] In a time of optimistic institution building, Americans shifted their confidence to facilities—whether hospitals, schools, or prisons—that professed the ability to improve life for all and to fulfill public responsibility to care for society's dependent.[100] Together, those factors ushered in an era of public asylum building.

While Dix played the lead role in expanding and founding public asylums, some church leaders advocated similar solutions. Surveying the state of care of sufferers in the first years of the nineteenth century, the Congregational minister Jedidiah Morse voiced indignation that insane persons were "committed to close confinement, under circumstance of great wretchedness." He worried that others were "left, forlorn and friendless, to roam through the country exposed to the insults of the thoughtless and wicked; to hunger, cold, and various calamitous and fatal accidents, a terror to female delicacy, and a grief and a continual cause of anxiety to their relations."[101] In response, Morse called for the creation of a "hospital for lunaticks." Shortly thereafter, the Massachusetts General Court began fund-raising for the hospital. The largest donations came from Congregationalists, but ministers used denominational rivalries to their advantage in fund-raising appeals. Leaders in other traditions asked their flocks, "Shall the Congregational scion alone be barren of the sweetest fruits which the tree of Christianity had produced?"[102] Notwithstanding denominational competitiveness, Morse's account demonstrated some remaining clerical authority in solving social problems, not in prescribing cures directly but by calling for the formation of institutions to provide assistance.

For nineteenth-century clergymen, helping ensure institutional treatment seemed a fitting response to illness.[103] Rev. Thomas Robbins of East

Windsor, Connecticut, spoke at the dedication of the Hartford Retreat and equated its work to Christ's healing of those possessed with devils. As he did so, he displayed an Enlightenment-driven doubt in the miraculous. Robbins observed that while "the insane found a safe retreat in Christ" having exorcised demons, he felt that "this power to cure insanity through miraculous means '[was] now withdrawn,' and the insane could only be restored by natural means."[104] While ministers continued to offer private spiritual remedies, in public they asserted the need for the secular treatment, or at least the containment, that institutionalization provided.

Dix's work demonstrated that lay Christians also staked a claim in the provision of institutional care. Her efforts to expand asylum care to reach those of all classes followed the work of early advocates, including Horace Mann (1796–1859). Mann, a member of the Massachusetts house and senate, was an educational reformer who, after chairing a committee that surveyed the number of insane citizens in Massachusetts, urged the legislature to open a hospital. Mann, a Unitarian, grounded his efforts in his Christian faith, believing that "to be a social activist was to fulfill a religious mission."[105] Encouraging his fellow legislators to act quickly in the face of suffering citizens, Mann offered a plea:

> While *we* delay, they *suffer*—another year not only gives an accession to their numbers, but removes, perhaps to a returnless distance, the chance of their recovery. Whatever they endure, which we can prevent, is virtually inflicted by our own hands. . . . It is now . . . in the power of the members of this House to exercise their highest privileges as men; their most enviable functions as legislators, to become protectors to the wretched, and benefactors to the miserable.[106]

In 1833 Mann's efforts resulted in the creation of a new hospital in Worcester, Massachusetts.[107] Larger than prior private institutions, the hospital became a blueprint for facilities built in other states, in part because it reported recovery rates of more than 80 percent.[108] Through both clerical and lay initiative, Protestant interest widened, and efforts expanded beyond the pastor's study and Christian physician's sickroom. The cause, however, needed a champion.

DIX GOES PUBLIC

Dix's return from Europe in 1837 fell early in the initial public asylum-building boom. By that time, inheritance from her grandmother's estate and royalties from her books offered Dix a measure of independence. After a period of domestic travel, Dix returned to Boston and began teaching religious classes in a Massachusetts jail. It was there she found insane inmates confined with criminals. Time in Europe prompted Dix to learn more about the treatment of prisoners and the insane in American institutions. Her past scientific study equipped her to catalogue her findings. After visits and correspondence with nearby jailers, physicians, and officials, she spent a year travelling throughout Massachusetts chronicling the condition of insane citizens.

Dix found mentally ill men and women starving, chained (by waist, neck, leg), filthy, lacking fresh air, naked, exposed to the elements, without sunlight, and wondering what they had done to be deserted by God. Often having to demand that jailers and almshouse keepers let her inspect their facilities, she, with persistence, generated volumes of observations like these:

> *Lincoln.* A woman in a cage. *Medford.* One idiotic subject chained, and one in a close stall for seventeen years. *Pepperell.* One often doubly chained, hand and foot; another violent; several peaceable now. *Brookfield.* One man caged, comfortable. *Granville.* One often closely confined; now losing the use of his limbs from want of exercise. *Charlemont.* One man caged. . . . *Lenox.* Two in the jail, against whose unfit condition there the jailer protests.[109]

Dix recorded similar conditions each night of her journey. In addition to outrage over poor treatment in inadequate institutions, she worried about insane men and women she saw "wandering reckless and unprotected" throughout the countryside. She spoke compassionately about the tenacity of sufferers, amazed at their ability to survive amidst horrible conditions. Unlike past observers that described the mad as beast-like, Dix described the suffering of real women and men, hoping her readers would sympathize with their plight.[110] Dix admitted that visits left her "sick, horror-struck, and almost incapable of retreating," but it was the conditions the ill suffered through that she found despicable, not the mad themselves.[111] Though they were ill, Dix viewed mad Americans as fellow, beloved creatures of God.

With that initial tour, Dix's advocacy had begun. In January 1843, observations in hand, and encouraged by the Boston reformer Samuel Gridley Howe, she petitioned the Massachusetts legislature to expand the Worcester State Lunatic Hospital. The presentation, her thirty-page *Memorial to the Legislature of Massachusetts*, "struck and exploded like a bombshell" and launched her career as a public reformer.[112] "I have come to present the strong claims of suffering humanity," she announced. "I come to place before the Legislature of Massachusetts the condition of the miserable, the desolate, the outcast." She did not speak on her own behalf but spoke "as the advocate of helpless, forgotten, insane, and idiotic men and women; of beings sunk to a condition from which the most unconcerned would start with real horror; of beings wretched in our prisons, and more wretched in our almshouses."[113]

Part sermon, part graphic account, her presentation won the rapt attention of her audience: "I proceed, gentlemen, briefly to call your attention to the *present* state of insane persons confined within this Commonwealth, in *cages, closets, cellars, stalls, pens! Chained, naked, beaten with rods*, and *lashed into obedience*."[114] Dix's controlled yet assertive demeanor, paired with the content of her proclamation and the fact that she was a woman communicating to legislators, made her part prophet, part moral authority, part civic expert. She insisted that the state's obligation to provide asylum care was moral, humanitarian, medical, and legal.[115]

Although clear about the injustices she found, in her first appeal, Dix exempted wardens, keepers, and officers of institutions from responsibility. The conditions she encountered were not their fault, at least not directly: "*Most* of these have erred not through hardness of heart and willful cruelty so much as want of skill and knowledge, and want of consideration."[116] Prisons and almshouses, Dix argued, were simply not designed to care for the mentally ill. Instead of implicating leaders of those facilities, Dix blamed the commonwealth as a whole for the abuses. Dix accused her fellow citizens of "callous indifference to suffering and . . . lofty pretensions of Christian virtue that struck her as hypocritical so long as they tolerated such flagrant brutality in their midst."[117] Her findings demanded a response.

Dix suggested proper reactions. First, individuals should respond with thankfulness for their health, a recommended first response that mirrored Cotton Mather's advice more than a century earlier. Dix also hoped to invoke empathy as she invited Americans to picture themselves alone and deserted "in that dreary cage" and to imagine the care they would like to receive.[118] Above all, faithful citizens should devote themselves to ameliorating the conditions of sufferers.[119] While neglect and abuse might persist, she asserted that if the government and all individuals did "what they could"—what she herself was willing to do—then treatment could surely improve.

EXPANSION AND SPECIALIZATION

Dix's pleas occurred at an opportune time. By 1841 sixteen public and private mental hospitals incorporating Tuke's and Pinel's principles of moral treatment operated in the United States.[120] State institutions in Pennsylvania, New York, and Rhode Island opened in the following years.[121] Most of the first superintendents of those institutions—some formally trained, some apprenticed into medicine—were Protestants reared in small towns and rural areas. Like Dix, physicians believed they had a mission to help less-fortunate Americans. Those superintendents, men Dix befriended on her journeys, formed a tight-knit group, regarding themselves as "brethren" with much to learn from one other.[122] In 1844 their association, and the practice of asylum medicine, took formal shape with the creation of the Association of Medical Superintendents of American Institutions for the Insane.[123] The cadre of alienists met annually to discuss insanity and institutional treatment.[124]

Dix helped prompt the creation of institutions, but from 1840 to 1880, that group of men directly shaped the care of the insane in America. It took decades, though, for care for mental diseases to standardize. While Benjamin Rush's treatise on mental ailments proved outdated by the 1840s, no new American general psychiatric text appeared until 1883. Until then, each superintendent maintained comprehensive control of his establishment and dictated courses of treatment.[125] Before 1865, while asylum physicians hoped to present a common front, they also disagreed. Dix steered clear of those debates, but they occupied the alienists she befriended. Doctors debated whether mental disease stemmed from somatic or psychological origins. Each advocated a different mix of medical and psychological treatments. They moved—but at varied speeds—from an understanding that mental disease stemmed from inflammation of the blood vessels (as Benjamin Rush had asserted) to the conviction that irritation of the nervous system was at fault.

Alienists also differed in their understandings of how the mind and brain related, and Christian beliefs played a role in some of the most heated debates. Most doctors maintained an immaterialist conception of the mind and a view of the unity of the human soul consistent with their Protestant faith, but scientific advances prompted reconsideration.[126] Phrenologists, on the other hand, specialists who designated areas of the brain as responsible for different behavioral, cognitive, or emotional traits, presumed that insanity resulted from any imbalance in those faculties. Met with charges of being "atheistic materialists" that perceived minds as susceptible to being diseased, they "maintained that the mind and brain were intimately connected but separate and that the nature of their relationship was a mystery."[127] Opponents worried that their theories risked overturning the eternality (and imperviousness to disease) of the mind and soul. Pliny Earle (a Quaker and prominent asylum superintendent), for example, held tightly to traditional beliefs. "Were the arguments for the hypothesis that in insanity the mind itself is diseased tenfold more numerous than they are, and more weighty," he reflected, "I could not accept them." "My ideas of the human mind are such that I cannot hold for a moment that it can be diseased," he argued, because disease implied death, "but Mind is eternal. In its very essence and structure . . . it was created for immortality." Earle and others held that the mind proved "superior to the bodily structure, and beyond the scope of the wear and tear and disorganization and final destruction of the mortal part of our being," even if they failed to understand how.[128] Those alienists simply accepted that "psychological factors could irritate the brain and cause physical disorder," producing "emotional derangement" that characterized insanity.[129] Mind and brain, however, remained separate entities.

Despite a commitment to somaticism, physicians could only observe psychological symptoms and often relied on psychological explanations. Yet, alienists increasingly leaned toward somatic conceptions of mental disease, and for more reasons than adherence with their religious beliefs. As the rest of medicine moved toward somatic causes, alienists hoped they too could identify a "relationship between bodily lesions and symptoms." Somatic conceptions of illness also helped practitioners fend off demonological and superstitious definitions of insanity, views that created cases they were not qualified (or necessary) to treat.[130] Local physicians continued to treat sufferers, but when attending to mental maladies, the practices and treatments of general practitioners lagged behind their asylum counterparts.[131] Asylum-based physicians tried to educate general practitioners about the benefits of hospital care, but readership of the journal articles they authored proved limited.

Despite disagreements and still-elusive etiology, alienists held wide agreement on a number of topics. The classification of disorders remained simple and relatively unchanged from the prior century. Mania, monomania, melancholia, dementia, and idiocy formed the common diagnostic categories. Asylum doctors assumed physical causes—perhaps lesions on the brain—existed but focused on behavioral and moral causes that were easier to identify and treat, including "intemperance, masturbation, overwork, domestic difficulties, excessive ambitions, faulty education, personal disappointment, marital problems, excessive religious enthusiasm, jealousy, and pride." Such "deviations from acceptable lifestyles" remained suspect.[132] In addition, with causes still difficult to pinpoint, doctors increasingly suspected heredity as a factor in the predisposition to succumb to mental ailments. Even when a direct hereditary link seemed absent, some assumed illness resulted from "some bad and often sinful ancestral trait."[133] Finally, modern civilization itself was blamed as a cause. The psychiatrist Edward Jarvis, for example, concluded that insanity was "part of the price we pay for civilization." The trouble, he argued, was not "the increase of knowledge, the improvements in the arts, the multiplication of the comforts, the amelioration of manners, the growth of refinement, [or] the elevation of morals." Rather, those changes in society disturbed "men's cerebral organs" and created "mental disorders" because they brought "more opportunities and rewards for great and excessive mental action, more uncertain and hazardous employments, and consequently more disappointments, more means and provocations for sensual indulgence, more dangers of accidents and injuries, more groundless hopes, and more painful struggle to obtain that which is beyond reach, or to effect that which is impossible."[134] The presumed influence the forces of civilization had on causing illness varied. Less-civilized people of the world were thought to suffer less frequently. Physicians included slaves in the southern United States in that group but considered freed slaves in the north ten times more prone to mental distress. Poor and uneducated Americans, including Irish immigrants, doctors thought, were less able to control their minds and thus more susceptible. The greatest incidence of mental maladies, however, was presumed to exist in the northeast (where, not coincidentally, statistics on illness were gathered more assiduously).[135]

Despite much uncertainty, through 1850, those treating mental maladies remained optimistic that cures existed and that institutions were the best places for the administration of care. While some help could be offered in local communities, asylums provided a more controlled environment. Given the medical training of asylum physicians and the focus on moral causes, attention to prevention involving a "synthesis of medicine, religion, morality, and social activism" became popular. As the profession solidified and treatments standardized, alienists and asylums "reinforced and conferred legitimacy upon the other."[136] Dix counted many of the nation's leading alienists as her friends and coworkers in the campaign to improve care. She relied on them for medical expertise and access to asylums. They valued the visibility and funding she secured to grow their institutions.

SHIFTING PUBLIC PERCEPTIONS

Even with medical advances and Dix's advocacy, perceptions of mental maladies changed slowly.[137] A few elite members of society, Dix among them, helped increase access to asylum care, even while some citizens objected to receiving help.

The Bible, popular medical works, and newspaper reports each influenced common perceptions of mental maladies. The public proved more likely than physicians or the elite to deploy the supernatural in their understandings. Drawing on the Bible, the most widely available book in the early nineteenth century, many Americans continued to assume that demon possession caused insanity and that it was best treated by "exorcism" or "more drastic means." Relatives of the insane hesitated to discuss madness, fearing the work of the devil.[138] As a result, some shunned institutional and medical treatment, fearing exposure to demonic forces or opting for other solutions. The trustees of the Worcester asylum, for example, reported that a woman with a deranged son refused treatment for him because "an evil spirit . . . troubled him, and until the Lord was pleased to take it off, she was quite sure, that nothing any man could do would be useful to him."[139] Although alienists held alternate opinions, some Americans, like past generations, continued to assume that only spiritual cures and the will of God could remedy spiritual problems.

Published medical volumes also shaped public opinion and resistance to institutional care. In one of the most popular medical handbooks of the eighteenth and nineteenth centuries, *Domestic Medicine*, the Scotsman William Buchan acknowledged melancholy and mania as real ailments.[140] Yet, based on observations of the first U.S. and European asylums, he believed that those "institutions, as they [were] generally managed, [were] far more likely to make a wise man mad than to restore a madman to his senses." Instead of institutionalization, Buchan recommended soothing and diverting the attention of sufferers with amusements and good company, plenty of exercise, and a diet of vegetables.[141] Similarly, Rev. John Wesley's widely read *Primitive Physic* (1773) commended exercise, temperance, and proper eating habits.[142] For more severe illnesses, the founder of Methodism recommended "placing a violently mad patient directly under a powerful waterfall for as long as he could bear it."[143] Perceptions of the causes of illness shaped popular approaches to treatments as much as did suspicions about institutional care.

Citizens that approved of treatment preferred gentle approaches, but an exception appeared with insane individuals that committed violent crimes. Newspaper accounts portrayed such men and women as less than human. Physicians like Rush had hoped to subdue even violent patients, but "reporters and witnesses in criminal trials frequently expressed the opinion that the insane were beasts who deserved their fate and warranted no sympathy" because they were morally responsible for their crimes. The "loss of reason was seen as the loss of the soul and of humanity and God's grace." [144] If God had withdrawn support from such humans, were not other citizens justified in doing the same?

Though others speculated about causes, Dix proved more interested in cures. "I have been asked if I have investigated the causes of insanity," she wrote. "I have not."[145] When she did mention sources of mental distress, her views matched what she gleaned from asylum physicians, and she happily deferred to their medical expertise. While touring, she rarely recorded speculations about causes, but she did note the case of a woman who had once been "a respectable person, industrious and worthy." The woman from Danvers, Massachusetts, fell ill after "disappointments and trials shook her mind."[146] Undue stress might trigger illness, and all were susceptible. Mental maladies,

Dix argued, could befall the poor and the "most prosperous and affluent," including physicians and public officials.

Dix admitted that sin might play a role in insanity, but, even if sin caused illness, she pled for humane treatment:

> I have been told that this most calamitous overthrow of reason often is the result of a life of sin; it is sometimes, but rarely, added, they must take the consequences, they deserve no better care. Shall man be more just than God, he who causes his sun and refreshing rains and life-giving influence to fall alike on the good and the evil?
>
> Is not the total wreck of reason, a state of distraction, and the loss of all that makes life cherished a retribution sufficiently heavy, without adding to consequences so appalling every indignity that can bring still lower the wretched sufferer?
>
> Have pity upon those who, while they were supposed to lie hid in secret sins, "have been scattered under a *dark veil of forgetfulness*, over whom is spread a heavy night, and who unto themselves are more grievous than the darkness."[147]

Illness itself, she realized, provided just punishment in many cases. Sinners and saints alike garnered God's love and deserved care from their fellow citizens.

Salvation came from God, but Dix wrote that she found "no redemption but in action"—for herself or others.[148] Her understanding of religion showed not only in her motivations but also in her assumption that it should influence the responses of others. In pleading with the men of the Massachusetts legislature, Dix called on their Christian charity and religious responsibility: "Raise up the fallen, succor the desolate, restore the outcast, defend the helpless, and for your eternal and great reward receive the benediction, 'Well done, good and faithful servants, become rulers over many things!' "[149] She also invoked God and God's mission in her closing words to the lawmakers: "Gentlemen, I commit to you this sacred cause. Your action upon this subject will affect the present and future condition of hundreds and of thousands. In this legislation, as in all things, may you exercise that 'wisdom which is the breath of the power of God.' "[150] Care for the suffering formed a mission for Dix, one she believed all Christians should embrace.[151]

Dix's advocacy spread public awareness of mental illness. It touted the benefits of humane treatment more broadly among the lower classes and engaged the sympathies of the elite to fund better treatment. Her work played a large role in shaping public perceptions and bringing change in the years after 1843. Eventually, the public's desire for humane treatment, emerging awareness of gentle institutional care, and outrage over the reality of treatment of the pauper insane converged with Dix's desire to help and accelerated the growth of asylum care.

SUCCESS AND FAILURE

On January 25, 1843, just five days after the presentation of her *Memorial*, the Massachusetts legislature approved a $25,000 appropriation from state funds and $40,000 from an endowment to enlarge the asylum in Worcester. Whether the legislature was swayed by Dix's testimony or simply by the numbers—the 1840 census had identified 978 lunatics in the state (229 housed at Worcester, 124 at the Boston Lunatic Hospital, so 625 lived without asylum treatment)—Dix viewed the approval as "a brilliant victory" proving that she was indeed "doing God's work."[152] Elated by her success with the legislature, Samuel Howe asserted that he could not "but be impressed with the lesson of courage and hope" that Dix had "taught even to the strongest men." Horace Mann offered his thanks for her accomplishing "the Christian labor of doing good to those who cannot require you."[153] Affirmation from men, leaders she respected, emboldened her work. Dix relished success and the recognition of her efforts.

Nonetheless, some resisted Dix's work. A few legislators and local administrators questioned the accuracy of her observations. Some towns published rebuttals to her findings, defending the care they provided. Dix, however, remained steadfast about the truthfulness of her reports. Her social status and prominent acquaintances helped her deflect criticism. Those that tried to discredit her learned that "anyone who thought she could be brushed off as some meddlesome spinster vastly underestimated Dorothea Dix."[154] That proved true, in part, because she offered not a general, abstracted account, but one that profiled individual lives and particular horrors.

Taking her success in Massachusetts as a sign from God that she "was now an instrument of divine mercy," Dix moved on to make similar assessments and pleas in other states over the next decade.[155] In each location, she followed the same pattern—compiling research, presenting to legislatures, and often writing newspaper articles to garner public support. Citizens and lawmakers in other states met her campaigns with enthusiasm. After appealing for a new asylum in Tennessee, for example, the legislature printed four thousand copies of the memorial she presented. Local papers urged fellow Tennesseans to enact the suggestions of this "most distinguished philanthropist."[156]

Continued success meant that Dix shaped public policy throughout the country. Young physicians exploring the possibility of working in asylums consulted her. Hospital boards included the crusader in hiring decisions when hospital superintendent positions became vacant. Members of the

Association of Medical Superintendents counted on her "great influence" to strengthen solidarity among their geographically disperse group. Persistence and experience, coupled with her personal connections, meant that legislatures took her seriously.[157]

Within two years of her *Memorial* to the Massachusetts legislature, Dix's travels took her over ten thousand miles to three hundred county jails, eighteen state prisons, and five hundred poorhouses and other institutions.[158] Her journey also included determined conversation in the nations' sitting rooms. "You cannot imagine the labor of converting and convincing," she wrote to a friend. "Some evenings," she noted, "I had at once twenty gentlemen for three hours' steady conversation."[159] Though it may have taken effort, Dix put her gift of persuasion to good use. The Providence, Rhode Island, businessman Cyrus Butler "listened spellbound" to Dix's appeal for $40,000 to enlarge the city's insane hospital. "Madam, I'll do it!" he was reported to have answered. Butler, whose name the hospital soon bore, counted the gift as a philanthropic victory. Dix tallied this and other successful appeals as a "spiritual triumph."[160]

Traveling more widely than an itinerant preacher, by August 1847, Dix estimated that she had covered 32,470 miles.[161] Her treks mirror those of the Methodist Francis Asbury. Like the relentless bishop, Dix spent decades traveling throughout the country, with a clear religious mission; owning no home; and relying on the hospitality of friends and strangers for food and lodging. Throughout her journeys, Dix preached the gospel of humane treatment and remained convinced that asylum-based care formed the right solution to ameliorate suffering. "My conviction is continually deepened," she asserted, "that hospitals are the only places where insane persons can be at once humanely and properly controlled." Poorhouses "converted into madhouses," she lamented, "cease to effect the purposes for which they were established and instead of being asylums for the aged, the homeless, and the friendless, and places of refuge for orphaned or neglected childhood, are transformed into perpetual bedlams."[162] Violent, severe treatments only "exasperate the insane," but "kindness and firmness" brought recovery.[163] Dix's dogged labors paved the way for institutional alternatives.

Existing facilities expanded, new asylums opened, and admissions and resident populations rose steadily. The hospital in Worcester, for example, grew from 120 beds in 1833 to over 360 by 1846. In 1840 eight asylums admitted approximately 180 patients each. Ten years later, twenty-two institutions admitted nearly 329 persons, a five-fold increase in the population of insane patients.[164] What contributed to such rapid growth? Early public resistance to hospitalization waned, and the appeal of the asylum changed. Families were more willing to admit loved ones than in prior decades.[165] The availability of asylums also solidified the legitimacy of mental illnesses as medical phenomena best dealt with in institutions. That change crossed class lines and even enticed upper-class Americans to turn to mental hospitals for help.[166] New hospitals filled quickly with a mix of Americans.

As asylum building continued and hopefulness about society's ability to heal mental illness persisted, optimism about treatment effectiveness also helped fuel growth. The toolkits of asylum superintendents grew, and even institutions that once specialized in moral treatment began to address issues first with medical treatments before turning to psychological cures. Physicians believed that medical attention prepared patients for moral treatments and that the paired treatments formed the most potent medicine for madness.[167] As the range of treatments administered widened, reported recovery rates rose. In 1825 the Hartford Retreat, for example, cited a 91 percent cure rate of recent cases.[168]

Though treatment in institutions grew more palatable for a wider range of Americans, care still failed to reach all in need. The location of new asylums proved inconvenient for many. States most often built new hospitals in rural areas, under the assumption that centrally located facilities provided easy access for all of the state's residents. Urbanites, though, balked at travel to remote hospital locations. City populations remained underserved, and municipalities were left to find other solutions, often reverting to almshouses and prisons. Even after the first wave of public institutions launched, many mentally ill Americans continued to receive inadequate care.

Undeterred, Dix reacted to those realities and continued her campaign. Dix thrived on controversy, and difficulty provided deeper motivation. In a letter to a friend, while ill, she resolved, "I shall be well enough when I get to Kentucky or Alabama. The tonic I need is the tonic of opposition. That always sets me on my feet."[169] Recovered from her temporary illness, and with multiple successes on the state level, the reformer set her sights higher.

In May of 1848 Dix began preparations for an assault on Congress to secure a federal endowment for state hospitals.[170] Her efforts faced resistance. Because municipalities sometimes held responsibility for paying for their citizens' care in state asylums, they often opted for cheaper, local almshouses. In addition, superintendents still preferred private patients whose payments proved more reliable than those from municipalities. Opposition threatened to disrupt Dix's ability to help launch new facilities.

Undaunted, Dix fortified her argument. Echoing those that argued modern civilization caused mental maladies, she claimed, "Free civil and religious institutions create constantly various and multiplying sources of mental excitement." Further, she concluded that insanity was inevitable where "every individual, however, obscure, is free to enter upon the race for the highest honors and most exalted stations."[171] Because Dix assumed that the nation's freedoms could cause insanity, it seemed right to her that the federal government should support her proposal and fund asylum care. Confessing that "through God's good Providence" she and her "cause are now rather popular," Dix felt sure Congress would act quickly on her *Bill for the Benefit of the Indigent Insane*.[172] Federal legislators, though, had other priorities, including territorial expansion and the deepening sectional strife over slavery. The bill passed in 1854, only to be vetoed by President Franklin Pierce, who argued that states, not the federal government, held responsibility for social welfare.

Despite her failure in the nation's Capitol, Dix had turned the country's attention to the plight of the mentally ill.[173] Newly formed and expanding state legislatures had vast amounts of land and good funding available, which allowed them to grant wide approval to public infrastructure projects of all sorts, often without the detailed investigations that funding decisions required in the next century.[174]

Dix was a wise woman, unflagging in her mission. Biographer Gollaher argued that her work garnered such swift reaction because of the personal face she painted of madness alongside her clear compassion for those that suffered: "Her willingness to make simple human contact with these outcasts sparked flashes of unanticipated humanity and serenity. She was the first in America to identify with their plight and to invest the insane with the dignity of individual identity."[175] While Dix might not have been the *first*, she certainly became the most public. Her aloofness, "intellectual self-assurance and moral certitude" combined with "polished manners," and "implacable reserve" seemed to "epitomize upper-crust Boston" for many and affixed her as "a most improbably, and thus supremely compelling, guide to the geography of hell."[176] Dix appeared uniquely equipped for her mission.

That she was female played a role in Dix's effectiveness. Her gender let Dix approach men in power without seeming threatening, but because society assumed women "were the repository of morality and virtue," it also gave her an air of authority.[177] As society's moral guardian, Dix proved able to influence state and federal legislatures despite the fact that she could not vote.

From Dix's perspective, however, only God could be credited with her success. Though she rarely talked about her own accomplishments, in a 1850 letter to her English host, Mrs. Rathbone, the pious reformer asked, "Shall I not say to you, dear friend, that my uniform success and influence are evidence to my mind that I am called by Providence to the vocation to which life, talents, and fortune have been surrendered these many years?" Not only sure of God's call on her life, Dix proved confident that, with divine help, she had fulfilled her responsibility: "I cannot say, 'Behold, now, this great Babylon which I have builded!' but 'Lo! O Lord, the work which Thou gavest thy servant; she does it, and God in his benignity blesses and advances the cause by the instrument He has fitted for the labor.' "[178]

FAITHFUL ADVOCACY OR SOCIAL CONTROL?

Without question, Dix proved successful in her efforts to sway legislatures and rally public support. Many of the hospitals she helped launch still operated over a century later. One in North Carolina bore her name until it closed after 150 years of service. Whether the system of institutional care that she helped propagate benefitted the insane and society, however, was debated in the next century as conditions in mental asylums once again came under scrutiny. With hospitals bursting at the seams, the poor care, squalid conditions, and persistent incurability in the nation's mental institutions were far from Dix's vision. The optimism that once surrounded care for mental maladies slowly faded—first among physicians, and then in the public. Abhorrent conditions at asylums too large and crowded to offer humane care prompted one vein of criticism.

An additional line of critique surfaced in the twentieth century. Some surmised that in their efforts to make society better, nineteenth-century reformers sought social homogeneity. Such homogeneity required that citizens deemed abnormal, like the mentally ill, be moved out of sight. Coercive power, they argued, not a quest for humane treatment, motivated the growth of asylums and other social institutions.[179] The nation appeared more productive and more advanced when its deviant members were locked away. That darker motivation of the quest for institutionalization remained outside the conscious Christian motivations of Dix and others, but it warrants investigation.

Cotton Mather viewed madness as a part of every human. With the rise of asylums, social theorist Michel Foucault has argued, "madness had become a thing to look at: no longer a monster inside oneself, but an animal with strange mechanisms, a bestiality from which man had long been suppressed."[180] That European and American asylums became places for Sunday excursions to view mentally ill patients offers support for Foucault's assertion. Rather than sick citizens in the process of being healed, the insane were treated as public spectacles. With madness an external reality—something present not in oneself but instead in unfortunate others—insanity became easier to fear and more imperative to try to resist. After the Enlightenment, citizens viewed madness not simply as an inevitable consequence of human incarnation but as something dangerous, something needing to be avoided. The insane were deemed worthy of confinement because their illnesses demonstrated the dreaded power of unreason. With such logic, madness was dehumanizing, not a mark of humanity as Mather assumed. For Foucault, those like Dix, reformers who fought for the construction of asylums, were not "liberating heroes" but "agents of bourgeois repression and conformity" motivated by "capitalist development."[181]

It seems unlikely that Dix would have affirmed Foucault's line of thinking, but it is worth considering how such notions may have shaped her work and the actions of her contemporaries. With the rise of scientific medicine, and the increasing ability to prevent and cure disease, maladies that lingered drew suspicion. Were defects of character to blame for incurable madness? Perhaps. Foucault argued that Pinel's and Tuke's removal of physical restraints was replaced by the constraints of moral culpability.[182] Whether or not Foucault's assessments hold true, by the late nineteenth century, Americans increasingly believed that those that remained ill might be responsible for their illness or at least for not working adequately for its cure. Suspicions of individual guilt gave rise to deepened social stigma.

Eventually, changing conceptions of mental maladies in the antebellum period surrounded the afflicted with disgrace. The effect was far from intentional, but with heredity deemed as a likely cause, and with notions of irregular behavior as predisposing factors, the chronically ill seemed doomed—unable or unwilling to control their own fates. In addition, while scientific discoveries ushered in assurances of solving physical illnesses, cures for mental maladies remained undiscovered. That allowed suspicions of demonic possession, or sin and moral wrongdoing, to linger. Early institutions hoped to restore patients to health and return them to the community, but that became impossible as hospitals grew crowded and dedicated treatment transitioned into custodial care. Once hopeful retreats, asylums turned into institutions that left a taint on those admitted.

Public crusading, even when well intentioned, sometimes failed to bring desired results for Dix and other citizens. Regardless of the conscious and subconscious motivations for the establishment of asylums, their deterioration would shape the work of a later Protestant, Rev. Anton Boisen. By the time the mentally ill Boisen found himself hospitalized, American asylums had veered far from Dix's vision of gentle, curative, restful institutions.

As Dix crisscrossed the country, hospitals with friendly superintendents became her favorite resting places. In October of 1881, at age seventy-nine, Dix visited the New Jersey State Lunatic Asylum.[183] While there, she fell ill, complaining of a severe chill and a pain in her lung. For the next six years, she convalesced at the asylum, only sometimes feeling well enough to write and entertain visitors. Dix died at the hospital in July of 1887 and was buried in Mount Auburn Cemetery in Boston, just yards from the tomb of William Ellery Channing.[184]

In a letter announcing her death to her European friends, the asylum's superintendent proclaimed, "Thus has died and been laid to rest in the most quiet, unostentatious way the most useful and distinguished woman America has yet produced."[185] Throughout her public career, Dix was heralded as a "national symbol of benevolence" but rarely sought fame.[186] After her legislative triumph in Tennessee, for example, she declined the offer by "twenty-five society matrons" to have a sculptor portray her in "a permanent and pleasing form a countenance expressive at once, of feminine delicacy, and heroic firmness, sensibility and strength, compassion and courage."[187]

Dix journeyed as a Christian motivated by a need to discern her unique way to serve God, by the perfectionism she learned from her Methodist father, and by a desire to tend to the afflicted she gleaned from Unitarian outreach impulses. She lived in a rational, enlightened world that declared political, medical, and even religious men as ultimate authorities. A determined soul, she ventured into society and grasped unclaimed authority in advocating for care of the nation's insane citizens. She invoked public responsibility by relaying graphic details of her visits to public institutions. Dix appealed not to Protestants directly but to legislatures, the bodies with the power to do something about the problem as she identified it. She cooperated with politicians and medical professionals yet bore full responsibility for her mission. Indirectly, though, Dix called on all Americans to do their part, to fulfill their Christian duties to care for the least of these.

As Dix appealed for treatment on behalf of others, she and other nineteenth-century believers reclaimed lost authority in attending to mental maladies. Their declaration of authority in institution building revealed an attempt to compensate for spiritual authority lost by clergy over the prior century. As a result, Dix's work pioneered Protestant advocacy for institutional reform. In the years before the Civil War, Christians focused their concern on providing care for others, not advocating for themselves when ill.[188] By advocating on behalf of sufferers, Dix exemplified the faith of one who knew she could change the world. Her work altered the landscape of care for the country's mentally ill, but even her relentless advocacy and the purity of her motives were no panacea given the ongoing challenge of society's care for sufferers.

· internal failure
· to good to get good, do bad
  to get bad.

4

Reclaiming Religious Authority in Medicine

Anton Boisen

> The physician, as a result of his empirical method and his careful,
> systematic study of living men and women, has thus in very truth become
> a physician of souls, while the traditional "physician of souls," clinging to
> his traditional methods, has become merely the custodian of the faith.
>
> —Anton Boisen, 1923[1]

In the fall of 1920, the Presbyterian clergyman Anton Theophilus Boisen (1876–1965) found himself a patient at the Boston Psychopathic Hospital. Committed after exhibiting strange behavior, he transferred a few months later to Westboro State Hospital. Diagnosed with schizophrenia, the minister experienced five severe psychotic episodes in the next fifteen years. Boisen's hospitalizations turned his attention to the complexity of illness and the plight of those suffering with mental maladies. It also made clear to him the Church's responsibility.

Boisen referred to mental illness as a "little-known country," a place visited by a minority of Americans and understood by even fewer. His periods of psychosis provided—both literally and figuratively—a vision for his life's work. While sick, he conceived that he had "broken an opening in the wall which separated medicine and religion," and in that rupture, the clergyman found a "new mission" for his life.[2] In 1921, just a few months after emerging from his first episode, and still hospitalized, he named his hopes in a letter to a colleague. "My present purpose," he reflected, "is to take as my problem the one with which I am now confronted, the service of these unfortunates with whom I am surrounded."[3] Illness provided a personal cause with pastoral implications.[4]

89

Success navigating his own affliction gave Boisen confidence that he could remedy Protestants' lapsed attention to the suffering brought by mental distress. "The problem seems to me," he argued, "one of great importance not only because of the large number who are now suffering from mental ailments but also because of its religious and psychological and philosophical aspects." "I am very sure," he concluded, "that if I can make any contribution whatsoever [to the problem of mental illness] it will be worth the cost."[5] For the remainder of his life, he harnessed insight gained as a patient and a pastor to challenge both medical and prevailing Protestant attitudes toward mental illness and in doing so helped reorient the role of clergy in providing care.

Boisen's story demonstrates new developments in the relationship between Protestantism and mental illness from 1865 to 1930. By reflecting theologically as one who suffered, the minister introduced a new vantage point for Protestant consideration. Cotton Mather and Benjamin Rush had ruminated about mental distress, but not experienced it firsthand. To be sure, Dix lived in fear of illness and experienced depression, realities that likely informed her advocacy, but she never drew connections between her suffering and the plight of those she sought to help, at least not publically. Boisen's experience as a patient fueled his work. Undertaking his mission, the minister encountered the theological and medical systems established by Protestant clergy and physicians of prior centuries. He found neither adequate to bring healing but believed that the combined insight of religion and medicine could enable cures. He encouraged a deep investigation of the human condition and a reconfiguration of clergy training. He felt sure that recovery—for himself and for others—depended on a new understanding of the relationship between mental illness and religious experience.[6] The pastor/patient insisted that "many forms of insanity are religious rather than medical problems and that they cannot be successfully treated until they are so recognized."[7] Proper treatment, he held, started with correct diagnosis, and as he redefined some illnesses as spiritual problems instead of medical concerns, he challenged prevailing medical theory.

Though he brought new insight, Boisen drew on the work of Protestant forebearers who had shaped the country's approach to mental maladies. In some ways, his thought offered a return to the reasoning found in the work of colonial clergyman Mather. Like the Puritan preacher, Boisen saw a religious dimension in emotional disturbance and found illness purposeful in the spiritual life. Unlike Mather, or the physician Benjamin Rush, however, Boisen claimed no direct authority in medicine. Though he possessed medical knowledge, more important to him was the authority of experience, a claim made possible by the newly developed disciplines of psychology, the psychology of religion, the emergence of liberal theology, and his own struggles. Dix too had relied on experience to fuel her advocacy, but her authority came as a lay observer, not as a patient, social scientist, or member of the clergy. Like Mather, Rush, and Dix before him, Boisen felt a divine call to alleviate the distress of others and for forty years deployed his talents in the service of sufferers.

In the decades between Dix's advocacy and Boisen's hospitalization, much changed for the nation's mentally ill. The quality of institutional care degenerated, and although psychiatric practice continued to professionalize, cures remained elusive. In addition, new social theories touted the promise of human progress and decried the dangers of dependency. Combined, those forces entrenched social stigma toward the mentally ill and thwarted Christian responses to their distress.[8] Amidst waning religious attention, Boisen called fellow Christians to reconsider their attention to mental suffering.

The pious Presbyterian could enter the story of American Protestantism and mental illnesses from several perspectives, and that multiplicity demonstrates his importance to the account. Boisen knew firsthand the pain of mental disorder, but he also brought a range of professional expertise to bear. He was an ordained minister, and his background included service in several local parishes. He studied religion and psychology at Andover Theological Seminary and Harvard University, worked as a chaplain in mental hospitals, and pioneered the creation of clinical pastoral training for seminary students. In 1924 he was appointed to the faculty at Chicago Theological Seminary, where he taught for nearly twenty years. Boisen published extensively about mental illness, the psychology of religion, and the intersections of medicine and religion. The well-trained minister called for a restoration of clergy and church authority in attending to mental maladies, authority ministers had ceded to medical professionals in the prior half century. He felt the church gave far too little attention to mental illness, and he knew that properly trained ministers could reclaim their rightful position at the bedsides of those enduring mental distress. The pastor/patient remained sure his insights could improve not just clerical but also clinical care.[9] Boisen's efforts brought changes not only in clerical training but also in psychiatric practice and in medical-ecclesial relationships.

With clerical authority reasserted, the clergyman's work encouraged Protestant leaders to reconfigure their attention to mental maladies. Dix had done her part as a layperson by ensuring the creation of asylums. Boisen argued that believers must do more. Instead of handing off care to institutions (public or private), Christians, particularly clergy, needed to work directly with those hospitalized, both to attend to their spiritual needs and to understand suffering. Many American church bodies listened to his plea. They updated training requirements for ordination and expanded fields of ministry. Boisen's work shifted the course of theological education and seminary training. Key for the clergyman was adding "first-hand study of human experience"—what he called a reading of the "living human documents" to supplement classroom-based theological education.[10] Deploying social scientific methods in combination with religious insights, his work established Clinical Pastoral Education and mental health chaplaincy and paved the way for the new discipline of pastoral theology. Claiming religious authority and medical insight, Boisen's work helped cultivate a period of cooperation between many Protestants and medical practioners.

All told, Boisen's story signals that something had shifted dramatically in the two centuries since Cotton Mather's reflections on illness. Boisen's hospital stays followed six decades of sweeping changes in institutional life and in the profession of psychiatry. Perhaps in no other period did care for America's mentally ill evolve so rapidly or views of mental maladies shift so dramatically. In addition to clerical abdication of care to medical professionals, during this era, the social stigma affixed to mental illness grew intractable. If religion had still played the primary role in defining mental maladies and in directing care, Boisen could have remained silent. Instead, he felt something had gone awry with how America's Protestants responded to mental distress. Boisen longed to remedy those problems and in the process make his suffering purposeful.

Though healing concerned him, Boisen contended, "Sanity in itself is not an end in life." Instead, "the end of life is to solve important problems and to contribute in some way to human welfare."[11] Awakening to his opportunity to contribute, he shared that "if there is even a chance that" improving human welfare "could best be accomplished by going through Hell for a while, no man worthy of the name would hesitate for an instant."[12] Sensing a divine call and an urgent need to help, he served gladly.

WELL EDUCATED AND WANDERING

It took decades—and the experience of illness—for Boisen to settle into a career. Born in Bloomington, Indiana, he came from a family dedicated to higher education and experienced in church leadership. His maternal great-grandfather and grandfather each worked as ministers in Presbyterian churches. His maternal grandfather also taught as a professor of mathematics at Indiana University for forty-six years and served as the university's president.[13] His father, Hermann Boisen, earned a doctorate and taught botany and modern language courses at the same institution. His mother, one of the first women enrolled at Indiana University, instructed for a year at the University of Missouri before marrying. Both parents valued education, and his father passed on his interest and skill in scientific inquiry. Boisen idealized his father, and the elder Boisen's influence persisted even though he died of heart failure when his son was just seven years old. After his father's death, Anton, his mother, and his siblings lived with his maternal grandparents in their strict, devoutly Presbyterian household.

As a young adult, Boisen tested several career paths. After graduating from Indiana University, he briefly taught high school. In 1902, despite having started graduate work in modern languages, he decided to become a forester. Memories of his father's love of the outdoors, a desire for adventure, and a growing sense of restlessness influenced the shift. In 1908 his vocational plans changed again. While studying at Yale Forest School, Boisen experienced a call to ministry and matriculated at Union Theological Seminary in New York City, where his studies focused on the psychology of religion.[14]

Ordained as a Presbyterian in 1912, the minister initially failed to secure a church appointment. Without a parish to tend, Boisen combined his interests in science and religion and conducted surveys to document the economic, sociological, and religious landscape for the Presbyterian Board of Home Missions. After completing that work, he finally was appointed to a series of rural Congregational churches in Iowa, Kansas, and Maine.[15] During World War I, Boisen served as a chaplain with the Overseas YMCA and then returned to conduct religious surveys for the Interchurch World Movement. Like Dorothea Dix, at age forty, Boisen's most significant work had yet to begin.

Also reminiscent of Dix, Boisen's life included personal difficulty, although of different sorts. Beginning in adolescence, Boisen had "felt shame and guilt for his inability to control sexual feelings."[16] Similar ideas troubled him throughout his life and triggered his first severe depression at age twenty-two. Unrequited romantic infatuations also plagued Boisen and contributed to his mental distress. For decades, starting in 1902, he maintained a one-sided love affair with Alice Batchelder, whom he met when she spoke on behalf of the YWCA at Indiana University. Obsessed with the never-married woman, Boisen made career choices to try to prove that he would be a worthy husband. He pursued the uninterested, but occasionally friendly, Batchelder until her death thirty-three years later. Boisen's sense of failure, and his perception that "he was not good enough for her," led to at least two, possibly three, of his mental breakdowns.[17] In 1930 the death of his mother precipitated another collapse and hospitalization. Five years later, after hearing

the news that Alice Batchelder suffered from terminal cancer, he underwent
a third major psychosis. Repeatedly, personal distress interrupted Boisen's
vocational pursuits.

INSANITY AFTER THE RISE OF INSTITUTIONS

When breakdowns led to committal, the hospital system that Boisen experienced as a patient was far different from the idyllic haven imagined by Dix
in the prior century. By the close of the nineteenth century, asylum-based
care fell short of the ideals of earlier Christian reformers because of over-
crowding, underfunding, and the continued elusiveness of cures. Changing
perceptions of mental illness also played a role in shaping institutional care.

In the nineteenth century, medical, social, moral, and religious understandings of mental illness combined with deteriorating institutional conditions to shape the treatment offered to patients like Boisen. They also
influenced the willingness to access care. Laity, clergy, and medical professionals sometimes shared conceptions of illness and treatment, but not
always. Medical professionals took the lead in defining illness in the antebellum era, drawing on both medical and moral rationale. They viewed mental
illness primarily as a "somatic disease that involved lesions of the brain."[18]
Belief in such lesions, though, involved a leap of faith given that no diagnostic tools were available to confirm their presence, at least in living patients.
As a result, physicians suspected inherited and psychological causes in addition to physical ones. In most cases, professionals assumed mental maladies
involved human transgression of the proper created order.[19] While not all
mental illnesses were self-inflicted, doctors held that those ignoring moral
norms risked succumbing to disease. They found presumed moral causes of
insanity—"intemperance, overwork, domestic difficulties, excessive ambition, faulty education, personal disappointments, jealousy, pride, and . . . the
pressures of an urban, industrial, and commercial civilization"—easier to
identify and treat than organic ones.[20] Given that understanding, and despite
belief in somatic origins, psychiatrists focused as much on behavioral prevention and cures as on physical treatments.

The focus on behavioral causes, and presumptions about human responsibility, formed part of the deepening stigma associated with mental illness.
No longer did Americans view mental maladies as no-fault illnesses caused
simply by the legacy of original sin. Suspicions of personal responsibility
intruded into all cases, particularly incurable ones.

Physicians' views of illness dictated treatments, and in the late nineteenth
century, most formal care for mental ailments took place in asylums. While
treatment plans varied significantly between institutions, the majority of

alienists tried to restore a normal balance to patients through a combination of diet, exercise, and fresh air, along with tonics and cathartics, approaches that continued the practice of moral treatment adopted earlier in the century.[21] In addition, sedatives and hypnotics, including opium and morphine, became common remedies for calming patients. Restraint systems—created to prevent patients from harming themselves or others—remained controversial. Some understood those restrictive measures as protective; others saw nothing but repression.[22] Altogether, nineteenth-century care remained an inexact science.

Though debate about treatment methods emerged, professional optimism in the curative potential of institutions prevailed, at least throughout the period of institution building that Dorothea Dix helped prompt. From the 1830s through the 1870s, reports of high recovery rates fueled demand for asylum care. In 1834 and 1841, for example, the annual reports of Samuel B. Woodward of the state hospital in Worcester indicated recovery rates between 82 percent and 91 percent.[23] Other antebellum superintendents claimed similar results, and, with proper care, asylum physicians considered mental maladies more treatable than other ailments. In 1835 Woodward pronounced, "In recent cases of insanity, under judicious treatment, as large a proportion of recoveries will take place as from any other acute disease of equal severity."[24] Throughout the middle of the nineteenth century, reported high cure rates helped legitimize the care institutions provided and prompted continued government funding for treatment.

After 1851, growing professional coordination among alienists meant that care for patients began to formalize. One of the first measures of the recently formed Association of Medical Superintendents of American Institutions for the Insane was the publication of guidelines for design and construction of mental hospitals.[25] The twenty-six standards included recommendations for site selection, room size, lighting, and a basic architectural plan. The document advised a rural setting and a central administrative building flanked with long wings of patient wards on each side.[26] In those spacious facilities, physicians lived on site with their families, affording them direct, daily access to patients and tight control of all aspects of their institutions.

Despite emerging professional standards, human behavior, not medical definitions, dictated lay perceptions of insanity. Families often encountered symptoms first, and a range of odd behavior led families to suspect insanity. The loss of cognitive faculties, including the inability to speak coherently or remember the past, might cause concern, as would a disruption to basic living habits such as dramatic changes in eating, sleeping, and working patterns. Debilitating mental states and moods (excitement, melancholy, irritability), and delusions or bizarre beliefs, prompted loved ones to fret.[27] Not all strange behavior drew suspicions of insanity, though. If present from birth, odd behavior was labeled by families as idiocy; when present only during fever, it was considered delirium. Only when the behavior of loved ones changed suddenly and persisted did family members fear a more serious problem.[28]

While uncertain of exact causes, families assumed insanity stemmed from disorder in the nervous system. Much like physicians, they concluded that stressful events—physical or emotional—shocked the system and affected normal brain function. A severe physical sickness might lead an individual toward insanity, so could common bodily processes like constipation, menses, and menopause. At times, families suspected the habitual use of alcohol and tobacco in their relatives' distress. They described psychological causes too, including "grief, anxiety over the sick, business losses, intense application to work or study," and "unrequited love." Severe trauma might also precipitate insanity, as in the case of an uncle who never recovered from the "great shock" of witnessing the assassination of Abraham Lincoln at the Ford's Theatre.[29] Regardless of the suspected cause, disruptive, odd behaviors worried family members.

While comfort with institutional care grew with asylum construction, families still made the decision to commit loved ones reluctantly and only after exhausting other options. Relatives considered kin that acted bizarrely simply eccentric, but persistent behavior that interrupted normal life routines, or turned violent, forced them to consider a more significant problem. Only after failing to squelch odd behavior was the local physician called. When enlisted, local physicians deployed an assortment of cures including age-old remedies like bleeding, purging, and blistering. Doctors also administered morphine, chloroform, and other drugs. When physical treatments failed, family physicians recommended committal. The more controlled asylum environment, they reasoned, might help. Even then, families that could afford to do so sent men and women for extended stays at health resorts and spas before resorting to mental hospitals.

In time, the inability to provide care at home coupled with the carefully cultivated presentation of the asylum's capabilities by superintendents helped ease decisions to institutionalize loved ones. Though committal remained a last resort, violent, self-destructive behavior and suicide attempts accelerated decision making. Nonetheless, anxiety and guilt could accompany the decision to commit a relative, even when the asylum seemed the best hope for peace at home and recovery for the patient. Yet, eventually, many families trusted institutions to bring healing they, or family doctors, could not.

With medical treatment options growing more prevalent, nineteenth-century clergy, Boisen's predecessors, no longer served as lone experts on mental distress. An 1873 reflection by the physician D. A. Gorton showed the ground physicians had claimed from clergy in the provision of care. Mental health had always interested physicians, but only in the middle of the nineteenth century did doctors move beyond their "disinclination to intrench [*sic*] upon a department of study which the custom of centuries has wrongfully confided exclusively to the profession of theology." Gorton saw religion as good and true but found medical professionals more qualified to deal with matters of the mind. Many ministers and laity agreed.[30]

Though most clergy left no indication of their thoughts about mental illness, a few recorded their views.[31] Some, including those that ministered in asylums or campaigned for reforms, viewed illness as alienists did. Mental maladies, they agreed, were conditions requiring treatment by medical professionals. Rev. D. S. Welling's 1851 *Information for the People; or, The Asylums of Ohio, with Miscellaneous Observations on Health, Diet and Morals, and the Causes, Symptoms and Proper Treatment of Nervous Disease and Insanity* exemplified an approach that yielded authority to asylum physicians. Given his approval of institutional treatment, Welling, who served as the chaplain at a state asylum in Columbus, even relaxed his usual stance on vice and virtue in support of practices that aided patient recovery. He considered dancing and card playing—typically activities that could generate "great evil" or even induce "mania"—"very proper for lunatics in an Asylum to engage in" because they offered the possibility of recovery, if not cure.[32] Clergymen like Welling trusted the authority of asylum doctors in defining cures and even let medical prescriptions trump their usual spiritual counsel.

Clerical endorsement of psychiatric techniques also allowed asylum superintendents and religious men to work cooperatively. That relationship proceeded most smoothly, though, when ministers ceded ultimate control to physicians. Religious leaders sought advice from superintendents when they encountered parishioners acting strangely, counsel that family ministers had dispensed a century earlier. In 1840 some asylums hired part-time chaplains or allowed local clergy to preach Sunday sermons to patients, but despite the Protestant affiliation of most nineteenth-century alienists, they proved wary that clergy "would weaken their authority or disturb their patients." Concern—and professional debate—about the role of Christian ministers in hospitals notwithstanding, many asylum annual reports noted that "religious services aided greatly in therapy."[33] Productive medical and clerical cooperation appeared possible, under some circumstances.

While many ministers ceded virtually all authority to alienists, others called for separate jurisdictions. The Congregational clergyman and president of Yale University Noah Porter, for example, declared in his textbook *The Human Intellect*, "It is no part of our duty to give a scientific theory of insanity." Clergy like Porter remained "interested in the mind-body relationship and in psychology" but "considered psychiatry out of their purview."[34] Even so, they helped the ministerial ranks retain some authority on mental diseases despite the growing professional power of asylum physicians. In 1840 Harpers and Brothers commissioned Rev. Thomas C. Upham, professor of mental and moral philosophy at Bowdoin College, to write a book about mental disease geared toward popular audiences.[35] Upham hoped to show that the "public mind is but little informed, certainly much less than it should be, in relation to the true doctrines of regular or normal mental action; but it is, undoubtedly, much more ignorant of philosophy of defective and disordered mental action."[36] The minister noted that most writing about mental disorder proved complex and not designed for "popular circulation." As a clergyman and professor, he asserted the authority to translate the topic for popular consumption. Even with separate jurisdictions, clergy retained some authority by making medical thought accessible to the masses.[37]

Undoubtedly, ministers continued to counsel the distressed, but in their public discussions and debate, clerical attention to mental maladies in antebellum America proved more of an intellectual exercise than an exploration of the best methods for the direct provision of pastoral, congregational, or public care. When Boisen entered the conversation in the early twentieth century, he endorsed an integrated, cooperative approach between medical professionals and clergymen. His call to action, however, was still decades away.

As they jockeyed for authority, nineteenth-century clergy, laity, and medical professionals all pondered whether religious belief and practice could cause insanity. Ministers fought assertions that linked religious adherence and mental illness.[38] Families, however, more freely suspected that nonnormative religious beliefs and practices might trigger mental illness. In the wake of widespread early nineteenth-century revivals—"a time when universal salvation, the innate goodness of human nature, and the harmony between spiritual and secular concerns were becoming dominant themes in mainstream American Protestantism"—relatives concluded that "too pessimistic or otherworldly beliefs" and "unwarranted convictions of sin and damnation" might precipitate delusion instead of piety. Letters from family members to asylum physicians also claimed that "overzealous religious practices, such as excessive Bible reading, too exacting observance of Lent, and adoption of old-style Quaker dress," brought "mental instability."[39] Religious practice outside of customary limits, they argued, could cause illness. Though they may have suspected it, family correspondence gave no indication of a primary role for personal sin or the supernatural as an attributed cause of illness, a claim more common in the prior century. Instead, a variety of non-supernatural, behavioral explanations now seemed most plausible.

While few psychiatrists thought that religion caused mental distress, they agreed that "excessive religious zeal" could trigger illness.[40] Asylum superintendents also posited a role for misguided clerical action. They feared "depressing or condemnatory sermons" might further disturb hospitalized patients, an understanding that fed the reluctance of some to allow clergy to serve institutions. Worried that ministers would preach sermons that were "too austere, denunciatory, and prone to dwell on the 'terrors of the law' " instead of consoling and comforting in the face of distress, they rejected clerical involvement.[41]

Unlike their medical counterparts, ministers felt sure that Christian belief and practice brought solace, not illness. Frederick A. Packard, for example, an editor of Sunday school publications, argued, "Properly revealed religion warded off insanity by engendering obedience to God through fear and love."[42] Disbelief, though, proved problematic—if not dangerous—because it inhibited proper mental functioning.[43] Religious belief, ministers argued, was necessary for mental health, and popular morality played a role in that assessment. Without religion to ground morality and tame free will, people might lose touch with moral truths, leading to insanity or, more likely, to sin.[44]

Though united about the threats of false belief, differences in clerical opinions emerged as nineteenth-century revivalism prompted disagreement. Ministers who opposed revivals sometimes linked them with insanity. Correlating the increase in asylum populations with the rise of religious revivals, the liberal clergyman Otis A. Skinner pronounced, "Something like one sixth [of the insane] are made crazy by gloomy views of religion" and revival preaching. Even supporters of revivals feared that the hysteria, catalepsy, and epilepsy that sometimes accompanied them could prove dangerous to those prone to mental illness.[45] Others, like the revivalist Charles G. Finney, simply assumed that the future of religion and the conversion of souls made the risk of insanity worthwhile. "It is very desirable," he argued, "that the church should go on steadily . . . without these excitements. Such excitements are liable to injure the health. Our nervous system is so strung that any powerful excitement, if long continued, injures our health. . . . This spasmodic religion must be done away. . . . But as yet, the state of the Christian world is such, that to expect to promote religion without excitement is unphilosophical and absurd."[46] Ministerial affinity to revivalism informed assessments of its dangers.[47]

Clerical disagreement also stemmed from diverging theological perspectives within the broad nineteenth-century evangelical consensus. Those committed to a more conservative, literal interpretation of the Bible proved reluctant to relegate completely "demonic possession and miracle healing" to the past. Conservatives appeared more likely than their liberal counterparts to offer theological explanations for illness, claiming individual sin as a cause of insanity and thus repentance and redemption as the primary cure. Alternately, more liberal Protestant clergy—Boisen's forefathers in ministry—proved willing to see mental illness as a bodily illness subject to treatment by physicians.[48] Liberal clergy, "influenced in part by the higher criticism of the Bible, abjuring fundamentalism and talk of the devil, and eager to keep up with current scientific trends, came to ignore the subject of insanity altogether as a religious theological issue."[49] Instead, they gladly handed over authority on medical matters to medical professionals. Basic differences in clerical opinion appeared for the next century, and Boisen's work sought a middle ground.

In short, many ideas swirled around to form understandings of mental illness in the final half of the nineteenth century, and no one point of view proved dominant. In the face of mental distress, the public looked to educated leaders for definitional help and treatment, but more than in the past, medical professionals, and not clergy, proved the more trusted sources of authority on healing. After the rise of asylum medicine, never again did clergy hold lone expertise for care of mental illness. Even ministers that recommended spiritual cures needed to offer critiques of medical treatment options. By Boisen's time, the normative presumption about responsibility for treating mental illness had shifted firmly to the medical realm.

ASYLUM-BASED CARE: FROM SALVATION TO SQUALOR

As lines of professional authority shifted, asylums emerged as the widely approved location for treating mental illness. Decades before Boisen's hospitalizations, responsibility for insane persons increasingly fell into the hands of state agencies, not local jurisdictions or church institutions.[50] In the three decades after 1860, the U.S. population doubled, but the population of America's mental institutions increased ninefold, demonstrating that the assumed proper locale of treatment had shifted from the home and community to the public asylum.[51] By 1880, spurred by the legacy of Dorothea Dix's efforts, nearly 140 public and private institutions offered care to nearly 41,000 mentally ill patients.[52] Those institutions offered "restorative therapy for curable cases" and provided basic care (food, shelter, clothing) to those unable to survive outside of institutions.[53]

Impressive institutional growth coupled with the emerging professionalism of psychiatry seemed to indicate widespread success in asylum care, but problems emerged. Those troubles deepened the stigmatization of the nation's mentally ill population and, eventually, contributed to Boisen's plea for renewed religious involvement in caregiving. The presence of more mental hospitals (and almshouses and prisons) failed to prevent illness and dependency, and institutions proved unable to provide adequate treatment to all in need. Increasing patient populations placed stress on systems of care. The 1851 recommendations of the Association of Medical Superintendents of American Institutions suggested each institution house between 200 and 250 patients. Low limits enabled superintendents and their staffs to offer attentive, personal care, but shifting legislative funding shaped definitions of mental illness and increased asylum populations. Local jurisdictions, for example, identified elderly and senile patients as candidates for state asylums rather than local almshouses.[54] By 1875, "state and urban asylums founded before 1870 had an average resident population of 432," and a "third had between 500 and 1300 residents."[55] Despite recommended patient-to-staff ratios, the number of patients at individual hospitals grew quickly and exceeded manageable levels.

Larger institutional populations forced alterations to treatment protocols. The practice of moral treatment, popularized in the nation's first institutions, "assumed that hospitals—like families—would remain small, and that superintendents—like firm but loving fathers—would have the ability and flexibility to shape the environment in order to arrest and then reverse the course of mental disorders." Overcrowded asylums made that approach untenable. Instead, hospitals exerted "rigid and coercive" control. Maintaining order took precedence over providing cures, and personal care for each patient from physicians proved infeasible.[56] Packed asylums also forced superintendents to take on more administrative roles, leaving daily treatment, if it even occurred, to attendants with less medical training. Exacerbating institutional crowding, hospitals built shoddily by penny-pinching state governments offered inadequate treatment facilities. Writing to Dorothea Dix in 1880, J. P. Brown, superintendent of the Taunton Hospital in Massachusetts, complained that political battles reduced funding—"cheapening everything" and limiting "the expenses of our Hospital to Poor House Rates."[57] Finally, a growing percentage of chronic cases at hospitals, including senile residents, made it difficult for caregivers to devote as much attention to acute and less severe cases. As a result, many went without treatment. As early as 1862,

Dix had lamented, "No State Hospital provision has been adequate to the needs of the insane." "Old cases," she relayed, "are removed at present of a hard necessity to make place for recent and probably curable cases."[58] Conditions continued to deteriorate, and as institutions became more custodial than curative and discharged patients before they were restored to health, the institutions could no longer promise relief from mental illness.

Political responses to urbanization also prompted changes in institutional life. In the decades before 1900, the demographics of the country changed dramatically. While only 11 percent of the population lived in urban areas in 1840, that figure had grown to 20 percent by 1860 and 40 percent by 1900. Population growth (from 31,443,000 to 75,992,000 in the same period) sparked by massive immigration fueled much of the urbanization.[59] With greater population density in cities, problems of illness and dependency grew more prominent, and coordinated efforts to combat them appeared. Massachusetts, for example, centralized its welfare efforts with the 1863 establishment of the Board of State Charities. Five more states had followed suit by 1869, and others followed soon thereafter.[60] As the complexity of the nation's bureaucracy increased, public funding and decision making took place at a greater distance from those experienced with the care of the poor, dependent, and ill, and it diminished the authority of institutional superintendents over their domains and accelerated the shift of their duties from the medical to the administrative realm.[61]

Institutional changes reshaped perceptions of illness. With late nineteenth-century changes to mental hospitals, Americans increasingly viewed them as welfare institutions instead of medical facilities. In addition, accounts like the 1854 *Report on Insanity and Idiocy in Massachusetts*, commissioned by the state and led by the physician and statistician Edward Jarvis, contributed to suspicions of mental illness as a problem of social dependency. Jarvis reported a "higher incidence of insanity, idiocy, and crime among poor and pauper groups than among" others. He traced both poverty and insanity to the same origins, an "imperfectly organized brain and feeble mental constitution." Jarvis also linked mental disease to class and ethnicity, saddling those that suffered with the social stigma attributed to immigrants and the poor.[62] As state welfare systems developed, the result was the positioning of mental hospitals as just one of many institutions that cared for dependent Americans, citizens viewed with both compassion and suspicion.[63] And, while physicians diagnosed mental maladies as illnesses, increasingly, those maladies were also viewed as a social problem.

As the result of shifting patient populations and changing bureaucratic control, by the end of the century, life inside many asylums resembled care in the almshouses Dix once sought to eradicate. To be sure, many patients benefitted from hospitalization, even if institutions failed to live up to earlier ideals. But, with larger patient populations, strained facilities, less attentive care, and weary professionals, insane asylums operated as warehouses more than as hospitals.

Problems for the nation's mentally ill expanded beyond crowded facilities and deteriorating physical plants as professional confidence in the ability of asylums to cure illness diminished. Cure rates that hopeful alienists claimed earlier in the century proved exaggerated. Pliny Earle, the superintendent of the state hospital for the insane in Northampton, Massachusetts, exposed inconsistencies and errors in the calculation of recovery statistics. In what Earle diagnosed as a "period of apparent struggle for the largest numerical symbols," physicians reported increased treatment effectiveness, but he and others voiced concerns that statistics could mislead as easily as they could prove success. Addressing his peers at the New England Psychological Society in 1876, Earle urged them to reconsider recovery-rate calculations. Offering his colleagues the benefit of the doubt about past reports, he pointed to the desire of superintendents to "look upon the bright side of things" rather than pointing to statistical incompetence as accounting for exaggerated cure rates.[64] Sanguine physicians simply believed that new moral treatments would be effective given enough time, and their reporting reflected that optimism. Efforts to heal by altering patient behavior, though, brought limited success, and Earle's exposé of dubious calculations contributed to growing professional skepticism about nonmedical, moral treatment and to doubts about the "eminent curability" of mental diseases.[65]

Earle's suspicions proved true. While midcentury accounts from superintendents professed high, and sometimes universal, cure rates, a 1877 study of American and British institutions found that for every 100 patients admitted, only 34 recovered by year-end, 29 died, and 36 showed no progress or grew worse. Of the 34 reported as recovered, many relapsed.[66] Such evidence shattered optimism about the effectiveness of treatments and the possibility of universal cures. Reported recovery rates plummeted in the final quarter of the nineteenth century, and given lingering suspicions of personal responsibility for incurable illness, the public ascribed fault to patients as much as to medical professionals or inadequate facilities.

Alongside reassessments of recovery rates, as the century drew to a close, hope for medical cures for mental disorders waned. By 1900 changes in general medicine had colored mental institutions as remnants of the past, and a pall of disrespectability tainted both patients and asylum physicians. By the time Boisen was hospitalized, the paths of general medicine and attention to the mentally ill—long part of the same story—had diverged. While the earliest alienists were simply general physicians that chose to work in asylums, changes between 1860 and 1920 left them detached from the medical mainstream.

In addition, in the late nineteenth century, a general professional recon-figuration of medicine followed a period of disorganization and lowered public confidence in all medical practitioners. Medical schools proliferated, and dubious medical sects flourished.[67] In 1830 the country counted twenty-two medical schools, twice the number in similarly sized European countries. By 1860 the number of schools had doubled.[68] While each institution granted diplomas, the quality and length of instruction varied widely, as did the skills of graduates. Most states required only an M.D. degree as proof of compe-tency (independent of the granting institution), and "unhampered by legal prejudice, healers of every stripe assumed the title *doctor* and hung out their shingles."[69] Uncoordinated and contradictory treatment options dampened public confidence in all practitioners, including asylum physicians.

Because of the fragmented professional landscape, physicians worked to regain credibility. Reforms to the practice of medicine began with a focus on medical education and the reinstatement of legal barriers to entry.[70] In addition, between 1874 and 1900, every state in the union passed medical licensing acts, reversing the reluctance earlier in the century to regulate the practice of medicine. Those acts, combined with the 1889 Supreme Court decision *Dent v. West Virginia* (which upheld "the authority of the state medi-cal examining board to deprive a poorly trained eclectic physician of the right to practice"), fostered standardization.[71] Curricula also improved as medical schools aimed to prepare students for licensing exams.

Scientific medicine led to medical advancements, but in specialties other than psychiatry.[72] Innovations in anesthesia; the invention of stethoscopes (1819), ophthalmoscopes (1851), and laryngoscopes (1855); and the use of radiology revolutionized diagnosis and treatment and helped physicians attend to physical ailments.[73] While such improvements failed directly to affect care of mental disease, they encouraged many psychiatrists to pursue "scientific research rather than care or custody." And, as they shifted their focus to "disease rather than patients," they directed curative and preventa-tive measures toward all of society, not just those in the confines of mental institutions.[74]

Finally, population growth in urban centers brought the development of hospitals, which became the new focal point for medicine and medical research.[75] Charitable hospitals developed in the colonial era, but a more widespread expansion of general hospitals began in the 1880s.[76] Older facil-ities offered care for mostly indigent patients, but new hospitals catered to affluent groups that could afford new methods of care, and that provided higher incomes for their physicians.[77] New facilities became the seats of scientific study and physician training, and asylums, once viewed as the nation's most innovative and curative institutions, suffered a loss in prestige when compared to general hospitals. As a result, asylum physicians and mental patients endured a further loss of social status.

After the turn of the twentieth century, the professionalization of general medicine emerged with more force, leaving psychiatry even further behind. Membership in the American Medical Association grew rapidly as the organization coordinated with local medical associations, allowing it to exert more control over care. As the authority of "regular" physicians grew, it did so at the expense of medical sectarians, nurses, and pharmacists. Also left behind were psychiatrists and, even further behind, clergy. Rivals to orthodox medicine remained, with Christian Science, osteopathy, and chiropractic care appearing as the twentieth century dawned, but nonpsychiatric physicians had established their professional dominance.

Once drawing the interest of the nation's best physicians, tending to mental maladies lost appeal for later generations of caregivers. Challenging conditions and a sense that the rest of medicine had abandoned them pushed asylum physicians—now more commonly called psychiatrists—out of institutions in droves. They sought to reclaim public and professional respectability and to find new venues for plying their trade.[78] Their flight reinforced negative public images of asylums (and the insane) and simultaneously diminished further the quality of care received by institutionalized Americans. And, as psychiatrists ventured beyond asylum walls, "they were less and less prone to act—as their nineteenth-century predecessors had acted—as the representatives of the institutionalized mentally ill," particularly those with seemingly chronic cases.[79]

Not only did the professional status of psychiatrists fall; as the nineteenth century closed, asylum care and its practitioners drew criticism from several quarters. One line of critique came from other physicians. The neurologist S. Weir Mitchell's 1894 address to the American Medico-Psychological Association exemplified attacks on asylum medicine from their medical counterparts. Mitchell declared psychiatry deficient and too isolated from other medical specialties. "You were the first of the specialists," Mitchell observed, "and you have never come back into line. It is easy to see how this came about. You soon began to live apart, and you still do so. Your hospitals are not our hospitals; your ways are not our ways. You live out of range of critical shot; you are not preceded and followed in your ward by clever rivals, or watched by able residents fresh with the learning of the schools." Drawing a distinct line between psychiatry and scientific medicine, Mitchell claimed that mental hospitals failed to foster scientific inquiry, deployed distrusted therapeutics, and disregarded responsibility for educating the public about treatments and prevention.[80]

External critique of mental institutions and their leaders also emerged as vocal former patients decried forced committal and the treatment they received. Mrs. E. P. W. Packard, for example, led a public attack on forced captivity after she was institutionalized for three years in the Illinois State Hospital for the Insane by her husband, a Protestant clergyman.[81] Asylums throughout the country faced writs of habeas corpus that freed wrongly committed patients and generated negative publicity and suspicion about committal procedures.[82] Alongside such public exposés, increased government oversight meant that superintendents faced constant queries of their methods and approaches from state boards of charity. Citizens and bureaucrats alike perceived—and professed—that something was wrong with the treatment of mental disorders. Decades later, Boisen's laments added to that list of concerns.

As superintendents were attacked by both medical doctors and patients, internal disagreements weakened professional cohesion and deepened external criticism. With institutional crowding, for example, asylum physicians differed about whether states should establish separate institutions for the incurably insane (hospitals that provided custody but not treatment). Some argued that this move would improve care in "therapeutic" hospitals and use public funds most effectively. Others worried that distinguishing between curable and incurable disease invited error and that preventing the abuse of patients in custodial institutions would prove difficult.[83]

Despite disparagement from medical peers and disgruntled patients, most asylum superintendents held fast to the hope for cures, even as approaches to treatment diversified. As all doctors administered drugs more commonly in the final decades of the century, younger asylum physicians that experimented with medical cures and adopted purely somatic views of illness increasingly criticized moral treatments as unscientific and ineffective. Adopting a "therapeutic nihilism," some younger psychiatrists even claimed that mental illness would prove incurable until medical advances appeared.[84] They remained certain that cures lay just around the corner but believed they would stem from somatic solutions, and not asylums. In his 1917 presidential address to the American Medico-Psychological Association, Charles G. Wagner predicted that the hard work of a variety of approaches would "within the period of a decade or two . . . result in a much better understanding of the etiology, pathology, diagnosis and treatment of mental diseases."[85]

Such hopefulness, though, bypassed the chronically mentally ill to the extent that psychiatrists increasingly focused treatments, and hopes for cures, on those outside of asylums.

As the result of different treatment approaches, the field of psychiatry fragmented in the decades before Boisen's 1920 hospitalization. Not only had psychiatric practice moved beyond institutions, but practitioners also began to deploy a variety of scientific approaches to their craft. Some continued to search for physical causes of distress, while some relied on the newly published insights of Sigmund Freud to probe psychological causes. Others combined psychological and physiological approaches. A number even reached beyond customary medical jurisdiction to shape human behavior as part of the preventative mental hygiene movement.[86] With the professionalization of other fields of medical practice, scientific approaches to diagnosis and treatment garnered the most confidence.[87] As a result, no longer could someone like Dorothea Dix—or religious leaders—claim comprehensive authority over public asylums or mental illness. In 1898 Franklin B. Sanborn, the secretary of Massachusetts's Board of State Commissioners of Public Charities, affirmed that new reality as he reflected that past crusaders like Dix "lacked 'the special knowledge and discrimination required' to lead modern reforms." Scientific expertise and adeptness in public administration trumped Christian charity as public leaders rejected the "religious principles of moral treatment" inside and outside of institutional walls.[88]

Notwithstanding psychiatric professionalization, reforms at asylums were far from complete. Mental institutions in the years of Dix's campaigns offered the country's most dedicated medical care, but improvements and changes in medicine largely bypassed asylums. Just as reported cure rates for mental illnesses plummeted, other medical fields claimed success. Alienists remained specialists but were now detached from general medicine rather than being beacons of innovation. Without scientific advances in the care of mental illness, and because they continued to serve a socially and economically diverse population, a sense emerged that psychiatry and institutional care were "vestigial remnants of a pre-modern age" and leftovers of "an earlier social order."[89] Treating mentally ill patients not only became more onerous but also proved a less appealing profession.[90] Those realities—a dramatic reversal from the optimism that had fueled Dix's advocacy just a half century earlier—shaped the system that Boisen hoped to reform.

SHIFTING PROTESTANT ATTENTION

Changes in medicine and institutional care were the backdrop for a reconfiguration of Protestant attention to mental illness. Those at the helm of early nineteenth-century medical institutions had been motivated, at least in part, to pursue careers in medicine by their Protestant morality, but little evidence exists that Protestants in the antebellum or postbellum eras considered advocacy for the mentally ill of prime ecclesial importance. The rise of modern medicine and the authoritative administration of asylums by superintendents meant clergy ceded control of particular forms of suffering. To be sure, Christian belief influenced social action, but not all problems received equal attention. Clergy continued to attend to parishioners and call for care for sufferers, but by the middle of the nineteenth century, the majority of Protestants focused elsewhere. At a time when the nation's professionals were vying for authority, perhaps an attempt to hold onto—or regain—legitimate authority among other professions distracted clergy from attending to the mental distress of men and women as had earlier generations of ministers. Social stigma attached to mental illness may have also played a role. Caring for the nation's mentally ill seemed hopeless, and clergy may have been happy to let other professionals carry the load while they attended to other matters.

Following the revivals of the Second Great Awakening, American Christianity saw unprecedented diversification and growth. Believers focused on launching new congregations and denominations. Social causes including temperance, literacy, prison reform, the equality of women, and the abolition of slavery won attention too.[91] After the Civil War, some Protestants—like Boisen—embraced the ideas and approaches of German theological liberalism. Those attracted to the high anthropology and optimism of the movement assumed their efforts to prompt social improvement would help usher in the reign of God on earth.[92]

Religious changes took place among larger societal transformations. With a massive late-century spike in immigration, labor unrest, economic panics, and fears of degeneracy and widespread illness caused unease. Nonetheless, hopefulness persisted. Citizens assumed that solving the nation's problems was possible with hard work and the right scientific discoveries, and this outlook was central to an emerging sense of what it meant to be an American.[93] Enthusiastic and capable Americans hoped to solve the problems of a changing society, but progress seemed to pass some by. Mentally disturbed patients in the care of the state hardly fit the American ideal— they were "not quite right." In addition, the deterioration of institutional care meant that citizens viewed facilities—and sufferers within them—as outside of "normal" American society. Social stigma plagued both asylums and patients, and geographical separation exacerbated the taint of mental illness. Asylums were located on the outskirts of increasingly urban American life. Patients received treatment away from their families in rurally situated, fortress-like institutions, which fed a sense of uneasiness about those inside.[94]

All told, despite the work of many, care for the mentally ill proved no further along at the end of the nineteenth century than one hundred years earlier. The afflicted still suffered; facilities were inadequate; cures were far from guaranteed; professional debate raged. Many worked with good intentions, but the results remained dismal. Decades of deterioration in asylum life, changes in general medicine, shifts in psychiatric care, and deepened social stigma all shaped Boisen's experience in the "little known world" of mental illness and prompted his critiques of the institutional care he received.

SICKNESS OF THE SOUL

Boisen reflected on his own hospitalization in his 1936 *The Exploration of the Inner World: A Study of Mental Disorder and Religious Experience.* "To be plunged as a patient into a hospital for the insane," he observed, "may be a tragedy or it may be an opportunity. For me it has been an opportunity." What he named as his "brief but extremely severe period of mental illness" allowed him to witness the widest range of human existence, from "the bottommost depths of the nether regions to the heights of religious experience at its best."[95] The sympathetic pastor's immersion in an institution shaped by Dorothea Dix's legacy, but marred by a half century of unhappy change, provided a ready field of study that prompted him to pair theological insights and social scientific methods to bring healing, for both himself and others.[96]

Boisen's first hospitalization came as he struggled to rewrite a "Statement of Faith" for the New York Presbytery in hope of a pastoral placement.[97] His quest for a ministry position stemmed from a continued desire to earn the love and attention of Alice Batchelder. While writing the statement, he found himself obsessed with "a coming world catastrophe." His visions of destruction and evil frightened his friends and family, who eventually took action.[98] On October 9, 1920, six police officers "came marching into the room" where Boisen worked. After announcing that he "had better come quietly or there would be trouble," they whisked him away to Boston Psychopathic Hospital.[99]

During that first hospitalization, Boisen's severe psychosis included violent delirium, hallucinations, and delusions.[100] One vision held lasting significance. In what seemed to be a "prophetic delusion," Boisen was convinced that he had "broken an opening in the wall which separated medicine and religion."[101] He found the separation of the two realms over the prior century problematic, and the vision focused Boisen's attention, not only during time in the hospital but also for the rest of his life. The minister later reflected,

"The cure has lain in the faithful carrying through of the delusion itself."[102]
As Boisen delved into the meaning of his experience, he became convinced
that healing—for himself and others—required a new understanding of the
relationship between medicine and religion. He felt a divine call to make that
insight a productive reality.

Four months after his initial committal, Boisen transferred to Westboro
State Hospital. While often lucid, he occasionally relapsed into psychosis.
When his acute symptoms abated, Boisen drew on his knowledge of social
scientific methods and explored the institution's character, procedures, and
patients. As a result of his study, the minister concluded that most of the
other men were hospitalized with "spiritual or religious difficulties" rather
than organic illnesses. He also observed that purely physical treatment methods failed to address their problems.

As he worked, Boisen described his understanding of mental illness, in
part to understand his own distress. He defined two "main classes" of mental
illness, organic and functional. As he surveyed fellow patients and thought
about his own illness, he noted,

> In the one case there is some organic trouble, a defect in the brain tissue, some
> disorder in the nervous system, some disease of the blood. In the other there is no
> organic difficulty. The body is strong and the brain in good working order. The
> difficulty is rather in the disorganization of the patient's world.

The clergyman assumed his illness was of the functional variety. Such a malady, he argued, resulted when

> something has happened which has upset the foundations upon which his ordi-
> nary reasoning is based. Death or disappointment or sense of failure may have
> compelled a reconstruction of the patient's world view from the bottom up, and
> the mind becomes dominated by the one idea which he has been trying to put in
> its proper place.[103]

In a 1926 article for *Christian Work*, Boisen relayed that two-thirds of
the cases at Worcester Hospital lacked explainable physical origins and that
diminished intelligence or reason did not explain illness.[104] Rather than a medical problem, many functional mental illnesses, as Boisen understood them,
reflected acute spiritual trouble in need of religious ministrations. Unlike late
nineteenth- and early twentieth-century physicians that routinely presumed
physical causes, even if they could not identify them, Boisen pursued a different explanation. He believed that functional mental illness appeared when
conflict arose from an individual's personality seeking a reintegration about

one's purpose in life.[105] As a result, he contended functional mental illnesses were

> disorders of emotion and volition, of belief and attitude, rooted not in cerebral disease nor in the breaking down of the reasoning process but for the most part in the age-old conflict which the Apostle Paul so vividly describes, the conflict between the law that is in our minds and that which is in our members.[106]

The observant clergyman diagnosed such inner spiritual conflict as precipitating his first hospitalization.

In the coming decades, infrequent but debilitating breakdowns characterized Boisen's illness. At times, he suffered with symptoms of depression ("It was a beautiful day, but there was no sunshine for me, and no beauty—nothing but black despair") and manic episodes ("I was tremendously excited. In some way, I could not tell how, I felt myself joined onto some superhuman course of strength"). When sick, he continued to experience grandiose and religious delusions. He envisioned, for example, finding "most sacred relics" wrapped in "white linen" that were "connected with the search for the Holy Grail" and heard beautiful voices that he professed were "the celebration of the Last Supper."[107] Those experiences strengthened the minister's resolve that some mental illness called for religious, not medical, ministration.

Mental breakdowns caused by functional mental illness, the clergyman believed, could serve a creative, healing role. They were efforts "at a new synthesis of life"—attempts "to become reconciled with the 'Man Above' in order thereby to become reconciled with one's fellows."[108] Though "some forms of mental illness serve a curative, problem-solving function for the individual," Boisen observed that not all conflict resolved "happily."[109] Some sufferers remained in a state of psychosis. Yet, attention to symptoms seemed to provide the possibility of cures. Boisen lived at a time when the spheres of medicine and religion were divided firmly. Boisen, like Cotton Mather two centuries earlier, blended his knowledge of the two realms to explain illness. Combining religious and medical terminology, he compared successfully resolved mental illnesses to conversion experiences: "Such conflicts, when they result happily, as in the case of Augustine, George Fox and John Bunyan, we recognize as religious experience. When they result unhappily, we send the sufferer to a hospital for the mentally ill and speak of him as insane."[110] Some types of mental illness, Boisen argued, appeared to be "essentially a desperate struggle for salvation, a manifestation of nature's power to heal which is analogous to fever or inflammation in the body."[111] For some sufferers, traditional religious conversion—" 'hit[ting] the sawdust trail' at the meetings of evangelists like Billy Sunday"—brought resolution, but others suffered in a way that required a different sort of conversion.

Any illness caused by spiritual distress, Boisen surmised, appeared curable. In a letter to his mother during his first hospitalization, Boisen shared, "In many of its forms, insanity, as I see it, is a religious rather than a medical problem, and any treatment which fails to recognize that fact can hardly be effective."[112] "It came over me like a flash," he recalled, "that if inner conflicts like that which [the apostle] Paul describes in the famous passage in the seventh chapter of Romans can have happy solutions, as the church has always believed, there must also be unhappy solutions which thus far the church has ignored." While some, like himself, managed to steer through those difficulties after their "inner world(s) had come crashing down," others remained ill. He understood his own ailment as "at once mental disorder of the most profound and unmistakable variety and also . . . of unquestionable religious value."[113] Religion, the minister concluded, could help bring healing even in the worst cases of functional mental illness, ones formerly considered incurable.

With newfound insight, it frustrated Boisen that his physicians possessed "neither understanding nor interest in the religious aspects" of experiences like his.[114] Claiming not only personal experience but also clerical authority and medical knowledge, Boisen saw a clear distinction between functional religious distress and organic mental disease. He noted, though, that psychiatrists often failed to "recognize with sufficient clearness the sharp contrast between them."[115] When psychotic visions seemed specifically religious, like many that he observed (and experienced), Boisen sought to discern the presence of God and not to presume delusion. Such experiences, he argued, were "*mystical* experiences in so far as they give the sense of identification with the larger fellowship presented by the idea of God."[116] Reflecting on the ability of some psychotic hallucinations to heal, he noted, "Perhaps, we . . . need to learn . . . that all auditory hallucinations do not necessarily come from the devil but may represent the operations of the creative mind."[117] With that assertion, the patient/pastor reframed mental distress as a divine invitation in need of exploration and not a demonic fetter requiring exorcism.[118] Boisen encouraged reconsideration of mental maladies and pondered how to draw clergy attention to an area where he felt they held rightful expertise.[119]

As Boisen continued to develop his thinking about mental illness and its significance in the religious life, he corresponded with Rev. Elwood Worcester, an Episcopal clergyman and professor of psychology and philosophy.[120] His second letter to Worcester included hope "for the day when cases of mental trouble which are not primarily organic in origin will be recognized and treated as spiritual problems, and that the church will develop physicians of soul of a type whose work will be based upon sound and systematic study of spiritual pathology."[121] After recovering, Boisen's first task was to prepare himself for such a position.

Boisen's hope to shift clerical perceptions prompted further formal study. Prior coursework had planted seeds of interest in suffering and religion long before his first hospitalization. After enrolling in Union Theological Seminary in 1908, he studied the psychology of religion, finding an affinity with the work of the psychologist and philosopher William James. With James, Boisen "believed that sickness of soul might have religious significance" and "proposed to employ the methods of science in attacking the problems involved." At Union, Boisen continued his exploration of the psychology of religion with George Albert Coe, from whom he learned the importance of the "living 'human document'" as an object of theological study.[122] In 1922, while an outpatient at Westboro State Hospital, and with the approval of his mother and physician, Boisen enrolled at Episcopal Theological School in Cambridge. He also took courses at Andover Theological School and Harvard. In addition to theological topics, Boisen explored social ethics and abnormal psychology. He used those new tools to prepare case studies, almost forty of them, from his observations of fellow patients. Documenting the human condition amidst suffering served as a first step in Boisen's theological assessment of mental distress. Additional study prepared him to share his revelations with religious and medical professionals. Both groups, he argued, needed his insight.

A CALL FOR PHYSICIANS OF THE SOUL

Having survived illness and undertaken further study, Boisen embraced the challenge of convincing fellow clergymen to adopt his newfound insights. With his conviction that mental illness was partly a religious problem came the realization that Protestant contemporaries failed to understand or attend to mental distress. Boisen observed, "As yet the church has given little attention to this problem."[123] He sought to fix the oversight and hoped leaders and churches would come to see things differently.[124] As a patient at Westboro, Boisen had attended weekly religious services. Initially hopeful that the local clergy leading those worship services might become conversation partners, he discovered that while they "might know something about religion . . . they certainly knew nothing about" mental maladies. Recalling a minister from the neighboring village who preached on the text "If thine eye offend thee, pluck it out," he feared that "one or two of my fellow patients might be inclined to take that injunction literally."[125] In Boisen's view, although willing to lead formal worship services, clergymen failed to understand both the suffering experienced by patients and the role they could play in healing (or deepening distress). Studying the religious symbolism in his delusions helped Boisen heal, and the determined minister hoped to share that insight. As he touted the healing role that believers could play by addressing spiritual distress, he admonished fellow clergymen for failing to apply such care.

The church, Boisen alleged, bypassed mental maladies despite its attention to other suffering. "It seems not inaccurate to say," he argued, "that if a man has a broken leg he can be cared for by the church in a church institution. But if he has a broken heart he is turned over to the state, there to be forgotten by the church."[126] Protestants, the former patient asserted, cared for the sick in church-affiliated general hospitals but took "no interest in cases of pronounced mental disorder." Of 381 religious hospitals in the United States, Boisen identified only three that focused on mental maladies. As a result, the care of the mentally ill—many of whom Boisen understood to suffer from spiritual, not physical, problems—was "left practically without Protestant religious ministration." Boisen rued, "The one chief piece of machinery that the Protestant Church has worked out for dealing with the man who is sick of soul, is the 'revival meeting,' and it is an open question whether this method in practice does not do almost as much harm as good."[127] Boisen found it "truly remarkable" that "a church which has always been interested in the care of the sick" confined "her efforts to the types of cases in which religion has least concern and least to contribute, while in those types in which it is impossible to tell where the domain of the medical workers leaves off and that of the religious worker begins, there the Church is doing nothing."[128] Having identified the problem, Boisen diagnosed its origins.

The church's failure to respond—he argued, drawing from his most recent graduate studies—stemmed from an inadequate understanding of the human condition. The minister observed that clergy "have made little attempt to study the human personality either in health or in sickness" even though "the human personality [was that] with which it was . . . [the pastor's] task to work." Ministers, he held, must undertake that work in order "to bring to bear . . . the forces of healing and of power which lie in Christian Religion."[129] Alongside that assertion, the minister scolded fellow clergy for abdicating their authority for the care of souls to physicians. "The physician," he declared, "as a result of his empirical method and his careful, systematic study of living men and women, has thus in very truth become a physician of souls, while the traditional 'physician of souls,' clinging to his traditional methods, has become merely the custodian of the faith."[130] Boisen bitterly lamented the loss.

Despite "waning [clerical] influence," Boisen listed items of "fundamental importance" that ministers could bring to the treatment of mental illness. Religion, as mediated by clergy, provided a sense of the "ultimate realities of life," which offered comfort, hope, and strength to the afflicted. Because he understood that functional mental illness resulted from being "out of adjustment" with one's perceived purpose in life, the minister named advantages from prayer and the inclusion in a Christian community a "wholesome environment" for those in distress. Given those benefits, Boisen also cited a preventative role for religious workers—their participation might help sufferers work through problems before they became severe enough to require hospitalization.[131] Reflective observation served as a first step. Using social scientific methods of participant observation, Boisen felt sure that clergy could gain insight into human nature and suffering that would enable them to bring healing that medical professionals could not.[132]

Writing near the height of the early twentieth-century Fundamentalist-Modernist controversy that divided American Protestants, Boisen spared neither Fundamentalist nor liberal Protestants in lambasting the church's failed attention. On one hand, conservatives, with their focus on saving souls, undoubtedly brought comfort to many through a hope in a "new purpose in life" and a fellowship with other believers. But ultimately, the conservative evangelical Protestant response to mental illness was simply "treatment without diagnosis," for fundamentalism "has no clear idea of what salvation means nor of what people need to be saved from." And, Boisen feared, "its hell is a future affair and it has been blind to the hell which was right before its eyes." Liberals, on the other hand, "supply neither treatment nor diagnosis. . . . For the soul that is sick they have no gospel of salvation." Distracted by their focus on religious education and social reform, liberals were "all too ready to turn" the mental patient "over to the doctors and then forget about him."[133] Boisen hoped to inspire changes in practice for Christians of all stripes.

Liberal or conservative, Boisen faulted seminaries for allowing clerical abdication of authority to medical professionals. After studying the course catalogues of theological schools, he discovered that most focused on the traditional disciplines of Scripture, church history, systematic theology, philosophy of religion, and preaching, with very little focus on "the human personality either in health or in sickness, or the social forces that affect it."[134] Simply supplementing instruction would prove insufficient. Instead, he argued that future clergy needed education beyond the seminary classroom, training that deepened their attention to human experience. Few current pastors, he observed, possessed the skills for such work, but supplementing classroom instruction with clinical experience in mental hospitals could enrich that basic preparation. The clergyman hoped, "through the empirical approach, to call attention back to the central problem of theology and the central task of the church—the problem of sin and salvation." "What is new," he reminded his fellow clergymen, "is the attempt to begin with the study" of human experience.[135] Boisen's direct encounter with illness revolutionized his understanding. Facing it, even secondhand, would offer needed wisdom to seminary students.

The "person in difficulty," Boisen argued, served as the proper focus of theological training and practice. Mental hospitals, full of such individuals, proved a perfect location for a new form of education. Encountering complex human experience and suffering firsthand would help unleash what Boisen understood as "the potential power of the church to contribute to the solution of this problem."[136] If theological students witnessed "struggles in their dramatic vehemence, in their nakedness of panic and despair" at mental hospitals, then they "might be more sensitive to the little hints and small signs by which" their parishioners indicated a "need for help and salvation."[137] Clear about the problem, Boisen was optimistic about a solution.

In 1924 the recent mental patient persuaded William A. Bryan, the superintendent of Worcester State Hospital, to hire him as a full-time chaplain.[138] Bryan's interest was therapeutic, not religious. The physician, Boisen reported, was not a "churchman," yet he allowed that spiritual care might help patients recover. Though Bryan received "a good deal of chaffing from his fellow superintendents" for permitting a full-time chaplain, he countered, saying "that he would be perfectly willing to bring in a horse doctor if he thought there was any chance of his being able to help the patients."[139] And so, Boisen gained entry to the asylum, but this time as a professional instead of as a patient.

Hospitals sometimes employed clergy to lead worship services, but Boisen's role proved novel.[140] He offered religious services but also worked directly with patients "in which the religious problem . . . [was] an outstanding feature."[141] Serving as a chaplain offered both "a contribution toward the solution of the problem of insanity and the service of the class of unfortunates," like himself, that suffered from mental maladies.[142] His goal remained making changes—not just in institutions, but beyond. Continuing the study he started while a patient, Boisen focused on " 'charting and exploring the little-known country in which [patients] wander,' and with gaining 'some degree of mastery in the difficult art of helping the mind distressed,' for 'then and only then may we speak with authority in regard to the laws of spiritual life which affect us all.' "[143] The former patient saw spiritual distress as a universal condition.

Boisen sought change in more than just religious administration and staked a claim for the role of clergy as part of the overall caring process. He asserted, "Only as mental disorder and religious experience are studied the one in the light of the other will it be possible to understand and to deal intelligently with either."[144] Clerical cooperation with medical professionals was essential, with each professional deploying different expertise: "The functional group of mental disorders are of peculiar interest to the religious worker; those with religious authority should attend to such inner conflict in hopes of 'happy' resolutions." But, he also professed that, at times, "the provinces of religious and medical workers overlap." Attending to spiritual care was the only way to assure full healing. In addition, observation of the human condition by the theologically trained deepened the understanding of the human condition, providing a benefit to medical personnel. Admitting that clergy had ceded care for sickness of the soul to medicine, Boisen acknowledged that the religious worker functioned as a "mere beginner." But, the enthusiastic clergyman proclaimed, they needed to step forward and claim the authority that was rightly theirs.[145]

Boisen's passion extended beyond assessment of the religious significance of suffering, the training of seminarians, and how religion and medicine should influence each other. He also remained attentive to practices of the life of faith, including how suffering and worship intersected. Aware of the possible "therapeutic significance" of Christian worship, his work included the compilation of *Hymns of Hope and Courage*, first published in 1937. He developed the hymnal for use in worship services at mental hospitals. Boisen hoped it would anchor individuals in their faith, helping them find healing in Christianity. Selecting hymns, he carefully avoided topics and tropes that might have proven harmful to the therapeutic purpose of worship. Reminders of the love and forgiveness of God, courage and action, and consciousness of sin alongside aspiration for a better life helped the sufferer. But, allusions to enemies, hearing voices, magic, and things that might intensify helplessness, isolation, and fear Boisen avoided.[146] Religious practice contributed to healing, but only when attentive to the realities of mental distress.

The driven pastor sought a holistic medical and religious approach to asylum care, and, once established in his work at Worcester State Hospital, Boisen trained others. In 1925 the clergyman recruited four seminary students for a program of clinical training. Participants worked ten-hour shifts, serving most of their time as attendants on the hospital's wards. They also ran recreational programs, observed patients' experiences, and attended regular medical staff meetings. The students gained direct experience observing the relationship between religion and mental illness.[147] Five years later, thirty-five students had served as interns at Worcester. Most entered parishes after graduation, which pleased Boisen. While he extolled the virtues of the mental hospital as a place of learning, the patient-turned-teacher remained convinced that the lessons learned there proved useful in congregational ministry. He felt that a "clinical year" for clergy was equally important as the time physicians spent training in general hospitals before beginning private practice.[148] Only with adequate training—including deep study of human suffering—could clergy serve effectively in congregations.

Boisen also hoped increased contact between seminarians and patients could help curb social stigma affixed to mental illness. He recalled that during his first hospitalization some of his friends thought "it was [his] duty to remain in the hospital as a patient for the rest of [his] life. Others assumed that something in the nature of simple manual work was all that would now be open to [him]."[149] Hopeful and dedicated, the fellow minister proved them wrong.

Despite, or perhaps because of, his experience with mental illness, Boisen never stopped reflecting on the religious meaning and the social context of human suffering. The optimistic clergyman hoped that Christians, especially ministers, would learn to read experience with the "same reverence, respect, and depth, with which they read biblical texts." That "empirical theology" marked his teaching and writing, and it shaped a generation of theologians and caregivers.[150] Boisen's efforts bore fruit when he and his first students expanded clinical pastoral training. By January 1930 the Council for the Clinical Training of Theological Students had formally organized and developed standards for Clinical Pastoral Education.

LEGACY

Boisen's experiences as a clergyman and as a patient shaped his pastoral agenda. Not until his 1960 autobiography, though, did Boisen share the depth of his suffering. He offered his "own case record" as an account "of valid religious experience which was at the same time madness of the most profound and unmistakable variety."[151] The reflective servant of Christ discovered his vocation in suffering. He confessed that "the purgatorial fires of a horrifying psychosis" had allowed him to "set foot in his promised land of creativity" and thereby help others.[152] He resisted thinking of his illness either as incurable or as a sign of moral deficiency. Instead, "he spent a lifetime arguing the opposite," using both theological insight and scientific methods.[153] The minister's work convinced religious leaders of his era to reclaim mental illness as part of the church's purview and to adopt the view that, in cooperation with medical professionals, spiritual and medical care of mental disease could improve.

That Boisen claimed professional insight from his illness, however, proved problematic for some. A three-week psychotic break in 1930 persuaded some of his Council for the Clinical Training of Theological Students colleagues of his "unfitness to be involved in the Council's training programs." Despite a loss of confidence from peers, in the next few years, his productivity continued with the publication of nine articles, a revision of his hymnal for mental patients, and a book analyzing 173 case studies. In 1932 he moved to Illinois to serve as the chaplain of Elgin State Hospital and to be nearer to Chicago Theological Seminary and Alice Batchelder.[154] In 1938 Boisen left his chaplain duties at Elgin to teach and write full-time about religion and mental illness. He returned as chaplain at Elgin for three three-year stints between 1942 and 1955.[155] During that time, he consulted with clinical training centers around the country and continued to teach.

After a 1935 psychotic break, Boisen was never again hospitalized, but his most significant and enduring influence stemmed from insight gained during his hospitalization and recovery in a system that failed to provide for his needs. He spent decades working to change the provision of care. Like Dorothea Dix, Boisen's final resting place was beside the patients he cared for most deeply. In 1965 friends buried Boisen at Elgin State Hospital's cemetery after an "unremarkable state hospital funeral."[156] Decades later, Robert C. Powell—a professor of history and medicine, and a former student who helped found the Association of Mental Health Clergy—offered an overview of Boisen's life and work at the group's meeting. Powell hoped his account would remind a later generation of clergy attending to mental maladies of Boisen's influence as their "founding father." The former student called for his fellow mental health workers to take Boisen "completely seriously, and holistically, delusions and all."[157] Suffering, as Boisen had hoped, brought productive insight.

Boisen never wavered from the belief that treatment for mental distress must change. Ministers benefitted from the additional training he pioneered, but, as Boisen feared, pastoral use of psychological methods became the focus instead of more thorough theological reflection. Eventually, clinical pastoral training expanded beyond mental hospitals to general medical centers. Some saw that as a productive widening; others knew it shifted the focus from the problems of mental illness. Perhaps social stigma affixed to mental maladies made general hospitals more palatable locations for ministerial training than asylums.[158] As the twentieth century progressed, the mental hygiene movement and world wars brought some attention to mental maladies. For most Protestants, though, persistent stigma made it all too easy to aim attention elsewhere, realities that Boisen would have lamented. Only a few twentieth-century Protestants continued Boisen's focused advocacy.

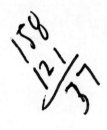

5

A Passionate Plea to Engage Finds Lukewarm Reaction

Karl Menninger

> It is doubtless true that religion has been the world's
> psychiatrist throughout the centuries.

—Karl Menninger, 1938[1]

> The basis of all religion is the duty to love God and offer our help to
> His children—and psychiatry, too, is dedicated to the latter duty.

—Karl Menninger, 1964[2]

INTRODUCTION

For the sake of those suffering with mental illnesses, Rev. Anton Boisen sought cooperation between Christianity and medicine, and many took up the charge. After 1930 Dr. Karl Menninger (1893–1990), the most revered American psychiatrist of the twentieth century, led the way. A life-long Presbyterian, the Kansas physician's advocacy spanned seven decades and, in many ways, exemplified the mainstream Protestant approach to mental illness in the twentieth century.[3] For the betterment of the world, Menninger drew together scientific knowledge, deep compassion, a Calvinist sense of vocation, and a dose of Christian realism. Tireless, he offered an active Christian witness in the face of mental distress. Few twentieth-century Protestants, though, achieved Menninger's level of involvement, even if they aspired to.

"Dr. Karl" was as comfortable talking to the readers of *Ladies Home Journal* and the *Saturday Evening Post* as to members of the American Psychiatric Association, and his commitment to help others took him around the globe

as he treated patients, debated colleagues, trained professionals, and campaigned for his version of holistic psychiatric care. As a physician, Menninger
attended to the suffering of the afflicted, and as a well-respected one, he was
able to influence colleagues and the public as he raised awareness about the
nature of mental disease and the need for proper treatment. In doing so, he
saw little need to keep medicine and Christianity at a distance. "The basis
of all religion," he argued, "is the duty to love God and offer our help to
His children—and psychiatry, too, is dedicated to the latter duty."[4] For Menninger, psychiatry and religion formed part of the same whole, responding
faithfully in the face of suffering.

Menninger's résumé brimmed with accomplishments. In 1941 he served
as president of the American Psychoanalytic Foundation. As a scientific con-
sultant during World War II, he toured the European theater of operations
to assess the need for psychiatric care among soldiers. A decade later, the
trainer of physicians copublished a textbook, *A Manual for Psychiatric Case
Study*. In 1965 the American Psychiatric Association awarded the doctor its
Distinguished Service Award. The same year, he founded the Villages, Inc.,
a nonprofit organization that provided homes for children declared wards of
the state, hoping to prevent their fall into delinquency. In 1979, along with
his father and youngest brother, he was pictured in the Wilson Memorial
Healing Arts Window of the Washington National Cathedral in Washington, D.C.[5] Two years later, President Jimmy Carter granted Menninger the
Medal of Freedom, the nation's highest civilian honor. Along the way, the
devoted physician published more than ten books and dozens of articles and
gave countless lectures that delivered his opinions to psychiatrists, psychologists, social workers, clergy, and homemakers.[6]

Menninger earned a living in medicine, but a sense of Christian vocation animated his endeavors. As a result, some heralded him as a "classical
Protestant moralist." Well into his old age, he decried mistreatment of children, prisoners, Native Americans, and the environment.[7] Menninger—like
Mather, Rush, Dix, and Boisen before him—was a pious Christian, sensing
God's call to attend to suffering and injustice. Though he never hid his religious identity, Menninger's primary claim to public authority came from his
training and practice as a medical man, not his faith. Regardless, Menninger
used the national stage to advocate for the well-being of others, and of central
interest to him was the welfare of those afflicted with diseases of the mind.

Other twentieth-century Christians held similar concerns. In the decades
after World War II, many imagined roles for themselves in caring for mental

illnesses. As they investigated ways to help, Protestants readily accepted scientific solutions for mental distress. While psychiatry had suffered a lull in confidence around the turn of the twentieth century—both from the public and from its medical peers—the specialty reclaimed its respected position during the world wars. With renewed approval, and with figures like Menninger at the helm (figures that combined scientific expertise with Christian morality), willingness to let medical practitioners lead the way in attending to sick minds seemed logical.

Although mainline Protestants ascribed nearly unqualified authority in matters of mental health to medical professionals, they hoped to cooperate with physicians to bring healing. Clergy sought advice from medical officials and added psychological insights to their ministerial toolkits. Laity advocated for quality institutional care and helped launch new hospitals. Yet, by the 1960s, when individual believers sought help with severe—or even minor—mental distress, they found themselves more comfortable in medical offices than in clergy studies.

Many social issues occupied twentieth-century Protestants. For a short time, mental illness appeared a top concern. In the decade after World War II, support for mental health initiatives—more so than any other public health concern—filled the pages of the *Christian Century*, the publication that best reflected the mainline Protestant ethos. By 1970, though, despite the past hopes of Mather, Rush, Dix, and Boisen, and notwithstanding Karl Menninger's best efforts, other pressing public needs occupied clergy and laity. Perhaps, the authority of medical science was too entrenched, and the social stigma that affixed to mental illness too powerful, to sustain engagement. By the century's final decades, Protestants were undertaking other causes. And, when they did consider mental illness, they relegated themselves to caring from the sidelines.

The forces that shaped care for mental maladies in the nation evolved dramatically in the twentieth century. Alongside attempts at professional cooperation came new wartime insights about mental distress, the popularization of psychoanalytic theory, national legislation of mental health provision, massive mid-century deinstitutionalization of mental hospitals, and the development of grassroots advocacy groups in support of sufferers. The voice of Karl Menninger proved audible throughout those changes and amidst the evolution of twentieth-century Protestant engagement. His story proves central in the cooperative and optimistic, but ultimately detached, Christian response to mental illness from World War II through 1980.

A FAITHFUL SON OF TOPEKA EARNS
NATIONAL ATTENTION

Medicine and faith shaped the life of Karl Augustus Menninger, the first of three sons born to Charles Frederick and Flo Menninger. Five years before Karl's birth, his parents moved to Topeka, Kansas, where Charles established a medical practice. The eastern Kansas town was home for generations of their descendants. Church involvement was central for the Menningers, and the family matriarch molded their devotion. Reared by Prohibitionist Mennonites, Flo Menninger found her way to the Presbyterian Church after teaching Bible classes there. In 1891 she convinced her husband to depart from his German Evangelical and Catholic roots and join Topeka's First Presbyterian Church. For decades thereafter, the family was deeply involved in the church's educational programs, worship life, and ministries.[8]

Christian discipleship in the Menninger home proved a combination of study, devotion, and action. From his mother, who patterned a life of Christian reflection and service, Karl gained a "commitment to missionary benevolence" and a sense that the Bible should be understandable and practical in daily life.[9] Flo led the family's "tradition of social service." As part of her sons' religious inculcation, for example, she taught them to sing the Fanny Crosby hymn "Rescue the Perishing" and put her convictions into practice as she welcomed long-term boarders into the family's home.[10] In many ways, Flo's approach to faith prefigured Karl's future.

The Menninger's oldest son did not set out to become a psychiatrist, but the wishes of both parents eventually influenced that decision. As a young adult, Karl entertained religious vocations. Exploring a clerical future, and to defray the costs of his undergraduate studies, Menninger preached at Sunday church services in nearby rural towns while enrolled at the University of Wisconsin. The pious college student also participated in the Student Volunteer Movement for Foreign Missions. In 1914 he attended the organization's national convention, where he pledged to put his talents to missionary use.[11] Given his college activities and his mother's influence, ministerial or missionary work called. Yet despite her evangelistic impulses, Flo found ministry "insufficiently practical" and hoped her son would pursue a career in business. Karl's father had other dreams. Longing for company to quell the loneliness of serving as a sole medical provider, and with the Mayo family's Minnesota clinic as his inspiration, Charles pictured launching a family medical practice.

Karl's eventual occupational pursuit pleased both parents. A career in medicine appeared an acceptable alternative to ministry for his mother and an answer to prayer for his father. While it was a secular career, faith played a role in the choice. Karl's sense that "the central purpose of each life should be to dilute the misery in the world" shaped even his more "practical" vocational path.[12] As much as an occupation or job, medicine formed a vocation—a Christian mission and a "solemn responsibility"—for the oldest Menninger son.[13]

While medicine led to Menninger's renown, Protestantism remained an influence. Menninger and his youngest brother were lifelong members of the same Kansas congregation discovered by their parents before the turn of the twentieth century. As adults, Karl served on the church's session, and Will led the congregation's Boy Scout troop to national recognition.[14] For many years, the elder brother taught a weekly Sunday morning class at the family's hospital to adult patients that professed interest in theology, philosophy, ethics, and biblical study. And, although nurtured in Topeka, Karl's Christian service extended beyond the walls of his hometown—he lectured at seminaries and spoke at churches around the country. Protestant faith and practice served as an anchor throughout the doctor's life.

Menninger gladly identified with his "fellow Presbyterians" and was happy to talk about his religious beliefs. He professed belief in God and prayer, yet, in public statements, lived-faith seemed of higher importance to him than particulars of Christian doctrine. The emphasis on practice over belief placed Karl firmly within the Protestant mainline, a fit recognized by some of his medical colleagues. Writing in the *Journal of Presbyterian History* in 1981, for example, a Menninger Foundation professor, Dr. Paul Pruyser, painted Menninger as a devout, intellectually curious believer. To locate him in the American theological landscape, Pruyser listed the doctor's long-held periodical subscriptions to *Christian Century, Theology Today, Commonweal,* and *Biblical Archeologist.*[15]

The fact that Christian convictions shaped the psychiatrist's medical work was no secret. Pruyser—not only Menninger's medical colleague but also a fellow Presbyterian—noted that Presbyterian faith shaped Menninger's life in a number of ways. Menninger, Pruyser observed, was "both theologically and psychologically first of all a realist who [knew] . . . that man has an uncanny proclivity toward an unduly flattering self-perception, and worse: toward vice, crime, violence, hatred, vengeance."[16] Dr. Karl refused to shy away from the presence of evil in the world. As a Calvinist, he revered the Old Testament for its thundering laments, lyricism, prophetic voice, and especially its "realistic portrayal of evil." Pruyser speculated that Menninger's Calvinist assessment of sin and evil "almost certainly aided him in embracing with great vigor" Austrian neurologist Sigmund Freud's controversial thesis that "a death instinct must be postulated to account for otherwise puzzling phenomena of self-destructiveness."[17] Later in his career, Menninger's religiously rooted realism spurred him to write his 1973 lament, *Whatever Became of Sin?*, where he decried the disappearance of sin as a category deployed in religious and public life.

Alongside a recognition of evil, love animated Menninger's thinking. The doctor was a realist, but, as Pruyser observed, "his Calvinism, insofar as it derives from the Pauline writings (especially 1 Corinthians 13)," prepared Menninger "for seeing love not only as a desirable condition, but as a forceful cosmic reality."[18] Dr. Karl held that love should dictate the shape of human relationships, including the relationship between physicians and mental patients. He saw the tension between love and hate as what "made human life so ambiguous, so turbulent, so contradictory."[19] Belief in the power of love allowed the doctor to remain full of hope despite his ready acknowledgment of sin, evil, and suffering in the world.

Alongside Menninger's sense of the power of evil and the role of love, his colleague observed that the "two Calvinist motifs" of vocation and curiosity shaped the physician's "obligation-imbued lifestyle." While Pruyser relayed no knowledge of the doctor's specific views on the doctrine of election, he observed in the whole Menninger family "a sense of being elected, if not to God's grace then to the shouldering of duties." Karl, his parents, and his brother Will "acted as if they were called, not only to perform meliorative work, but to do so with initiative and zest, even with a degree of pleasure in overcoming obstacles." Their sense of energy-infused divine vocation came with the compulsion to produce change in people's attitudes, a mission Pruyser equated with "the smashing of idols." Menninger's intellectual ability and knack for framing situations innovatively aided that undertaking. For example, at times when the culture around him looked with "fear, hopelessness and . . . pity at the seriousness" and irreparability of mental illness, the doctor called "attention to the healthiness of the patients' struggles" and asserted that health and illness existed on a spectrum and that all humans were ill to a degree.[20] Menninger's religious convictions shaped his understanding of the world and his role within it.

As a mainline believer, the Kansas physician presumed God was at work in the world, but he spoke mostly about the benefits of religious involvement rather than divine activity. For example, Menninger valued worship—for himself and others. Dispensing advice similar to that of Rev. Anton Boisen, the doctor noted that—for those living with mental maladies—religious ritual, hymn singing, and prayer held therapeutic value.[21] Thinking of patients and his colleagues, he asserted, "Going to church appeals to many psychiatrists as a prescription for patients, if not for themselves."[22] Using psychological language to profess the value of worship (which he referred to as "group assemblage and some kind of formal ritual"), the doctor commended the "mutual stimulation, reinforcement, and encouragement" present in congregational worship. He found "singing together" had "great and obvious a value in furthering interpersonal linkages and enthusiasm in a common purpose."[23] Menninger believed routine religious practice aided emotional health. Altogether, the call and practice of faith and the inspiration of Christian hope proved ever present in the Menninger family's life and in Dr. Karl's work.

Flo Menninger's Christian outreach inaugurated not only her oldest son's faith but also his medical specialty. Many of the individuals Flo welcomed into the family home were "mentally unbalanced," and Karl saw the effects of mental distress firsthand.[24] Later, formal study provided scientific tools for attending to the suffering he witnessed as a child. While Menninger was a student at Harvard Medical School, a lecture about Freud's ideas given by Louisville Emerson, a founding member of the Boston Psychoanalytic Society, deepened his interest in matters of the mind. A postgraduation internship at the Kansas City General Hospital cemented his vocational pursuit. Menninger felt drawn to patients with neurological ills, many of them "derelicts" brought to the hospital by police because they proved unable to survive without assistance. In 1918 he returned to the Atlantic Seaboard and put his interests and skills to use in the residency program in neuropsychiatry at Boston Psychopathic Hospital.[25]

The newly minted doctor's stay on the East Coast ended shortly thereafter, and in 1919 he returned to Topeka to enter medical practice with his father. A year later, Charles Menninger's dreams for a family medical practice came true when he and Karl formed the Menninger Diagnostic Clinic for the practice of general medicine and psychiatry. At first, the clinic treated a variety of ailments. A broad reach allowed both men to earn a living, but Karl continued to seek out cases of mental distress and travelled around Kansas to treat patients in need of neuropsychiatric care. Not all Topekans welcomed the junior Menninger's interests, and, in the first years after the clinic's launch, "alarmed citizens went to court to stop him from operating a 'maniac ward' at the local hospital." Undeterred, the eager young physician for a time smuggled in patients, often "disguising them under erroneous diagnoses."[26] Despite early reticence, decades later the clinic emerged as one of the largest employers in town and a source of local pride.

While settling in, in Topeka, Menninger continued to feel the tug of Christian missionary service. In 1921 he reflected, "I am not altogether relinquishing the hope that I may sometime develop neuropsychiatric work in

China."[27] Eventually, though, demands in Kansas and around the country satisfied his vocational goals. Six years after returning to his home state, he formalized efforts to care for mentally ill patients when the clinic opened a residential psychiatric hospital, the Menninger Sanitarium. Situated on a twenty-acre farm on Topeka's northwest side, the new facility admitted thirteen men and women suffering with "nervous and mental diseases" and provided optimistic and attentive psychiatric care, not merely the sort of sequestered institutionalization that had grown common throughout the country.[28] In 1925 the facility branched out to serve another population with the opening of the Southard School for emotionally disturbed children. The same year, Menninger's youngest brother, Will, joined the family practice.

The oldest Menninger son held that mentally ill Americans deserved good care. He found it "painful" and "paradoxical" that in America—a "rich, busy, idealistic, sympathetic, growing country"—the physically ill garnered more compassion than the mentally distressed, despite their "ofttimes greater suffering." "Let a man be taken to a hospital because he has a broken leg, crying out with pain when he tries to walk," Menninger observed, "and he will be surrounded by nurses, physicians, and technicians and within a few hours, his suffering eased and his leg so held that it can begin to mend." But, he reflected, "let a man's mind begin to wander or his memory to fail, his perceptions to become confused or his fears to overwhelm him, and he is likely to be conveyed in a dilatory fashion through the county jail . . . to the wards of what was once called the 'asylum.'" About the plight of the mentally ill, Menninger lamented, "Few know, few care, and fewer do anything about it."[29] That injustice motivated his efforts.

The doctor's passion for helping spurred further institutional growth. In 1933 the American Medical Association approved the Menninger Sanitarium as a provider of psychiatric residency training, and in the following decades, the Menningers launched educational initiatives for a wide range of professionals. From 1940 to 1951, their facility operated training programs in clinical psychology, social work, marital counseling, and pastoral care and counseling. In 1935 *Fortune* recognized the clinic as one of a small group of new, innovative facilities.[30] Along the way, the family physicians recruited other professionals to join their treatment team, and during the Nazi era, many Jewish European psychoanalysts who had fled their home countries settled in Topeka to work at the clinic.

Karl's publications contributed to the clinic's prominence. His first book, *The Human Mind* (1930), proved popular both among medical professionals and with the public. The text defined mental illness, discussed symptoms, considered causes, recommended treatments, and advocated for the broader usefulness of psychiatric theory for a "healthier-minded" humanity. In a review of the widely read volume's second edition, the University of Kansas professor of psychology J. F. Brown noted that with nearly two hundred thousand copies in circulation, it "must have been read by nearly all members of the [psychological] profession since its appearance" eight years earlier.[31] Broad scholarly readership was impressive for a text created out of class lectures on mental hygiene given to freshman at Topeka's Washburn College, but the book's accessible tone helped the Literary Guild selection became the best-selling mental health volume in American history.[32] Menninger continued to publish for decades, and, whether writing about psychiatry or social issues, his writing kept the doctor in the public eye.[33]

Faithfulness, not fame, however, continued to motivate the oldest Menninger son's work. Though he garnered international attention, attending well to suffering retained a larger purpose. When he toured East Coast psychopathic hospitals in the 1910s and 1920s, the care provided there impressed him. Steep fees, however, meant that the hospitals served only a small number of wealthy patients. Menninger hoped to offer top-notch care, but to a much wider population. And, by all accounts, he succeeded.[34] In 1935, despite the impact it had on profitability, he opened a free clinic for needy Topekans.[35] Six years later, father and sons formed the Menninger Foundation, giving their individual assets to the foundation in order "to be of greater service to the nation and the world."[36] In response to a sense of Christian vocation, Menninger and his family developed competencies that fostered worthy care for as many as possible.

The aftermath of war opened even more avenues for expansion. Following the Second World War, veterans sought psychiatric services, and the Menninger Foundation filled the need. In 1946, working with the federal Veterans Administration, Menninger established a psychiatric training program at a former army hospital in Kansas, and in the mid-twentieth century, "the Menninger School of Psychiatry became the largest training center in the world."[37] Three years later, one hundred of the eight hundred psychiatric residents in the United States had trained in Topeka.[38] What began as a spark of faith around the family dinner table grew into a wide-reaching medical organization that not only treated patients but also trained others to provide care.

MENTAL INSTITUTIONS AND TREATMENTS IN THE TWENTIETH CENTURY

Though a handful of private clinics for mental patients like the Menningers' Kansas hospital emerged in the first decades of the twentieth century, nearly 98 percent of the nation's institutionalized patients remained in public facilities. By 1940 state mental hospitals housed 410,000 Americans, and 59,000 additional patients lived in veterans, county, and city hospitals.[39] While founded as restorative institutions, those facilities were rarely—any longer—sites of productive therapeutic care. States continued to fund asylums, though, because no alternatives appeared to meet the demand for care. Deteriorating physical plants and insufficient staffs meant that for most patients, hospitalization brought containment more than a cure.[40]

A wide range of ailments led to institutionalization. In the first four decades of the century, the majority of the patients admitted to state hospitals were severely mentally ill, diagnosed with ailments such as schizophrenia and manic depression. Those suffering from paresis (the third stage of syphilis, which brought neuropsychological symptoms) also occupied hospital beds, as did sufferers with somatic conditions including epilepsy, alcoholism, mental deficiency, and pellagra (a disorder caused by a deficiency of niacin). Still others were committed as the result of behavioral symptoms without identifiable somatic causes.[41]

Through the end of World War II, the nation's mental institutions also accommodated a growing number of chronic and elderly patients, citizens relegated to hospitals when alternative methods of care, like almshouses, disappeared. In 1920 in New York, for example, 18 percent of first admissions to state mental hospitals were diagnosed as psychotic because of senility or arteriosclerosis. By 1940 those categories accounted for nearly 31 percent of all first admissions. By the 1930s chronic and aged patients occupied nearly 80 percent of the beds in American mental hospitals.[42] With few exceptions, causes and cures remained as elusive as they had for centuries.[43] To be sure, some patients in public facilities fared well, but, more often than not, sufferers experienced impersonal care at best and abusive treatment at worst.

In the 1940s, details of those horrible conditions reached many Americans. In May of 1946, the journalist Albert Q. Maisel's "Bedlam 1946" exposé in *Life* magazine compared the conditions in two state institutions to those in Nazi concentration camps. Shoddily clad or naked, patients, he revealed, were fed "starvation diets" and crammed into "hundred-year old firetraps" where some were forced to sleep on the floor. Others were restrained by "thick leather handcuffs" and in poorly lit rooms "reeking with filth and feces."[44] Similarly, when the journalist Albert Deutsch visited the Philadelphia State Hospital for Mental Diseases, he found it housed 6,100 patients, 75 percent over its stated capacity. Although the American Psychiatric Association standards called for 1,100 attendants for a patient population of that size, only 16 served. The rest of Deutsch's account in *The Shame of the States* (1948) sounded eerily similar to Dorothea Dix's observations a century earlier.

Buildings swarmed "with naked humans herded like cattle and treated with less concern." A "fetid odor so heavy, so nauseating that the stench seemed to have almost a physical existence of its own" pervaded the filthy, bug-infested hospital.[45] More than just a muckraker, Deutsch advocated for reform and voiced his concerns to local and national legislatures, hoping to bring change by restoring institutions as sites of therapeutic treatment and not just custodial care.

Occasionally, media coverage pointed to bright spots amist harsh realities. In 1946, for example, Mike Gorman, a reporter for the *Daily Oklahoman* and a health lobbyist, contrasted poor conditions in Oklahoma state hospitals with the superior care provided at Menninger Foundation facilities.[46] That same year, the writer Mary Jane Ward's *The Snake Pit*, an autobiographical novel about a young woman hospitalized after a nervous breakdown, described her miserable stay at a state institution but did so alongside hope in professional competence to treat mental disease.[47] Nonetheless, stagnating hospital populations and deteriorating conditions proved exasperating for patients and physicians.

Despite the realities of subpar care, in the years following the First World War, a "spirit of therapeutic innovation" generated optimism about the ability to treat mental illnesses. Newly discovered treatments including malaria fever therapy, insulin and metrazol shock therapy, and prefrontal lobotomy offered hope for some patients.[48] Early twentieth-century psychiatrists also deployed new drugs to calm and restrain agitated patients.[49] Therapeutic and pharmaceutical interventions not only offered hope to patients but also promised doctors treating mental maladies the ability to keep up with their medical peers that specialized in biological ailments.[50] New treatments, however, failed to bring lasting change. With sporadic use, and without standardization in treatment protocols (in part because psychiatrists disagreed about their effectiveness and safety), new medical technologies largely failed to improve care for the mentally sick and rarely brought cures. In addition, innovations proved difficult to deploy widely in overpopulated hospitals.

By 1943, with public funds diverted to support war and recovery from economic depression, care worsened. Staffing levels in state institutions dropped again, and physical plants deteriorated further.[51] As a result, use of the "moral" treatments popular in the prior century, therapies that called for carefully constructed therapeutic environments and individual care, faded. Dispensing such personal and labor-intensive care proved unmanageable, at least in large, public facilities.[52] Menninger and his family, however, tried to balance principles of past moral treatment with new medical theories.

In his first years of practice, Menninger broke new medical ground. He identified, for example, the reversibility of depressive and schizophrenic illnesses triggered by influenza. And, as he treated his first patients in Kansas, the doctor realized that biological treatments helped many patients suffering emotional distress, but not all of them. Victims of the later stages of syphilis, for example, benefitted from the newly discovered drug known as "Salvarsan" and "compound 606." Cases with no detectable organic origins, however, presented a challenge. Having "prodigiously" studied the theories of Sigmund Freud and read the works of Freud's adherents, Menninger found hope for those patients in emerging psychoanalytic techniques. With the right combination of treatments, he was hopeful that nearly all patients could recover, an optimism that deepened over time.[53]

Although Menninger held firm opinions about treatment protocols, in time, his brother William most strongly influenced the Menninger Clinic's approach to care, but always with his older brother's approval, or at least acquiescence.[54] The family's clinic sought to offer holistic mental health care, and with his brother's support, William Menninger deployed the moral treatment approaches of his nineteenth-century predecessors, including Dorothea Dix, Thomas Kirkbride, and Samuel Woodard.[55] Menninger operations remained small enough for an attentive, individualized approach to care to succeed. In a well-controlled hospital environment like the Menninger Clinic, for example, patients "could learn to cope with the past associations" that contributed to mental illness. Working closely in trusted relationships with staff, patients "would learn to master" their emotions in a "protected, instructional setting." In addition, drawing on the work of the Swiss-born psychiatrist Adolf Meyer, William Menninger rejected assumptions that mental illness stemmed from hereditary defects or from cerebral lesions. Instead, Meyer's "psychobiological" methods took into account the relationship between the patient and the patient's detailed social environment. The value his father, Charles, placed on working with good medical assistants undergirded William Menninger's sense of the importance of interpersonal relationship in the provision of care.[56] Suspicion of the new pharmaceutical and surgical treatments led William, like Karl, to favor psychoanalytic approaches based on Freud's theories.[57] Altogether, those influences shaped a scientifically informed, community-like "milieu therapy" at the Menninger Clinic. With a treatment protocol established, their earlier religiously based missionary drives made their clinic a "missionary outpost" in a shifting psychiatric landscape and a counterpoint to custodial care.[58]

The Menningers were not the only Protestants to provide alternatives to public institutions. While the majority of American mental patients received treatment in public facilities, private hospitals—including some of the nation's original, church-founded institutions—also offered care. Less burdened by chronic populations and motivated by religious convictions, a handful of Christian asylums retained a focus on moral treatment methods. Pine Rest Christian Hospital in Cutlerville, Michigan, serves as an example. Founded in 1910 by members of the Dutch Reformed tradition, Pine Rest's small size and commitment to "Christian mercy" enabled its adherence to moral treatment. Based on the conviction that "Christ's concern for undeniable dependents—widows and orphans, together with the blind, deaf, and demonically plagued—signaled a clear and continuing obligation to nurse and, if possible, cure such unfortunate people," church leaders felt called to provide an alternative to the secular care provided in state hospitals.[59]

A church-run hospital that included "spiritual counseling" as part of treatment efforts, Pine Rest offered another option to the incomplete and "neglectful care" reported in state facilities.[60] The hospital admitted 20 patients in the summer of 1912, and by 1940 it accommodated 270. True to the philosophy of moral treatment, patient regimens included occupational therapies ranging from housekeeping to maintenance of the hospital's 220-acre farm; weekly worship and pastoral counseling supplemented the routine. Sure that "all disease and suffering originated in humanity's corporate rebellion against God," but equally certain "God's grace and Christ's example demanded his disciples exert every effort to alleviate the consequences of sin," the hospital's staff responded with alacrity.[61]

Though motivated by different convictions, American Mennonites forged a similar path. As pacifists, Mennonites declared conscientious objector (CO) status during World War II and served as aides in public mental hospitals as an alternative to combat duty. The conditions they encountered prompted action. In the institutions where 1,500 Mennonite COs labored, they observed "damp and peeling plaster walls and dripping ceilings, rotten plumbing, filth-soaked wooden floors, dungeon-like bedrooms, inadequate sanitary facilities" that were "the normal situation" in such hospitals.[62] They also found overworked and undertrained staff members that were negligent and violent in their provision of care. Mennonite COs doubted those realities maximized the chances of patients regaining health.

Horrified by deplorable conditions and compelled by their faith, Mennonites responded quickly. During the war, they worked to improve conditions in state hospitals, and postwar they opened church-run facilities. Elmer Ediger, a founder of the Mennonite Mental Health Services, explained that, in the face of suffering, COs felt called by God to respond, sensing that "if God has exposed *us* to this need and *we* don't do anything, how can we expect anyone else to do so?"[63] Mennonites understood their response to the plight of the mentally ill as peaceful, loving, and Christlike.[64] Other Protestants took note of the work of those COs and urged all of "Christian America" to take up the work they had begun "in behalf of the mentally ill."[65] While Mennonite efforts garnered praise from mainline believers, their witness failed to inspire institution building by other denominations.[66]

The experiences of war not only created avenues for expansion of Menninger facilities and prompted Mennonite institution building, they also changed approaches to treatment and provided new opportunities for Protestants to attend to mental distress. During the Second World War, the U.S. military recruited physicians, many without prior training in psychiatry. They were initially hired to screen potential recruits for neuropsychiatric disorders that made them unfit for service, but attention turned quickly to attending to battlefield-induced mental distress.[67] With the unfit presumably screened out, and men still suffering, physicians concluded that environmental stress and the horrors of war—and not the preexisting structure of the personality—precipitated mental illness. William Menninger, then chief of the army's Neuropsychiatric Division and the first psychiatrist named brigadier general, played a key role in publicizing those discoveries.[68] As a result, prevention became a focus of wartime mental health efforts: leaders limited combat time, added "measures to promote group cohesion," and mandated "regular rest periods." Military psychiatrists also discovered that when environmental stress in war zones contributed to "mental maladjustment," treatment outside of hospitals proved helpful.

Similar tools soon became part of the broader psychiatric arsenal. After the war, as physicians shifted from military to civilian practice, combat zone experience shaped a new system of thought, and the science behind wartime discoveries about prevention built on a new, "dynamic psychiatry" that gained popularity after 1900.[69] The new model of disease "suggested that behavior occurred along a continuum" from normal to abnormal, took more seriously prior patient history, and called for psychiatric involvement well before mental disease became acute.[70] As medical professionals searched for clues to causes of illness in life histories, psychiatric practice outside of asylums was a logical result.[71]

Karl Menninger played a leading role in the professional adoption of that new psychology, which he described as "an articulate science of human misery and travail, human failure and triumph."[72] In 1944 he chaired the American Psychiatric Association's Special Committee on Reorganization. While doctors did deploy new physical treatments, committee members favored a turn to psychodynamic approaches. Menninger endorsed Sigmund

Freud's theories and credited the Austrian thinker with allowing mental illness finally to begin to yield to science. Like earlier medical "discoveries" of
internal organs and, later, technologies to view and diagnose illness (the dis-
secting scalpel, microscope, and X-ray), he argued, Freud's discovery of the
"vast organization of mental functioning of which our conscious experiences
are only a small part" and his methods for "looking behind the surface of
conscious thinking" helped diagnose and treat "mal-functioning personalities."[73] Yet, not everyone greeted Freud's psychodynamic theories and the
committee's work warmly.

Conflict emerged in the century-old American Psychiatric Association. Proponents of traditional psychiatry rooted in institutions—physicians
who were "committed to a somatic pathology and organic and directive
therapies"—rejected both Freud's theories and responsibility for broad social
concerns, and they focused their efforts on severely ill patients in hospitals.
Alternately, the younger wave of psychiatrists, including the Menningers,
"believed that institutional psychiatry," at least as it had been practiced,
"was obsolete." Instead, they "favored psychodynamic and psychoanalytic"
approaches and "endorsed community treatment and social activism." In
the 1950s and 1960s, proponents of psychodynamics dominated the American Psychiatric Association and most university departments of psychiatry,
and the approach of the Menningers prevailed. Yet, despite heated internal
debate, and jockeying for position, psychiatrists worked to keep their arguments inside the guild, lest their professional public image suffer as it had in
the past.[74]

Notwithstanding disagreements, wartime success of "local" (on the
battlefield) treatments meant professional efforts turned to reducing environmental stressors in civilian life through initiatives in mental hygiene.
Psychiatrists still cared for acutely ill patients, but their interests broadened.
Wartime experiences accelerated both the professional and the public interest in prophylactic care. Preventative measures proved popular with psychiatrists seeking work outside of institutions and sounded beneficial to the
public. Psychiatrists took the lead in preventing and treating "pathological
behavior." By doing so, they hoped to "create a better society" and enhance
"the welfare and happiness of all citizens." They quickly attracted other
professionals (social workers, occupational therapists) and laypeople to their
cause.[75] Optimistic about the progress of the nation, and with professionals
leading the way, Americans assumed they could eliminate weak traits and
ensure the country's continued success.[76]

A proponent of the broadened role for psychiatric care, Menninger
supported mental hygiene initiatives.[77] In his 1930 *The Human Mind*, he

commended the work of the National Committee for Mental Hygiene.[78] The doctor appreciated that mental hygiene philosophies investigated environmental causes instead of rooting mental illness in human sin, "orneriness," or a "feeble will." The goals of mental hygiene, he concluded, assumed that "mental health is attainable" and that "failure to attain it and retain it is to some extent dependent upon our ignorance of general principles."[79] Education formed a vital component of mental hygiene efforts, and much of Menninger's own work fell under an educational umbrella.

The doctor also lauded work preventing "unhealthy-mindedness" in a world that, while aware of physical health, seemed to ignore mental well-being. "Few people," he reflected, "give any attention to . . . brushing their mental teeth or to giving their minds a bath or their memories a cathartic." He found attention to the prevention of mental distress particularly important for children: "The teeth, the tonsils, the eyes, and the ears of thousands of schoolchildren are meticulously examined each year . . . and much clatter and fuss are made over elaborate statistical reports of the damage found, repaired, or averted." "Meanwhile," he asked, "how much thought is given to the examining of the *minds* of these same children? Are teeth and tonsils more important than minds?"[80] For many psychiatrists, mental hygiene provided an opportunity to distance themselves from institutions and the care of chronically ill adults. The same did not prove true for Menninger, who, while endorsing mental hygiene efforts, continued to assert a central role for institutional care and attended to all types of mental distress.[81]

COLLECTIVE PROTESTANT RESPONSES

Mental hygiene proved an easy point of entry for nonmedical professions to attend to the prevention of disease and human suffering. In 1940, for example, the parents' group of the Presbyterian Park Central Church in Syracuse, New York, sponsored a series of six lectures on "Mental Hygiene in the Family." An average of 150 individuals attended each talk. Similar events took place around the country, often jointly sponsored by congregations and mental hygiene organizations. Together, church leaders and public officials hoped to train parishioners to spot and treat nascent emotional troubles before they worsened.[82] Preventative care opened a new channel for Protestant engagement, one Menninger encouraged.

Some congregations claimed great success. In 1950, for example, the First Community Church in Columbus, Ohio, touted that of the "646 men and women from the church who were in the armed services during [World War II,] there was not one instance of mental breakdown." They credited that victory to their mental hygiene efforts that began before "the child is born." Premarital counseling was followed by careful monitoring for "deviation or abnormality" in the church nursery school and by psychological testing of adolescents. In the case of military servicemen and servicewomen, the church kept in close contact during deployments and after their return home through letters and clergy visits.[83] Menninger praised the work of First Community Church, calling it "the best example of organized mental hygiene that" he knew of or had ever seen.

Many believers were optimistic, but mental hygiene efforts also revealed a darker side of the American, and the American Protestant, ethos. With growing support of preventative measures, suspicion about individual culpability for those who continued to suffer deepened, as did stigmatization. In addition, fearing "that an alleged increase in degeneracy in general and mental illness in particular threatened the biological well-being of the American people," some promoted "interventionist measures, including marriage regulation, immigration restriction, and involuntary sterilization."[84] While fears of "socially undesirable" individuals were not new, in prior eras Protestant faith, grounded in an optimistic sense that "individual will and volition could surmount character imperfections," had mitigated concerns about intractable social deviance. But, as a new century dawned, interpretations of Darwinian evolutionary theory that assumed hereditary instead of environmental flaws spurred some not to seek the redemption but rather to limit the reproduction of "unfit" Americans.[85] The cost of preventative, "eugenic" measures eliminated the need to spend money housing and caring for "degenerates" later. Between 1907 and 1940, eugenics initiatives resulted in the surgical sterilization of more than eighteen thousand patients in state hospitals. While members of the psychiatric profession and the public held mixed views of the value of eugenics, those approaches shaped, and perhaps reflected, public perceptions of mental illnesses, particularly lingering and chronic cases.

Some Christians weighed in against eugenics campaigns. The Roman Catholic Church, for example, opposed voluntary and involuntary sterilization as a violation of natural law, but wider public concerns failed to appear until news of German Nazi sterilization practices emerged during World War II.[86] Not all mental hygiene initiatives focused on preventing reproduction, but efforts to remedy "difference" deepened suspicions about those that varied from a healthy and productive American ideal.

Though some Christians spoke out against eugenic measures, Protestant believers often endorsed "scientific" efforts.[87] To be sure, not all clergy and laity supported drastic practices to make the world a better place, but a cultural pervasiveness appeared, and lasting impact of eugenic thought among Christians emerged, even before the changes brought by World War II. In 1926, for example, the American Eugenics Society sponsored a eugenics sermon contest. The third-place winner—Rev. George Huntington Donaldson, a Methodist from New York City—argued, "The strongest and best are selected for propagating the likeness of God and carrying on his work of improving the race."[88] God's favor, by implication, was withheld from society's weaker members. The contest winner—Rev. Phillips Endecott Osgood, rector of St. Mark's Unitarian Church in Minneapolis—claimed that Jesus "was superlatively concerned to better the qualities of human living," and Osgood urged Christians to take up the responsibility of "refining" the human race through the sterilizing of criminals and through responsible reproduction. Instead of heralding a Christian impulse to attend to suffering, Osgood proposed creating a more perfect humanity by weeding out those whose handicaps meant the human race remained impure.[89] Menninger, who never hinted at approval of eugenics or sterilization, likely would have refrained from venturing that far in his assessment, but, in the hands of some, "Jesus' parables regarding the kingdom of God swiftly became parables for the eugenic separation of human wheat from human chaff."[90] Among the "chaff" were those deemed inferior because of race, poverty, moral laxity, or mental illness. Because such assessments required acceptance of Darwinian theories of evolution, eugenic views resonated with many mainline Christians who were supportive of scientific advancement.[91] With a prevalent sense that Americans, and Christians in particular, had a responsibility to demand that "every child born is worthy of a place in our midst," those admitting to mental distress or those institutionalized were considered defective.[92] Menninger supported many mental hygiene efforts, but he lamented that the movement deepened stigma for those that remained outside of the perceived healthy norm.

While preventative efforts captured the attention of some Protestants, others turned their attention to patients in state facilities, an impulse that matched Karl Menninger's desire to attend to those who suffered most severely. Albert Q. Maisel's *Life* feature, which included pages of "ghastly photographs," prompted Protestants to claim, "With continued publicity of this sort, an aroused public opinion is certain to demand sweeping changes."[93] Christians, and especially clergy, argued a *Christian Century* correspondent, should be aware of needed changes and, more important, take action. Public institutions, after all, were well within the purview of presumed Protestant responsibility.

Demonstrating that sense of ownership of state-run medical institutions, a 1946 *Christian Century* article titled "State Hospital Scandal" began with reference to "our state psychiatric hospitals." Both mistreated patients and overworked staff members drew the concern of Rev. John M. Gessell, an Episcopal priest and later professor of Christian ethics at the University of the South. Outraged, he lamented the "general indifference to the plight of these unfortunates" and implored concerned readers to "insist that state legislatures make sufficient appropriations for the care of the mentally ill." Gessell rooted his concern in two places. He pointed first to the societal cost of inadequate care measured in broken homes, ruined businesses, and the loss of gainful employment. After expressing those more secular concerns, he cited direct religious motivation, reminding his readers that "our Lord demonstrated repeatedly his concern for mental health" and, thus, so should modern believers. The clergyman also hinted at an "intimate relationship between religion and mental well-being." Not only should believers follow Christ's example and care for others, but religious practice might also bring healing.

In addition to promoting individual action, Rev. Gessell called for congregations to play a role in "fostering understanding of mental health in the community" and in advocating alongside secular organizations for adequate care. Desiring to see hospitals transformed into "places of refuge," the minister pointed readers toward involvement with advocacy organizations such as the National Mental Health Foundation.[94] Offering education and a means for getting involved, those groups provided a logical locale for Christian participation.[95] While not acting from religious motivations exclusively, Protestants like Gessell urged advocacy, education, and direct involvement in care in the face of mental illness. Less clear, however, was the breadth of response that such pleas motivated.

A number of public health concerns attracted Protestant attention in the twentieth century, including polio, leprosy, tuberculosis, and alcoholism. Measured by frequency of coverage in flagship periodicals like *Christian Century* and *Presbyterian Life*, however, none garnered as much interest as mental health. Mentally ill patients, mainline Protestants observed, occupied more than half of the nation's hospital beds.[96] Acknowledging the growing number of portrayals of mental illness in literature and drama, Protestants pointed to the "responsibility of gigantic proportions for the church and ministry" to attend to those ills before they reached "epidemic" proportions.[97]

Some believers organized to take collective action. The year after Gessell's plea, the Chicago Church Federation "launched a campaign to bring about action by the state legislature to remedy the deplorable conditions" in state institutions. The ecumenical group lamented crowding, inadequate staffing, and insufficient funding. Christians were encouraged to send away to the commission to receive materials that would prepare them to be knowledgeable advocates.[98] The federation's work also brought the plight of Illinois' mentally ill population into Chicago pulpits. "Almost with exception," a correspondent reported, "Protestant pastors last Sunday called upon their congregations to unite in demanding correction of the deplorable conditions in the nine state hospitals for the mentally ill and the two institutions for the mentally deficient."[99] Protestants, at least a few in Illinois, heeded calls to action.

Others advocated care outside state hospitals. Instead of "casting off" sick Americans to faraway institutions, they argued that "church people," more than any others, bore responsibility for the "welfare of mortal beings" and should work with public agencies to find local alternatives to the "vestige of the Dark Ages" of institutional care.[100] The Greater Minneapolis Council of Church Women, for example, stepped up to help. Partnering with the state Departments of Vocational Rehabilitation and Public Welfare, they formed the "Church F Club," at Wesley Methodist Church, to create a "circle of friendship" that promoted the health of discharged mental patients.[101] Similar initiatives sprouted up around the country, and in the wake of public exposés of conditions at public facilities, the decade after 1945 proved a time of heightened Protestant attention to mental maladies and, in some pockets, action.

Though riddled with problems, public institutions persisted as the most common venue of treatment for the severely mentally ill. By the early 1960s, however, national and state policies began to shift to favor community-based care options, and a massive deinstitutionalization of public facilities ensued. Before 1965, mental patients spent years or decades hospitalized. After 1970, inpatient treatment more likely measured days or weeks, with still-unstable patients left to find continued treatment elsewhere after discharge. As a result, patient populations decreased dramatically, with the number of public mental hospital beds falling from 413,000 to 119,000 between 1970 and 1986.[102] Community mental health providers, though, proved unable to provide care for all in need, and as a result, many former patients ended up homeless and cycled in and out of prisons and the psychiatric wards of general hospitals. The period also saw the discharge of chronic, aged patients from mental hospitals, causing nursing home populations nearly to double.[103] Changing locations for care eliminated large public mental hospitals as a focal point of interest and advocacy, and it coincided with a shift in Protestant focus from the plight of sufferers to the adequacy of preparation of clergy to prevent and attend to mental distress. Menninger's publishing, speaking, and training efforts supported that transition.

Though some hope surfaced for the treatment of mental illness in the twentieth century, overall, it is difficult to describe anything but a troubled treatment system. Locating good care proved difficult, and notwithstanding the desire to help and a handful of church-run institutions, in the twentieth century, congregations and church leaders had little sustained involvement in public mental institutions. Nor did they participate actively in deinstitutionalization efforts or in the provision of community-based care. Despite clarion calls to advocacy early in the century, Protestant efforts had much more limited influence than the advocacy of Dix a century earlier might have inspired and that Karl Menninger hoped for. Most believers simply cheered caregiving efforts on from the sidelines.

MODERN PERCEPTIONS OF MENTAL ILLNESS

Amidst a struggling system of care, evolving treatment protocols, and persistent stigma, Menninger played a lead role in shaping both public and professional views of mental illness and those that suffered from it. The doctor described illness—whether physical or mental—as "pain, disability, bodily deformity or disintegration." He saw it as "an adventitious state of being which impairs or hurts or threatens to destroy us" because it "interrupts, to some extent, the ordinary, 'normal' course of life." Illness, he argued, "impairs or threatens to impair comfort, effectiveness, and even life continuance." It "is always an unwanted, feared, dreaded, detested, avoided 'thing,' a state of being for which palliation or removal is imperatively desired."[104] Whether bodily or emotional, sickness proved a matter of chance, disruptive for the one who suffered, and it demanded remedy.

Turning his attention to mental illness, Menninger refused to define it as a " 'thing'—like a specimen in a museum—for which a label must be found." Rather, he saw mental illness as "a state of functioning" or a "way of behaving." Using the analogy of a trout gyrating wildly after being caught on a hook, he saw strange behaviors as "efforts [on the part of the sufferer] to get rid of the affliction," behaviors that sometimes succeeded and sometimes failed.[105] Menninger named mental *health* as "the adjustment of human beings to the world and to each other with a maximum of effectiveness and happiness. Not just efficiency, or just contentment—or the grace of obeying the rules of the game cheerfully. It is all of these together." The doctor described mental well-being as "the ability to maintain an even temper, an alert intelligence, socially considerate behavior, and a happy disposition."[106] In addition, rather than seeing mental illness as a binary state where one was either well or sick, Menninger assumed that mental health occurred along a spectrum, a view that included the sense that all humans suffered from mental maladies at one time or another. "If one has a mind at all," he argued, "his mental processes are subject to some of the faults and failing that characterize the human mind."[107] Using accessible, nonmedical language, the doctor pronounced that mental health enabled humans to function productively in the world; mental illness inhibited that ability.

Going deeper, Menninger described two basic categories of "mental sickness." First, he outlined "afflictions which cause anguish and pain primarily in the persons who suffer them. They suffer depression or fear, uncontrollable anger or bitterness, and sometimes this anguish drives them frantic or drives them to drink or drives them to the doctor and he drives them to the hospital."[108] The most commonly recognized form of mental illness, he asserted, manifested itself in pain, oddness, isolation, discouragement, ineffectiveness, disagreeableness, idleness, isolation, despoliation, and defilement.[109] The doctor also identified "a kind of mental illness from which individuals may suffer but the people around them suffer a great deal more." With this type of emotional distress, he reflected, "whether one calls it vandalism or psychopathy or criminality," the mental abnormality of others "results in *our* suffering."[110] In many ways, that twofold typology reflected the prevailing twentieth-century lay and professional categorization of mental illnesses as either neuroses or psychoses.

While offering definitions, the nation's leading psychiatrist also acknowledged uncertainties about mental distress. In a 1951 lecture delivered at the Chicago Theological Seminary, for example, he confessed that "mental illness has long been a mystery" and remained so, even with greater scientific insight. Paradoxically, however, Menninger knew mystery persisted despite the fact that mental illness was "enormously prevalent—more abundant than all other forms of illness put together."[111] Alongside the desire to attend to human suffering, the intellectual challenge of understanding and solving the long-standing problems of mental illness captured the faithful physician's interest.

Menninger detailed causes of mental distress. To begin, he dismissed deeply held presumptions. Convictions about supernatural origins were the first target of his reeducation efforts. In an interview with L. M. Birkhead, minister of All Souls' Unitarian Church in Kansas City, Missouri, Menninger observed that in the past, human misbehavior was often explained by demonic possession. He rejected supernatural causation, but he admitted, "sincere devout people still exist who regard the misbehavior of mankind as nothing but evidence of sinfulness and the cure as religious salvation." Others, he noted, refrained from blaming God (or the lack of God, or the Devil, or witches), but instead pinned culpability on human behavior, linking mental illness with immorality.[112] Assumptions of moral causes, he argued, were no more valid or helpful than supernatural ones. Finally, Menninger pushed aside thoughts that sufferers inherited mental defects. Education about illness, treatments, and preventative measures, he asserted, trumped theories of familial disposition, or "hereditary damnation."¹¹³ Whether supernatural, moral, or hereditarian, earlier theories, Menninger concluded, "all assume that something mysterious and malignant floating in the ether or transmitted in the germ plasm gets into the individual and makes him go wrong." The result, he regretted, was that the afflicted one "gets called names." But "calling people witches or devils or psychopathic personalities," he argued, "doesn't help" bring healing.

When exploring the origins of mental maladies, Menninger also looked past purely biological views of causation. Instead, he insisted that ailing should be viewed in terms of "psychodynamics, psychoeconomics, development, biology and adaptation."¹¹⁴ While adopting theoretical constructions from those like Freud, Menninger reserved a role for sin in causing some abnormal human behavior. He drew a distinct line, however, between sin and illness. In commenting, for example, on the 1978 mass suicide in Jonestown, Guyana, where Rev. Jim Jones led nearly one thousand people to their deaths, Menninger's Protestant moral sensibilities appeared. "Some of my colleagues," he observed, "persist in believing that coining Greek and Latin names and slapping them on accused individuals enables them to disguise depravity and to make the committing of evil (sins) something pardonable because it is something psychiatric." The event in Guyana "is not a psychiatric problem: it is a moral problem," Menninger contended. "Jones was a wicked, corrupt, unscrupulous, and evil man. Why call him by euphemistic 'scientific' names? What do we gain by throwing around words like *paranoia* and *dementia*?"¹¹⁵ Menninger's Protestant faith attuned him to the realities of human suffering and the reality of sin. When appropriate, his medical training allowed him to frame mental distress in scientific terms. Because his assessments rang true with professionals and proved understandable by laity, Menninger's view of illness held broad influence.

Alongside widely read descriptions of mental illness by Menninger, journalistic and cinematic exposés of institutional life played a role in shaping public perceptions about the causes of mental distress. Portrayals by those like Albert Deutsch and Albert Q. Maisel generated public outrage; they also demonstrated that presumed links between mental illness and sin continued to fade. In the preface to his 1948 *The Shame of the States*, journalist Deutsch declared that while "insanity was once considered a sin or the consequence of sin . . . we no longer regard our mentally sick patients as criminals, witches or paupers." Instead, Deutsch named mental illness a sickness that rendered "a person socially inefficient" and necessitated treatment that provided "some form of social control." In addition, the term "insane," he argued, "is fast becoming obsolete in modern medical parlance," instead replaced by notions of disease.[116] Two decades later, a study in the *Journal of Health and Human Behavior* revealed "the virtual disappearance of ideas that mental illness is a result of sin or the devil." No longer did Americans think of mental distress as "merely evil or willful misbehavior" or that "punishment was the only solution."[117] With mental distress no longer linked to the demonic, at least not explicitly, twentieth-century Americans tended to view mental maladies medically, as illnesses.

Public reactions to sufferers, however, remained mixed. Differing levels of comfort and knowledge about the afflicted were evident in the Methodist minister John B. Oman's 1952 observations. Oman—who served the First Methodist Church in Trenton, New Jersey, and worked as a prison and asylum chaplain—assessed that "those who understand" mental illness "react toward it the same as toward physical illness." But, those who do not understand "usually react toward it with a feeling of awe (more or less natural when something is beyond one's comprehension) or are morbidly curious." The "most ignorant," he observed, tend to ridicule, a response he named "a defense mechanism resorted to by many to cover up their own lack of knowledge, and therefore not a true expression of their real emotions." Rarely were the sick at fault for their illnesses, but, even so, they found themselves "banished from society" once they crossed the threshold of a mental hospital.[118] For Americans, illness prompted public sympathy, but dependency did not. In the case of mental illness, the difference between the two was not always clear.[119]

NEGATIVE STEREOTYPES OF SUFFERERS

By mid-century, social scientists began to survey public perceptions about mental illness, and one of the earliest studies suggested that public and professional perceptions did not always match. By the 1950s, "the public defined mental illness in much narrower and more extreme terms than did psychiatry." The results also showed that whether warranted or not, "fearful and rejecting attitudes toward people with mental illnesses were common."[120] Over the next four decades, views shifted, but stigma persisted. A later study indicated that between 1950 and 1996, "conceptions of mental illness . . . broadened somewhat . . . to include a great proportion of non-psychotic disorders." By the end of the century, the public differentiated between severe mental illness and less severe disorders, showing deeper knowledge of medical diagnoses. During that time, though, "perceptions that mentally ill people are violent or frightening" increased substantially. Negative stereotypes drove that change—perceptions often generated by media coverage of the underlying mental conditions of individuals committing heinous crimes.[121]

While suspicions of links between sin and mental maladies may have eased, patients and the institutions where they sought care remained tainted by stigma that painted sufferers as different, if not dangerous.

Evidence demonstrated that Protestants understood what mental illness was and who suffered from it. Definitions of mental illness in Protestant publications, though, were brief, general, and without medical detail. As a result, they offered a limited portrayal of suffering. Believers pointed frequently to the vast reach of mental maladies, and while they affirmed the U.S. Public Health Service's pronouncement that mental illness was "America's number one health problem," rarely did they admit to knowing sufferers or being those who ailed.[122] And not until the end of the century did some step forward and admit their own afflictions. In 1968, for example, when a Presbyterian elder shared his experiences in churches related to his wife's mental illness, he did so pseudonymously.[123] In almost every case, the afflicted were generalized, unnamed, institutionalized others, far from local church communities.[124] Protestants did acknowledge categories of people that might be in need of care. Stressful working conditions turned "defense workers" and government clerks in Washington, D.C., into "nervous wrecks and psychopathic cases."[125] Soldiers returning home from war should prompt churches to prepare to deal with "deep psychic wounds" inflicted on the battlefields.[126] Protestants also suspected that mental illness played a role in juvenile delinquency. The identity of other burdened and sick souls, however, remained elusive It seems likely that continued social stigma kept Christians hesitant to name those that suffered or to share their illnesses, even while acknowledging that many did.

Ordained Protestants held opinions too. Though some sufferers remained anonymous, given the prevalence of mental illness, attending to them was surely a central task for ministers. Less obvious was whether leaders understood themselves to be susceptible to mental maladies. Some thought "the very fact that a man has chosen the ministry for a vocation may indicate some sort of inner disorder," perhaps a "neurotic need for helping other people." Clear that clergy "as a group probably have as good a *physical* health record as any other group in the community," they wondered, though, how to assess the emotional health of men of the cloth.[127] Alternately, others asserted that clergy, at least well-behaved clergy, lived beyond the grasp of mental illness. A reflection titled "Are Ministers Cracking Up?" found it acceptable for some to suffer mental anguish, but not clergy. Taking an only thinly veiled defensive tone, the Presbyterian minister William Hudnut rebutted a *Life* magazine exposé of rampant "mental and emotional illness among the clergy" that asserted "the number one problem of American clergymen is mental health."[128] He argued that the few ministers that did "crack up" did so because they lacked the "discipline to crack down" on themselves, implying that clergy should be more adept at controlling their mental health than laity.[129] Hudnut provided practical stress-reducing techniques for religious leaders, but behind that tactical advice lay a fear of vocational failure and reluctance to name clerical vulnerability.

While Americans no longer explicitly connected mental illness to demonic possession, original sin, or individual transgression, they still struggled to understand its appearance. That even medical literature speculated when talking about the causes of and cures for mental maladies gave the public good reason to question, and it meant that a cloud of uncertainty and suspicion surrounded those that ailed. Proximity to sick friends and relatives may have eased discomfort about abnormalities, but even nearness provided no immunity from stigma. The public and professionals, however, continued to seek cures.

SHARING THE PROVISION OF CARE

Insanity was once the sole domain of asylum physicians (and before then simply the purview of the parish priest), but, by the 1930s, a gaggle of health professionals—psychiatrists, psychologists, psychoanalysts, mental hygienists, and social workers—declared their authority to help.[130] Clergy too staked a claim, but they were forced to find ways to cooperate in the provision of care. As a result, they asserted pockets of expertise. Of central concern for ministers was assessing psychiatry, psychology, and psychoanalysis and determining how those tools could and should interact with Christianity and the resources of religious communities. Menninger addressed those questions enthusiastically.

Though Menninger harbored few reservations, opinions varied about the wisdom of cooperation between medical and religious professionals. Sometimes physicians eschewed blended approaches to care. In 1936, for example, a Methodist minister asked the Canadian psychiatrist C. M. Hincks "about training that would enable him to deal with the mental problems of his parishioners." The doctor bluntly dismissed the clergyman's question. Instead, he responded that "the practice of psychiatry is so rooted in medical science that it could not possibly be entrusted to the hands of a layman, no matter how wide his readings on the subject had been" and that "only the trained psychiatrist is qualified to examine," diagnose, and treat mental disease.[131] Unlike Hincks, Menninger heralded cooperation. He "recognized that suffering human beings transcend the perspective of any single vision [of diagnosis and treatment] or even of all visions taken together."[132] Health necessitated joint efforts.

Specifically, Menninger saw an affinity in the work of psychiatrists and clergy. Both professions, he asserted, were "aware of the vast extent of misery and suffering in the world." In addition, each felt "impelled to do something to diminish this suffering" through "advice to the individual" and "proclamation of principles of living."[133] The trained physician knew that religious leaders stood on the front line of response. "Every priest, pastor, and rabbi," he observed, "spends a considerable amount of his time, I am sure, listening to parishioners who are in distress because of recognized or unrecognized mental illness." "Clergymen," he observed, "more than most people are aware of the vast extent of misery and suffering in the world. They and the psychiatrists are together on this."[134] Likely, Menninger's willingness to cooperate stemmed from his religious upbringing and continued church involvement.

Though many of Menninger's medical colleagues disagreed with him, the Protestant physician framed psychiatry and psychology as endeavors with connections to religion, if not direct links to Christianity. In 1951 he spoke to a group of Protestant ministers at the University Church of Disciples of Christ in Chicago. An observer at those Alden-Tuthill lectures noted that Menninger "stressed the similarities" between religion and psychology. Menninger "pictured the psychiatrist as one who is putting Christianity into practice" and translating "psychoanalytic theories and principles into theology." He also found "the psychiatrist's acceptance of his patients' hostilities while refusing to act against those hostilities . . . akin to Christian love" and reflected, "There is in the theory and practice of psychiatry a basic attitude of faith."[135] Downplaying clashes between faith and science, Menninger argued, "The life work of the psychiatrist does not conflict with either the usefulness or the content of religion."[136] Even when others denounced religious connections between faith and medicine, Menninger presumed them. The doctor's credibility with clergy was no surprise.

At times, it appeared that Menninger even resisted differentiating between ministerial and medical roles. Psychiatrists and clergy used many of the same tools—both attended to emotional distress by "listening, comforting, correcting, and reassuring."[137] He even understood (and perhaps experienced) the work of physicians as a form of ministry. Menninger named psychiatry a "ministry of care to the most miserable, the most unloved, the most pitiable, and at times the most offensive and even dangerous of human beings."[138] The doctor proclaimed that psychiatrists "ministered" to patients just as clergy ministered to congregants. Psychiatrists engaged in a "ministry of care" in the form of being the "friend, the guide, the protector, the helper, the lover of" sufferers.[139] He understood compassion, like that dispensed by doctors, as "a sentiment worthy of divinity."[140] Clergy and psychiatrists could be of one mind.

Yet, Menninger also drew distinctions. He defined a unique role for clergymen as moral prophets. Clergy, through preaching, had a venue to promote mental health: "No psychiatrists or psychotherapists, even those with many patients, have the quantitative opportunity to cure souls and mend minds which the preacher enjoys. And the preacher also has a superb opportunity to do what few psychiatrists can, to prevent the development of chronic anxiety, depression, and other mental ills."[141] Properly used, the doctor observed, the pulpit encouraged mental health. "Like the psychiatrist," Menninger argued, "the minister feels impelled to do something to diminish this suffering, not only by advice to the individual, but by proclamation of principles of living. In their sermons they endeavor—most of them—to hold out hope, comfort, encouragement, and reassurance to congregations in which there are many who need this help."[142] In some tasks, the doctor ascribed authority to ministerial colleagues.

Though clergy played a role, Menninger presumed that "the injunction of Isaiah to 'Comfort my people,' rest[ed] heavily upon psychiatrists."[143] Medical professionals, he claimed, undertook the essential part in bringing healing. Others noted similar professional demarcations. In 1955 mainline Protestants in St. Louis welcomed the assertion by the rabbi Joseph R. Rosenbloom at a meeting of the Institute on Religion and Psychiatry that it was "fatuous to believe that [religion and psychiatry] seek the same things with the same methods. Religion is religion and psychiatry is a branch of medicine. And while they frequently move along parallel lines, they are distinct. Psychiatry seeks to reconcile the patient to circumstance and to himself. Religion seeks to reconcile him to spiritual values and disciplines." Rosenbloom further forecast that "the greatest failure that may come in these two fields is not that they will not come together—become one great movement—but that they will not be used to bolster one another." Despite identifying separate roles, hopes for productive partnering fostered continued conversation.[144]

Menninger recognized, and seems to have supported, the transfer of authority from clergy to psychiatrists in matters of mental health that had cemented by the twentieth century. The doctor reflected that, with the rise of science, "the clergyman's morally burdened parishioners became the psychiatrist's complex-laden patients; sin became symptom, and confession became psychotherapy."[145] Though Menniger held that clergy should participate in the provision of care, he reserved the most important role for medical professionals. "It is not accident," he reflected, "that the highest social esteem, once reserved for princes and royalty, for high priests and prophets, is now accorded to physicians."[146] Some agreed. Pastors in Wisconsin, for example, were asked not to provide care directly but rather to "acquaint their congregations with the services being rendered by the state society for mental health" and to "work with other community agencies in hosting educational programs." Even church leaders affirmed that, sometimes, care and counseling were best if left to trained medical professionals.[147]

Nonetheless, many clergy were eager to incorporate psychiatric and psychological insight to strengthen their care of souls. From 1940 through 1970, advertisements and book reviews from the *Christian Century* teemed with texts aimed to help them do so. A sample of titles that drew clerical attention included *The Church and Psychotherapy*, *Psychology for Pastor and People*, and *Pastoral Psychology: A Study in the Care of Souls*. Ministers also assessed purely medical volumes, recommending secular books like *Steps in Psychotherapy*, *Culture and Mental Disorders*, and *Today's Neurotic Family* as resources. Often, clergy gathered in person to learn from medical professionals. In 1944, for example, "a large percentage of Denver ministers" attended the first in a series of four lectures on psychiatry. Topics included "The Relation between Mental Disease and Religion" and "A Psychiatric Interpretation of the Golden Rule."[148] Similar sessions took place around the country in the 1940s and 1950s. At work in those publications and gatherings was a suspicion that medical professionals possessed knowledge and authority that clergy needed and perhaps coveted.

Clerical adoption of psychiatric, psychological, and psychoanalytical techniques generated decades of debate, and little resolution. Many saw benefit in conversation and urged dialogue. In 1946, for example, Rev. John Gessell argued that while psychiatry was a "highly specialized science," it was not necessary that "we, as Christian laymen and ministers, let the church's function of ministry to the ill in mind and spirit atrophy."[149] According to Gessell, the church had a role to play in the care of those suffering from mental illnesses, and from his vantage point, those newly emerging scientific and medical disciplines offered resources. Protestant support was also apparent for organizations that enabled dialogue between the medical and religious communities. A *Christian Century* editorial from April 1956 noted that "an auspicious star brooded over the launching of the National Academy of Religion and Mental Health." Beyond the "threat of atomic annihilation," the editors of *Christian Century* saw no greater need than addressing mental health.[150] Willingness on the part of the medical establishment to engage with religious leaders, however, developed more slowly. In a May 1956 editorial report on a joint meeting of the American Psychiatric Association and the American Psychoanalytic Association, the *Christian Century* called for renewed cooperation between pastoral and psychiatric efforts.[151] Both disciplines, the American Psychiatric Association acknowledged, shared concern and responsibility for "human well-being," and thus greater understanding of each other's approaches provided mutual benefit. But the editorial also noted that "in the persons of some of its wisest men, the church has been putting its best foot forward for some time, looking for just such cooperation, and finding [only] a little."[152] Many welcomed the American Psychiatric Association's call for reciprocity.

Other church leaders were less enthusiastic. In 1940 John Wright Buckham, professor of Christian theology at the Pacific School of Religion, worried that adoption of secular medical insight might signal trouble. Psychology, he argued, had supplanted ethics, degraded reason, belittled religion, and attempted to displace philosophy. While his concerns extended far beyond the impact of psychology on Christianity, in all things he urged, "Let psychology be servant, not master."[153] Though not calling for cooperation to cease, Buckham urged caution.

Notwithstanding skeptics, Menninger worked to bring physicians and clergy together. In 1954 his hope for cooperation sparked the first Gallahue Conference on Religion and Psychiatry, a forum for the discussion of common concerns. Attended by theologians and psychiatrists, the gatherings, which continued annually through the end of the decade, "led to the establishment of training programs at Menninger for scholars in theology and psychiatry and for clergy in pastoral care and counseling."[154] As part of those initiatives, Karl, along with his brother William, worked with Rev. Dr. Seward Hiltner and other leaders of the Clinical Pastoral Education movement begun by Anton Boisen.[155] They hoped joining forces would alleviate suffering caused by mental illness.

Clergy had counseled parishioners for centuries, but a "new" field of pastoral counseling emerged with clerical adoption of scientific techniques. Mainline Protestants were happy to seek answers to problems related to illness outside of the church, understanding God as working in the church and the world.[156] In 1955 the journal *Pastoral Psychology* published *The Minister's Consultation Clinic: Pastoral Psychology in Action*, a text that exemplified the exploration of the new field. Geared toward clergy, the volume compiled questions from ministers and other professionals. Readers sought advice about a wide variety of topics: "The Limits of Counseling with Neurotics," "The Pastor and Suicide," "Unpardonable Sin and the Psychopath," "The Interrelationship of Theology and Counseling," and "The Relationship of Preaching to Pastoral Counseling."[157] Inquirers wondered about their work as caregivers, about the relationship of theology to psychology and psychiatry, and how scientific disciplines should inform ministry. Respondents weighed in with psychological, ministerial, and medical insight. Early the next year, subscribers shared their reactions to the book.

Menninger, who was also one of the volume's respondents, endorsed pastoral counseling in his contribution. In addition to training ministers at the Menninger Clinic, he served on the editorial boards of *Pastoral Psychology* and the *Journal of Pastoral Care*.[158] A half century after Anton Boisen's prophetic vision, the Presbyterian clergyman's hope of cooperation between religion and medicine in attending to mental maladies was a reality for a number of clergy and medical professionals. Although not all of their colleagues agreed, Boisen and Menninger were among many that saw great possibilities for cooperation between religious leaders and mental health professionals. By 1964 the Menninger Clinic's Pastoral Care programs had trained more than 120 seminarians and clergy. Menninger felt that "his mother would have been pleased with its success as an exercise in 'practicing Christianity.' "[159]

Despite widespread interest in pastoral counseling, clergy failed to reach a consensus about the practice.[160] But, even with diverse approaches, by 1950, pastoral counseling was embedded enough in mainline Protestantism that those without training feared incompetence. Reflecting on his first nine years in ministry, Rev. Robert E. Luccock, for example, confessed that he "came out of seminary poorly trained to handle a counseling ministry." The Congregational minister encouraged men in seminary to seek the training he lacked so that they could "avoid regrettable fumbling of the cases that are sure to come to [them], and to equip [them] to be helpful."[161] With scientific techniques viewed as the most authoritative, clergy felt they needed nontheological training to serve well.

Although enthusiasm for training as psychologically and psychiatrically informed pastoral caregivers prevailed, some continued to recommend caution. Rev. Dr. John Oliver Nelson, for example, urged balance in training ministerial candidates. "It has become a plain necessity that the minister be able to spot a neurosis or sense of insecurity," he declared. The Presbyterian professor of Christian vocation at Yale also acknowledged that pastoral caregivers should be competent deploying the latest secular techniques. Echoing the language of his medical peers, Nelson argued the minster should "make his pastoral counseling largely nondirective," should "use group dynamics where they will work," and should "keep aware of what goes on within his own mind and emotions." But, Nelson counseled, "in the best balanced approach, seminarians are kept aware that clinical techniques merely provide therapy for a set of ills which Christianity, through the life of conviction and devotion, has long been concerned to prevent."[162] These were simply new tools for a task that had been undertaken by clergy for centuries.

Others voiced stronger concerns and worried that psychological methods would obliterate theological reflection. In 1951 the professor of pastoral counseling and pastoral theology at Wartburg Theological Seminary, Dr. William E. Hulme, cautioned that pastoral counseling without a theological framework was like unenriched, bleached flour—devoid of life-sustaining nutrients. For Hulme, theology should not be used dogmatically or with an air of authoritarianism. However, for the professor, the centrality of the atonement—recognition that "God was in Christ, himself suffering in man's stead to redeem him"—was critical to any pastoral counseling endeavor. Even while adopting secular resources, staying grounded in the doctrines of the Christian church remained crucial in the eyes of those like Hulme.[163]

Despite moments of cooperation, tension between religious and medical workers emerged and garnered public attention. A 1951 *Time* feature on "Psychiatry and Religion" began by observing, "psychiatrists and clergymen, meeting over the ailing psyche of modern man, still eye one another suspiciously." Hopes of cooperation often failed to materialize. "Rare is the churchman," the article continued, "who makes systematic use of psychiatric techniques in his ministry to souls; rare is the [psycho]analyst who lives and works upon specific premises of religious faith." The magazine, though, declared Menninger an exception, a man who "practices Presbyterianism as well as Freud" and "sees no irreconcilable conflict between the two."[164] The same could be said of Menninger's brother William.

The younger Menninger acknowledged that some found "psychiatry, especially psychoanalysis . . . anti-religious and destructive of religious faith."[165] Aware of opposition, Karl and William both worked to refute such claims. The older Menninger rejected commonly voiced views that psychiatrists "persuade their patients to a Godless, immoral philosophy," that they "repudiate the conscience" and "advocate irresponsible self-expression to the disregard of the moral law," and that they "attempt to thwart the design of the Creator, whom they deny while they themselves play God."[166] William affirmed, "Psychiatry is no more pro- or antireligious than is surgery." While some suspected that psychiatrists might not be believers, Karl Menninger claimed otherwise, even when they outwardly eschewed faith. "Referring to the agnosticism of some modern psychiatrists," the older Menninger brother explained, "'I suspect that this refers more to conceptual nonconformity than to deep reverential emotion.'" He even characterized Freud as "more religious than he [Freud] realized."[167] Both brothers fought opposition to the type of religion and scientific integration that marked their own lives.

Clergy sometimes pointed to concerns about the impact of psychology on morality. The most commonly voiced concern about secular professionals claimed that "psychoanalysts favor sexual promiscuity and that they encourage people not to have any sense of guilt about it." Karl Menninger decried such assumptions as "false" and stated that their "reiteration is a lie, a slander, and canard, and a misrepresentation of facts, and a piece of dishonest and dishonorable" aspersion. Medical professionals, the doctor argued, attempted to solve the abnormal personalities associated with sexual irregularities, not to promote them.[168] Menninger lamented those misunderstandings, arguing that they perpetuated the suffering of mentally ill persons that could otherwise receive treatment.

Clergy both cooperated and competed with secular professionals through the 1950s, and Americans continued to endorse the work of Protestants in healing. In 1946 Harmon Wilkinson of the National Mental Health Foundation appealed to the religious community for help with "mentally defective" Americans. He imagined Protestants engaged in "full-time Christian service" with needy mentally ill patients.[169] More formally, in 1950 Minnesota governor Luther W. Youngdahl appointed seven (of an eventual eighteen) full-time chaplains at the state's mental hospitals.[170] Three years later, the state of California mandated chaplains on the staffs of state mental hospitals.[171] Public organizations and institutions seemed to value the role of clergy with mentally ill Americans, but chaplaincy service lacked direct connections to congregational activity and caregiving.

Though Menninger was clear about the role of clergy in mental health care, he had little to say about wider congregational participation. Church members sensed some responsibility but rarely detailed plans of action. Most often, they did more thinking than acting and simply articulated something close to Rev. Seward Hiltner's 1943 assertion: "In the field of mental health, [the church] has a twofold task, curative and preventative."[172] Some envisioned more specific roles for churchgoers. In 1952 Rev. John B. Oman urged churches to educate members *and* the public about the prevention, treatment, and research necessary to combat mental illness. Providing "proper facilities" for prevention and treatment, for example, helped the church put "legs on its prayers." "To do less," he argued, "is to miss completely the spirit of Christ." The "healing of the demoniac" by Christ was, for Oman, "sufficient proof of our Lord's concern for the mentally sick. His church can have no less an interest and still be Christian." He placed the "future of millions who are mentally sick" squarely on the shoulders of nation's Protestants.[173] Thirty-two years after his original statement about the church's role, Hiltner worried that "excessive emphasis on positive mental health" on the part of Christians and others could "turn into a sneaky way of avoiding social responsibility for persons now suffering."[174] Despite some clear visions of paths Protestants might take in responding to suffering, the professor of theology and personality at Princeton Theological Seminary lamented the lack of progress—secular and religious—in attending to mental illness.

Perhaps, as clergy asserted their right to master scientific tools, laity felt incapable of stepping in. In a 1986 reflection, English professor Robert Drake recalled attending a worship service that included a young woman home for a visit from her lifelong stay at the local mental hospital. Drake found himself in the middle of a summer Baptist revival haunted by the words of the spiritual "Were you There?" He wondered if he, "like Peter, had denied [the] Lord, maybe even gone to sleep on him when he needed me."[175] Noting the "crazy" young woman was also moved by the song, Drake felt shock and wondered, "Would she have liked to talk about [her miserable lot as part and parcel of it all], would she have liked to ask other people, myself included, where they were when she had suffered her own affliction?"[176] Convicted by his own lack of action, Drake felt his faith challenged. The call to action, however, proved less clear.

STIGMA AND THE AMERICAN IDEAL

Despite advances in treatment, and some attention from Protestants, social stigma continued to plague those living with mental illness. Menninger lamented that the attitudes of "uninformed" Americans led to "cruel stigma . . . present in the minds of too many good people."[177] While he denounced stigma, he also feared psychiatrists helped propagate it. In a 1964 *Saturday Evening Post* article, the doctor asserted that "psychiatrists use dangerous words," labels that might stigmatize patients. Diagnostic terms like "schizophrenic," "manic-depressive," and "psychotic," he claimed, "frighten patients and worry their anxious relatives and friends" and even affect psychiatrists. Such labels led medical professionals "back into the pessimism and helplessness of the days when mental illness was thought to be made up of many specific 'diseases,' and when each 'disease' bore a formidable label and a gloomy prognosis."[178] Menninger worried that labels could "blight the life of a person, even after his recovery from mental illness." Although admitting that many of his American Psychiatric Association colleagues disagreed, he confessed that he avoided using terms like "schizophrenia" "just as" he steered clear of "words like 'wop' or 'nigger.'"

With his warning about diagnostic labels, Menninger hoped to prevent stigma's damaging effects. Reflecting on the mental distress of a college student, for example, he wondered, "Suppose she had been officially labeled?" Her parents and "the college authorities would have" more likely "reconciled themselves to probability that this girl would never return to college." And, if she had returned, "it would have taken extraordinary courage for her to face her comrades as a 'schizophrenic.'" Instead, concluding not that the young woman was afflicted with a specific mental illness but rather that she experienced a "moderate to severe personality disorganization related to certain exaggerated stresses" that was "amenable to treatment" allowed her to say to her friends, "I had a severe spell of illness; I was quite depressed but got it straightened out. I'm fine now and I think I learned a great deal from the whole experience."[179] Even while dispensing them, Menninger understood the burden of diagnostic labels.[180]

The doctor also recognized that the stigma associated with mental maladies minimized public funding of psychiatry and psychiatric research. "The enormous effect of a substantial investment in research pertaining to mental disease," he argued, "is like a dream of Aladdin's lamp." While citizens found themselves bothered by (and gladly attended to) poverty, the suffering of children, and racial and ethnic discrimination, they considered interest in the plight of the mentally ill "abnormal" and put it "out of their minds." The doctor also pointed out what sociologist Erving Goffman later named as "courtesy stigma," namely, the fact that people who choose to attend to mental maladies would themselves "be regarded by some as abnormal, a little crazy."[181] Perhaps the Kansas physician spoke from experience.

Rather than stigmatize those seeking psychiatric treatment—whether inpatient or outpatient—Menninger declared them courageous and more intelligent than others that needed help but lacked the wisdom to obtain it.[182] Besides, Menninger asserted, no one proved immune from mental maladies. In fact, he found "that curious emotional defense which impels some people to believe themselves exempt from all failure, from all weakness, from the taboo of 'abnormality,' is perhaps the greatest enemy of healthy mindedness."[183] He put little stock on the societal definitions of normality against which stigma was generated:

> The adjuration to be "normal" seems shockingly repellent to me; I see neither hope nor comfort in sinking to that low level. I think it is ignorance that makes people think of abnormality only with horror and allows them to remain undismayed at the proximity of "normal" to average and mediocre. For surely anyone who achieves anything is, *a priori*, abnormal; this includes not only the geniuses,

but the presidents, the leaders, and the great entertainers. I presume most of the people in *Who's Who in America* would resent being called normal.[184]

Menninger found emotional distress, even if occasional, more normative than health.

Undeterred by stigma, Menninger operated with a personal sense of responsibly to attend to mental maladies, and he hoped to remove obstacles for others to do the same. Perhaps Christian hope in healing and redemption as ever-present possibilities drove his willingness to see things this way. From the days when he watched his mother's service to those in need, Menninger understood the power Christian faith and physical proximity could have in slashing social stigma in order to enable the perishing to be rescued.

Nonetheless, stigma deepened, and perhaps because the nation took its cues from Protestants. If Christians failed to attend to suffering, who could be expected to do so? With only sporadic Protestant involvement in caring for mental maladies in the first half of the twentieth century (and waning attention by the 1960s), believers, unlike Menninger, lacked the proximity to sufferers that would ease their own entrenched stigma. To be sure, because mental illness was prevalent in the population at large, chances are Christians did know those who suffered. They simply refrained from talking about mental distress—their own or that of family members—publically.

While Menninger found the "normality" defined by society dangerous, the same cannot be said of twentieth-century mainline Christians at large. Baseball, hot dogs, apple pie, and happy, well-adjusted, healthy Protestants proved normative in the 1950s, 1960s, and 1970s. Cultural normativity brought societal prestige and power, benefits that mainline believers relished. In the face of mental illness, the risk of being abnormal, and even the curse of "courtesy stigma" generated from committed advocacy for mentally ill Americans, proved obstacles too great for Protestants to climb.[185] Or, at least, most chose not to.

"BY THEIR FRUITS"

Menninger believed God called Christians to offer help in the face of suffering and evil. "By their fruits," he reflected, "ye shall know them."[186] He found not reacting sinful: "Caring. Relinquishing the sin of indifference. This recognizes acedia as the Great Sin; the heart of all sin. Some call it selfishness. Some call it alienation. Some call it schizophrenia. Some call it egocentricity. Some call it separation."[187] For few twentieth-century Protestants did the divine call to attend to mental illness seem as clear as to Menninger. While sure that medicine could remedy suffering, and confident of the work of physicians, the Kansas Presbyterian left the ultimate healing to God. "By the grace of God," he observed, and through help from caring physicians, "*most* psychiatric patients get well."[188] A realist, the doctor knew that sometimes healing would not arrive.

In 1965, after growing tensions with senior staff members, Karl Menninger was ousted as CEO of the Menninger Foundation. His brother William stepped into the lead role but died of cancer the following year. William's son Dr. Roy Menninger then took the reins of the family practice. Karl Menninger, while no longer atop the organizational chart, continued to be involved and exert influence on the foundation and in mental health care around the country. In 1975 *Time* described the then octogenarian as propelled by "encyclopedic knowledge, insatiable curiosity, moral strictures and unflagging energy."[189] Years later, a medical colleague painted Menninger as "brilliant" but also "quixotic, volatile, challenging, demanding, ruthless in the pursuit of truth. He was unaware of how hurtful he could be. And yet he was the mobilizer of great feelings of loyalty and admiration."[190] Menninger left an indelible mark and helped many. By the mid-1980s, *Family Circle* considered the Menninger Clinic the nation's top psychiatric hospital, and the American Psychiatric Association named Menninger "America's greatest living psychiatrist." He served as the face of the new public psychiatry but also as a representative mainline Protestant in his desire to serve and his willingness to blend the secular with the sacred to achieve the desired ends.

Protestant responses to mental maladies had evolved as the century progressed. In the 1940s and 1950s, rooted in early twentieth-century Social Gospel influences, believers called for church support for, and cooperation with, emerging organizations (often secular) that sought to care for those with mental illnesses. They understood God at work providing care through the church and the medical establishment. By the 1960s, though, believers adopted a more reflective tone and lost their prescriptive call-to-action in the world. They continued to hope that the afflicted would find comfort amidst suffering, if not in the church, then through secular providers. Mental illness, however, was simply one form of suffering among many, and despite the focus of those like Menninger, it failed to spark dedicated efforts at amelioration as it had in the past. Other pressing social concerns—including communism, the Cold War, threat of nuclear war, and civil rights—occupied Protestant agendas.

Centuries earlier, the colonial clergyman Cotton Mather had assumed that sickness was part of life and a reality that prompted believers to turn toward God. When they fell ill, twentieth-century believers turned first to medical professionals. The Revolutionary-era physician Benjamin Rush hoped that science would enable healing. In some ways, he was right, but, as more professionals grasped for authority, and as cures for mental maladies remained elusive, providers squabbled with each other as much as they attended to patients. The reformer Dorothea Dix hoped that establishing solid, caring institutions would ease suffering, but, within decades of her death, mental hospitals looked more like the places she hoped to reform than her vision of redemptive facilities. The early twentieth-century sufferer Anton Boisen saw a way forward in affirming experiences of mental illness as useful and therapeutic, and while some adopted his approach, his hope for a leadership role for clergy and the church failed to materialize. Likely, Mather, Rush, Dix, and Boisen would have been dismayed by the suffering that persisted for those living with mental illnesses, even if they would have commended Menninger's life work.

On July 18, 1990, Menninger died of cancer in Topeka. With his death, hope disappeared for a unifying figure for Christian action in the face of mental illness. Perhaps no one individual could have effected large-scale change or navigated the diverse theological landscape to do so. As early as 1948, the journalist Albert Deutsch had declared that "the day of the individual crusader [on behalf of mentally sick Americans] is over." "Our time," he stressed, "calls for organized, persistent effort in behalf of desired social change."[191] Many Protestants concurred, but few lasting efforts to do so prevailed.

The closing sentences of Menninger's *The Human Mind* included his hope that "surely there is a balm in Gilead." Taken from the lines of an American spiritual, it reflected the doctor's confidence that healing would come, whether through science or from God. Within the nation's twentieth-century Protestant congregations, those living with mental illnesses may have been more comfortable with this Old Testament formulation: "Is there no balm in Gilead? Is there no physician there? Why then has the health of my poor people not been restored?" (Jeremiah 8:22). Despite Menninger's efforts, many remained ill, with comfort provided only infrequently by Protestant churches. Many, however, continued to long for healing.

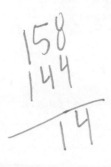

Conclusion

Suffering, Stigma, and Hospitality

> Only a community that is pledged not to fear the stranger—
> and illness always makes us a stranger to ourselves and others—
> can welcome the continued presence of the ill in our midst.
>
> —Stanley Hauerwas, 1986[1]

INTRODUCTION

Hope for healing formed a consistent theme in Christianity. Despite inattention by most believers, a few Protestants attended to mental illness and affirmed a sense of divine call to attend to those in need. Theological beliefs and practical considerations shaped responses as churchgoers wondered why mental illnesses existed, how Christians should engage, and who bore responsibility for responding.[2]

American Protestants offered an array of reasons for the presence of mental illness, often appealing to multiple explanations simultaneously. Rarely did the presence of mental illness surprise churchgoers—they accepted sickness as part of what it meant to be human and finite. Under continual debate was whether mental illness was a physical, spiritual, social, or moral problem, or some combination thereof. Believers pointed to sin—original or personal, corporate or individual—as the culprit of all illness, including mental disorders. A few even insisted on direct links between individual behavior and mental maladies. Suspicions of demonic possession and illness as divine punishment appeared, but, in America, those explanations diminished as the centuries progressed.

Believers pinned illness on individual and social failures. Persistent mental illness prompted suspicions of personal culpability. Women and men who refused to abandon willful wrongdoing, moral laxity, and deviant behaviors (like homosexuality or masturbation) perpetuated illness.[3] Resisting treatment brought condemnation from fellow believers, but churchgoers also faulted secular and ecclesial institutions for providing inadequate care. An increasingly complex society made mental distress inevitable, especially for populations deemed vulnerable to illness, including minorities, immigrants, the poor, and women. American Protestants diagnosed individuals, society, and sometimes both as sick and in need of treatment.

Churchgoers explored the proper location and method of treatment. Healing efforts emerged in congregations and church-sponsored facilities, but Protestants also affirmed a role for state-run and private institutions, particularly for more acute cases. Confession of sinful behavior and intercessory prayers offered on behalf of sufferers supplemented medical care. Preventative measures, like early twentieth-century mental hygiene initiatives, also attracted Protestant attention. Regardless of treatment locations or approaches, Christians hoped to bring relief from suffering and enable cures.

Believers professed confidence in both human and divine agency in healing, although inclinations about who should lead caregiving efforts differed. Spiritual care seemed within the purview of clergy, but laity, asserting their place in the priesthood of all believers, identified ways to help. Serving at hospitals as chaplains, mental health professionals, and volunteer caregivers fulfilled a sense of Christian duty. Alongside lay involvement, both clergy and physicians claimed authority in the diagnosis and care of mental distress, but the formalization of scientific medical care brought tensions. Cooperation between religious and medical professionals appeared a logical harnessing of God-given resources to mainline Protestants, but, for some physicians (and more conservative Christians), religion and medicine formed necessarily independent spheres.[4] Ultimately, sickness and health were under God's control, but churchgoers assumed that humans, as servants of Christ, worked cooperatively to ensure both health and healing.[5]

Christian beliefs and social realities—including the state of medicine, the availability of institutional care, and negative media portrayals of insanity—determined individual Protestant responses to mental illness. Cotton Mather, Benjamin Rush, Dorothea Dix, Anton Boisen, and Karl Menninger reacted in ways rooted in their theological convictions, professional opinions, and social locations. Only Mather and Boisen were formally trained theologians, but each figure deployed formal and practical theological insight in their responses. While the five pursued different paths to bring healing, mitigating suffering remained their central concern.

As they labored, Mather, Rush, Dix, Boisen, and Menninger sought to discern God's leading, and such promptings formed a core Christian impulse. Following the example and command of Christ, in the face of illness and suffering believers felt confident in Christianity's healing power, and they envisioned roles they could take to diminish distress. Nonetheless, despite centuries of thought and practice, no normative Christian responses to mental illness emerged. The chronic nature of mental illness, the elusiveness of cures, the power of secular medicine, and the entrenchment of social stigma thwarted the standardization of Christian reactions.[6]

By the early twenty-first century, little evidence appeared that Protestant churchgoers spent time figuring out how to offer care or seek cures for mental illness. Initiatives appeared, but mental illness failed to top congregational agendas. Beyond attendance at weekly worship services, activities like Sunday schools, vacation Bible schools, youth groups, work with local social service agencies for the homeless, and short-term mission trips were more likely to occupy parishioner attention. In contrast to attempts to ameliorate the suffering of mentally ill parishioners and community members, other activities proved easier to plan and recruit volunteers for; they were also less fraught with complexity and stigma.[7]

THE MODERN CONTEXT

Yet, for Christians, suffering demands a response. The centuries inhabited by Mather, Rush, Dix, Boisen, and Menninger offer insight for ongoing conversation about mental illness and the possibility of reshaping Christian responses to mental distress.

The Christian practice of hospitality serves as an antidote for Protestant paralysis in the face of mental illness.[8] Joining theological reflection to insight into past and present Christian practice, a practical theology attends to human responses to suffering, given God's redemptive mission in creation, and aims to enable Christian action in the face of mental illness that has been disabled by social stigma and the abdication of care to scientific medicine.[9] For congregations, the practice of hospitality precipitates the relief of suffering by encouraging churchgoers to ask "what?" and "what now?" instead of focusing on "why?"[10]

Whether or not twenty-first-century believers respond to mental illness, mental distress remains prevalent and affects many inside and outside of sanctuary walls. Navigating mental illness troubles sufferers and bewilders family members, congregations, and clergy. Though each experience of mental distress is unique, common themes surface: the pain and discomfort of illness, isolation, sadness, exhaustion, reluctance fully to voice the nature of ailments, and a desire for care. The relationships within faith communities for those who suffer and their families remain deeply ambiguous. Men and women affected by mental illnesses long for God's presence and the comfort of fellow church members, but distress rarely prompts the provision of casseroles, public intercessory prayers, or spiritual care as quickly as do other ailments, if at all. Fear, stigma, and aversion shape—and often inhibit— reactions that witness to hope and offer healing.

SUFFERING AND THEOLOGY

Mental illnesses bring suffering in many ways. Unwanted symptoms include stifling depression, crippling anxiety, and frightening delusions. With medical attention, symptoms sometimes yield formal diagnoses like chronic depression, obsessive-compulsive disorder, or schizoaffective disorder, and receiving a diagnosis focuses treatment efforts. Pharmaceuticals relieve symptoms, but they also bring unpleasant side effects. Diagnoses may feel reductive instead of helpful. Receiving a diagnostic label brings further distress, as sufferers are labeled "a schizophrenic," "a manic depressive," or "crazy." Medical diagnosis can make those who ail feel as if they handed over the ability to define their own experience of suffering to physicians.[11] Even productive medical care proves complex—diagnosis and care remain far from an exact science, and inherent flexibility and ambiguity in treatment protocols sometimes exacerbate suffering.[12]

Suffering, though, proves deeper than frightening symptoms and diagnostic complexity. Because treatments are not always available or utilized, and because in many cases cures prove elusive, many who suffer face chronic distress. Not only do sufferers despair, but family members and friends also find themselves weary and at a loss for ways to help. Sometimes, loved ones exhaust their ability to care and sever ties with those in need of help to maintain their own health or safety. Disease causes discomfort and disorientation, but estrangement and isolation deepen that distress. And, for sufferers, the prospect of chronic affliction can disable hope and disrupt a sense of connection to family, friends, and God. Mental illness casts doubts on a meaningful existence. Suffering, including mental illness, disrupts a sense of the rightness of the created order and one's place within it; much suffering seems inexplicable.[13] Mental illness can cast adrift those who suffer, in visible and invisible ways.

Severe mental distress presents existential difficulties, and for Christians it also prompts theological reflection. A core set of claims sparks theological inquiry and offers insight in the face of suffering. Christians profess the presence and name creation as good, creation is not perfect, and suffering is to be expected. This "shadow side" of creation includes the "finite, limited, and vulnerable" realities of human life and assumes that "challenge, risk, and growth are part of creaturely existence as intended by God."[15] Inherently, even if paradoxically, creation, including human existence, is simultaneously good yet imperfect and finite.[16]

Christians also hold that though sin brought (and continues to bring) brokenness—and thus suffering—into the world, God through Christ entered the world to bring healing and redemption. Suffering proves part of human reality, but Christians refuse to concede that it has the final word. Through the incarnation, Christ entered into and overcame human suffering, for and with creation. The healing brought by God in Christ takes many forms and occurs both in the present and in the world to come.

Finally, an understanding of divine creation assumes the interconnectedness of all of creation.[17] With or without brokenness and suffering, God created humans to stand in relationship with God as Father, Son, and Spirit, and with one another. Divine and human interdependence grounds Christian identity and calls Christians to work for the wholeness and flourishing of one another.[18]

It seems, then, that distress, like that stemming from mental illness, would spark action. Christian doctrine affirms the goodness yet brokenness of creation, the hope that suffering does not have the final word, and the promise of facing distress as a community, but, in the face of suffering associated with mental illness, believers often fail to act as if those assertions are true. Given the scripturally based understanding of a call to love God and neighbor and to continue the healing and caring work of Christ, the inability to attend to the suffering caused by mental illnesses seems curious. It might also be labeled unfaithful or sinful—whether a sin of omission or commission.[19] Belief and practice appear incongruent, in large part, because the logic of social stigma vies for attention with—and often overpowers—theological convictions and stymies action. Social norms and fears rooted in stereotypes trump Christian professions and, as a result, bring theological disorientation and distort practice.

THE POWER OF STIGMA

Because it undermines core theological claims, social stigma proves powerful, even within the walls of congregations that profess God's love and the promise of the redemption for all of creation. Christians, for example, often accept cultural definitions of created-ness and humanity—ones open to social stigma. Instead of theocentric or Christocentric logic, Christians are prone to deploy culturally shaped and anthropocentric logic. While Christian doctrine asserts that God created the world and named it good, Protestants ingest and adopt modern American social norms that indicate that only *some* of creation is good. Instead of biblical understandings that place all of creation in relationship with God and name creation as good, albeit finite, cultural definitions of created-ness name the potential for economic productivity as the primary designation of human value to society. Some parts of creation, including those living with mental illnesses, are deemed "diseased," "inferior," and "unproductive."[20]

Similarly, the logic of stigma resists the paradox of the good yet finite and limited nature of creation. Instead, it categorizes social realities and names conditions, events, and even some people as defective. Mental illness becomes an unwanted anomaly, something to be hidden, shunned, or avoided. While theology draws attention to God's saving work in the world in and through Christ, the logic of stigma asserts that humans are responsible for bringing change and ensuring salvation. The healing of human distress is presumed to rest on human effort alone, and medical professionals are invested with that responsibility. Finally, while Christian belief affirms the interconnection of all of creation, the logic of stigma dictates that men and women, as independent actors, hold individual responsibility for bearing suffering. God and faith communities, under those presumptions, have little help to offer.

In total, the logic of stigma declares those living with mental maladies as "other," "frightening," "dangerous," "unwelcome," and even "contagious" rather than as fellow children of God. Stigma clouds theological wisdom and misshapes Christian reaction to mental illness. However, awareness of the reach of stigma's tentacles brings conflicts between belief and practice to light, allowing a reconsideration of social stigma and theological claims that helps undergird a reshaping of Christian practice.[21]

Stigma theory helps describe the dynamics that enable stigma to overpower theological convictions and to interrupt the experience of God's love and the Christian call to care in the face of mental illness. As formulated by the sociologist Erving Goffman, stigma theory describes the construction of social identities and explores how stigma infuses human interactions.[22] Humans, living in societies, develop ways to understand themselves and others, and the construction of social identities enables this process. When meeting someone new, stereotypes ("normative expectations" of identity) help decipher and categorize who and what a person is. For example, a woman wearing a suit? She must be *a professional*. A young white man with dreadlocks? He must be *a free spirit*. A disheveled older man sleeping on a city park bench? He must be *a bum*. Stigma surfaces in human relationships when the attributes of an individual vary from what social norms tell us one "should" be. "While the stranger is present before us," Goffman observed, "evidence can arise of his possessing an attribute that makes him different from others in the category of persons available for him to be, *and of a less desirable kind*. . . . He is thus reduced in our minds from a whole and usual person to a tainted, discounted one."[23] Stigma introduces a wedge between one's "virtual social identity" (based on characteristics that a person is *assumed* to possess) and "actual social identity" (based on characteristics that a person *actually* possesses). Perceptions and reality often differ, and a human attribute triggers stigma when it is, in some way, "deeply discrediting" as the result of a preexisting stereotype held by others. As an example, consider a young man hospitalized after a call to the police from his congregation, where his behavior frightened fellow congregants one morning. If the hospital released him and he complied with his treatment plan, he might live a life free of symptoms of illness. Yet, based on their experience, fellow congregants continue to view him as erratic, unreliable, and potentially dangerous. The stigma of mental illness proves difficult to shake. Similarly, a veteran diagnosed with severe post-traumatic stress disorder might encounter resistance leading a church youth group, long after symptoms abate.

Stigma originates from a variety of sources, physical and nonphysical. In Goffman's system, attributes like missing limbs, facial deformities, and other very visible characteristics generate presumptions of "abominations of the body." In addition, "blemishes of the individual character" generate stigma when, for example, a "weak will" or "dishonesty" that is inferred from "a known record of, for example, mental disorder, imprisonment, [or] addiction" appears. Finally, racial, national, or religious affiliation can generate stigma.[24] Regardless of its origin and strength, stigma appears in contrast to what is considered "normal"; thus, stigma marks both normalcy and its alternative, "deviancy." For the stigmatized, including those living with mental health problems, this division between "normal" and "deviant" creates distance in social relationships as those who suffer are defined as "other" and "not like us." A mental illness visible through strange behavior, an unkempt appearance, or an unreliable presence, for example, marks the one who suffers as an undesirable person who is not to be welcomed into a church community rather than as a fellow congregant and child of God to be embraced.

For many stigmatizing attributes, the visibility of the trait determines its impact. Stigmatizing qualities may be visible and discrediting (i.e., readily apparent to all, such as race or physical deformity) or discreditable (i.e., hidden, but risking possible exposure, such as sexual orientation or mental illness). A man with a speech impediment (discrediting), for example, finds that strangers make assumptions about his intelligence and avoid conversation. A woman taking medication for clinical depression (discreditable) fears making this known, even to her closest friends. She may withhold this part of her identity from those around her, enabling her to "pass" as normal. Those suffering from mental illness, or those who have recovered from severe past mental distress, are often able to hide symptoms and treatments and limit knowledge of their past and present illness, and fear of the consequences of stigmatization prompts them to do so.[25] Often, shame, self-derogation, and self-hate follow decisions to hide illness and compound already painful experiences and conditions.[26]

Sometimes, however, symptoms are impossible to hide, and visible mental illness brings social consequences, as in the case of the young man who was hospitalized after strange behavior at church. Although the congregation's call to the authorities to remove him may have been appropriate for his protection and their own, church members likely foster a view of his ongoing danger to the group. In the future, whether or not his health warrants it, the young man may find himself unwelcome (or received coldly) in his community of faith.

Both visible and invisible attributes that prompt stigma deepen suffering. Invisible or hidden mental illnesses bring distress because they force sufferers to limit awareness of their plight.[27] A congregant who grieves alone following the death of her hospitalized brother because of her reluctance to share the details of his institutionalization demonstrates suffering generated from stigma-induced invisibility. In social situations, those who ail invisibly manage "undisclosed discrediting information" about themselves.[28] Hiding a potentially stigmatizing attribute requires effort (and sometimes careful planning), but it is an effort that those who ail and their families deem worthwhile.

Mental illnesses often remain hidden because "passing" for normal seems a path of least resistance.[29] Passing, though, poses tradeoffs. In the context of churches and mental illness, this means, for example, that sufferers present a public front that fails to match the reality of their experience. As a result of stigma, they choose to be known as less than fully themselves and hide their pain and desire for care.[30] The forces of stigma also convince those who suffer—or who are at risk of suffering—that the virtual social identities imposed by stigma are true. Through media portrayals and individual encounters, society tells those living with mental illness that they are "other," "useless," "dangerous," and "unwelcome," and sufferers begin to believe those messages. If churches, populated by the people of God, confirm those beliefs, sufferers wonder if God feels the same way.

For those with stigmatizing attributes, whether visible or invisible, not every location in society poses the same difficulties. *Out-of-bounds places*, where stigmatized people are forbidden, are locations where "exposure means expulsion." In the segregated Jim Crow era, for example, an African American woman who "passed" for white might be able to eat a meal at a southern restaurant, but only by concealing her ancestry; otherwise, the establishment would be out-of-bounds. *Civil places* are those where stigmatized individuals are "carefully, and sometimes painfully, treated as if they were not disqualified for routine acceptance, when in fact they somewhat are." A homeless man recently released from a state mental institution who arrives at worship at a prosperous suburban church might find a civil reception, but not a warm one. Finally, *back places* are locations where individuals need not conceal their stigmatizing attributes. *Back places* can be experienced involuntarily (institutionalized mental patients gathering for group therapy) or created voluntarily (recovering addicts gathering for a Narcotics Anonymous meeting at a local church).[31] Stigma shapes reception in each type of setting.

For those with mental illnesses, modern Protestant congregations often operate as *civil places*, places where those who suffer are not completely excluded but where stigma causes them (and their families) to navigate communal life carefully. Many conceal illnesses, pain, and the desire for spiritual, emotional, and physical care. When those living with mental illnesses hide their symptoms in order to belong in congregations, or when Christians deem—consciously or unconsciously—that mental illness is too difficult, complex, or dangerous for church help, stigma negatively forms, or completely inhibits, faithful Christian practice.

Congregations, however, engage and reshape distorted practice by acknowledging social stigma and norms, by noticing how they vary from theological claims, and by choosing to take action, even at the risk of being labeled culturally nonnormative. Churches, instead of perpetuating negative effects of social stigma, can choose to subject themselves to potential stigma, albeit of a different sort than that generated by mental illness.[32] In this way, congregations come to view religious stigmatization as evidence of faithful practice. Because religious people sometimes respond to situations in culturally nonnormative ways, religious affiliation and practice can generate stigma. During World Wars I and II, for example, thousands of pacifist Quakers and Mennonites refused military service. Some Americans stigmatized those conscientious objectors as unpatriotic, untrustworthy, and subversive.

Social stigma marks some as deviant and others as normal, but other social positions exist. Those who are free from stigma ("normals") take on the role of "sympathetic others" when in the presence of a stigmatized individual they "are ready to adopt his standpoint in the world and to share with him the feeling that he is human and 'essentially' normal in spite of appearances."[33] At times, sympathetic others share the stigmatizing attribute (fellow patients in a mental hospital), but they can also be outsiders (fellow congregants or close friends and family members of sufferers). Sympathetic others understand the plight of the afflicted. Further, sympathetic others who deepen their knowledge of the plight of the stigmatized become "wise." In relationship with "wise" contacts, "the individual with a fault need feel no shame nor exert self-control, knowing that in spite of his failing he will be seen as an ordinary other."[34] Sympathetic others gain this wisdom in a variety of ways. Some work "in an establishment which caters either to the wants of those with a particular stigma or to actions that society takes in regard to those persons" (a nurse or chaplain at a state mental hospital). Others are "related through the social structure to a stigmatized individual—a relationship that leads the wider society to treat both individuals in some respects as one. . . . The loyal spouse of the mental patient, the daughter of the ex-con, the parent of the cripple, the friend of the blind, the family of the hangman, are all obliged to share some of the discredit of the stigmatized person to whom they are related."[35] By sharing discredit—willingly or unwillingly— such individuals garner "courtesy stigma," a sort of guilt by association.

Following the witness of Christ, Christians, when identifying mental illnesses and other forms of suffering and injustice, are called to be wise, sympathetic others—aware of, but unconcerned about, the infliction of "courtesy stigma."[36] In the face of being stigmatized by association, congregations prove reluctant to risk care for those suffering from mental illness, and a natural impulse for many in the face of such stigma is to reduce potential social tensions by adopting more normative behavior. Making such adjustments, though, reduces the coherence between belief and practice, between theological convictions and resulting actions. However, to mitigate the suffering stemming from mental illnesses, congregations, like members of early twentieth-century peace churches, could choose to embrace a position of social difference, even if such a stance garnered stigma for church members.[37] Reorienting their perspective, Christians understand they are called to be a stigmatized people: to resist social norms contrary to Christian belief and practice, to eat with outcasts and tax collectors, with sinners, and with those who ail, and to remember that Christian identity is defined by baptism into the body of Christ, not by adherence (or lack of adherence) to social norms.[38]

Those society sees as "other" or "outcast," Christians claim as brother and sister, rejecting characterizations imposed by social stigma.

From the colonial era forward, those working most actively to enable care for those suffering from mental illnesses prioritized ameliorative work over avoidance of social stigma. Religious conviction, for example, prompted Dorothea Dix to transgress social norms for women in order to crusade on the public stage for adequate care. Anton Boisen fought for a role for pastoral care in the mental health system, even at the risk of exposing his own illness. Karl Menninger cast his vocational lot among deeply stigmatized patients, in what had come to be considered a nonpremiere medical field. Individuals like Dix, Rush, and Menninger took action, and the adoption of similar faithful, countercultural positions for modern-day communities of faith would serve as a reminder of their role in participating in God's mission in the world. Christians possess the resources and the power not only to reshape their practices but also to alter views of those around in their midst. Doing so, however, takes conscious effort and risks consequences.

Whether or not churchgoers endure courtesy stigma based on their responses to mental illness, they have a role to play in relationship with those stigmatized. Christian life calls for a willingness to engage with those in need, even those labeled by society as "other." Rarely do Christian congregations seek to *cure* illness; rather they hope to bring themselves and those who suffer into closer relationship with God and one another and to be a people who willingly enter into the suffering of one another. Christian doctrine acknowledges suffering as a universal experience. While the world offers different scripts, Christians remember that where suffering exists—*especially* where suffering exists—Christ remains in relationship with us. When the world deems those with mental illness as frightening, unproductive, unwelcome, and "other," Christians embrace them as suffering, frustrated, welcome, and "just like us." Being damned by association should be an expected part of Christian witness, but it is a reality difficult to embrace in a society, like modern America, where a safer, more sanitized Christian belief and practice are deemed normative.

RESHAPING CHRISTIAN PRACTICE

Mental illness causes suffering. Stigma exacerbates suffering. Christians deem suffering problematic but sometimes fail to respond.[39] For many Christians, suffering prompts both theological reflection and action, but not always. The forces of stigma that stymie the provision of much-desired care prove powerful in church life, and as a result, belief and practice do not always align. How should individual believers and congregations seeking to repair this breach, proceed? What theological considerations offer guidance?

While powerful, the forces of stigma can be averted and congregational practice reshaped. Even in light of stigma's pervasive power in forming social identities and social relationships, "purposeful social action" changes how stigma operates.[40] Framing reaction in light of congregational practice reasserts a role Christians are called to fill amidst suffering, one that is neither completely dependent on nor fully independent of secular medical care and one that recognizes that when a member in the community suffers, all suffer.

Identifying a hope or an end point—a telos—that reflects Christian beliefs will help reorient Christian practice and supplement the insight gained from exploring the dynamics of stigma and claiming a role for Christians among the stigmatized. Beginning to dismantle, or work around, the power of stigma calls for an alternate telos to the normative societal claim that humanity is good only when useful or productive. A more adequate telos will not exclude from understandings of God's good creation those who suffer, will allow for more faithful attention to suffering, and will help belief and practice align.

Christian attention to suffering hopes to alleviate distress and bring healing, and as congregations think theologically about health, a productive goal of Christian practice appears. Health can be viewed, simply, as the absence of disease.[41] But understandings of health vary by time and social situation, and given that subjectivity, if the goal of health is to be helpful in shaping the responses of Christian communities to suffering, then that understanding needs to be anchored beyond, or at least in addition to, medical and social conceptions. Christians hold that physical and emotional health, defined medically, is *a* good, but not the ultimate good.[42] If only medical notions of illness and health animate Christian responses, then the only solutions deemed appropriate are medical ones. Beyond working as medical professionals, Christians might see no role for themselves amidst the suffering that results from illness. The witnesses of Jesus and the broader Christian tradition offer—and require—more. As an alternative, if believers view health not as the absence of disease but as human flourishing (as defined through relationship with the Triune God and one another), then health may be present (and worked toward) even in the presence of illness.[43]

A fundamental feature of the suffering stemming from mental illness is that it disconnects the believer from others and from confidence in God's presence. A more theologically adequate understanding of health and healing, then, is the ability of humans to live in relationship—in communion—with the Triune God and with one other, to live as they are created to live.

Along these lines, John Swinton's definition of mental health as "the strength to live as a human being, the strength to maintain holistic relationships with God, self and creation, the strength to continue moving towards the restoration of the *imago Dei* irrespective of one's circumstances" proves useful.[44] Mental health understood theologically, Swinton argues, has little to do with the absence of disease diagnosis. Instead, health is the restoration of the image of God (the *imago Dei*) in those who suffer—both by those who ail and by those around them.

Central to the *imago Dei* that animates Swinton's proposal is an understanding of the mutual relationship (the perichoretic relationality) of the Trinity. Father, Son, and Holy Spirit exist in ongoing relationship and unity, similar to creation's ongoing relationship with the Triune God. As a result of that focus on the relational nature of the image of God, mental health, Swinton declares, "is a communal process" that "is the work of the whole people of God as they struggle to participate faithfully in God's continuing redemptive mission in and to the world." Suffering calls for action on behalf of all. Working toward mental health "has as much to do with the building of a community which can absorb pain and difference and grow in spite (or because) of it, as it has with the eradication of individual ailments."[45] With a theologically grounded understanding of health—rooted in cultivating divine and human relationship—Christians reorient their practice to achieve those ends (that telos).

Christian practices, including the practice of hospitality, are ongoing, transformative activities. The theologian Michael Warren calls on congregations to be both "communities of interpretation" and "zones of cultural contestation." Communities, as they search for faithfulness in practice, are reminded of their distance from their telos through reflection on sacred texts and the text that is the congregation itself. Warren argues that "those in a Spirit-resonant community are meant to develop a perceptive system attuned to the gospel the way a parent of an infant can be so physically tuned" to his or her child in times of need.[46] Communities of interpretation sense— consciously or unconsciously—suffering in need of redress. The challenge for congregations is to bring suffering to consciousness and then to explore means of healing, even if it risks challenging cultural norms. By doing so, congregations more fully become places of redemption and healing for all involved.

Theological reflection triggers not just intellectual but embodied responses. Cotton Mather, Benjamin Rush, Dorothea Dix, Anton Boisen, and Karl Menninger devoted energies to the provision of care for mental illness, and their work yielded lasting results. Yet, their dedicated efforts failed to refashion congregational practice, despite ongoing suffering. For congregations, hospitality constitutes a fitting embodied action in the face of the suffering and stigma generated by mental illnesses.[47] The practice of hospitality serves as a remedy to limited collective Protestant reaction by countering stigma and clearing the way for more attentive care in the face of suffering.

In their own, noncongregational, spheres of influence, each of the historical figures profiled advocated for a sort of hospitality for mental illness and those suffering from it. Mather's writing reflected a theological hospitality toward the topics of madness and melancholy. Rush made scientific medicine hospitable to mental ailments. The asylums Dix helped launch and expand provided institutional hospitality. Boisen hoped medicine would yield a sort of professional hospitality to religious ministrations. Menninger fought for hospitality both for sufferers in the world at large and for the discipline of psychiatry (within medicine and with the public). None of the figures, however, focused on how congregations received and attended to sufferers.

Intentional, theologically reflective hospitality within congregations witnesses to the love of God and incorporates both care providers and care receivers into God's ongoing, redemptive work in the world. Christian hospitality enables that work of healing. Offering such hospitality, however, requires an ethic that is, in many ways, countercultural, and rightly so. Stigma stems from societal norms that often differ from the divine intention for God's creation to be in relationship with God and fellow believers.

Despite the best efforts of those like Mather, Rush, Dix, Boisen, and Menninger, the provision of care for mental illness failed to form a central part of congregational life. Christian communities, however, need not wait for a theological beacon or noteworthy crusader to remedy the lack of attention. Instead, heeding a call to counter entrenched stigma through the provision of deep hospitality offers a way to continue their legacy.[48]

PRACTICING HOSPITALITY

> Contribute to the needs of the saints; extend hospitality to strangers.
>
> —Romans 12:13

Varieties of congregational practices appear in response to the suffering that stems from mental illness, including the provision of pastoral care, friendship, and worship services that acknowledge distress.[49] Affirming the value of such endeavors, the practice of hospitality subsumes those activities and offers a fuller response. Hospitality offers solidarity both *for* and *with* the one who suffers. In order to combat the forces of stigma, it draws together the work of the whole community, not just clergy or individual members of the church body. Hospitality orients the full life of the community, not simply liturgical or caregiving practices. In addition, hospitality connects theology and practice in order to help remedy the distance between belief and practice that persists in the face of mental illnesses.[50]

Often, twentieth-century Protestants think of hospitality as a secular activity as much as a Christian practice. Hospitality involves welcoming friends and not strangers. Hospitality is paid for (at distant resorts, hotels, and restaurants) and is not the gracious gift of care to those in need nearby. The hospitality of strangers is required only by those who are "weak" or "needy" and not by those merely journeying through difficulty.

Christian hospitality at the most basic level is the welcoming of strangers.[51] It is more, however, than a detached provision of care or nourishment. Hospitality is both the receiving of a stranger and a posture toward others.[52] Much more than a well-planned social hour with coffee and sweets following a Sunday worship service, Christian hospitality draws together guests and hosts into relationships of mutuality with one other and with God in Christ. In that way, Christian hospitality is "potentially subversive and countercultural."[53] A reclaiming of that sort of traditional hospitality, hospitality that defies social norms, thwarts the force of social stigma that shapes reactions to mental illness.

Theologian Letty Russell declares Christian hospitality "the practice of God's welcome embodied in our actions as we reach across difference to participate with God in bringing justice and healing to our world in crisis."[54] Russell makes clear that hospitality is the work of God, carried out by God's people. That work of God takes place through the people by the power of the Holy Spirit. Hospitality is the "witness to God's intention to mend" creation.[55] To those made "different" or "strange" by crises like suffering, hospitality offers healing and restores justice. In addition, hospitality, as a theologically informed practice, is more than a one-way action aimed at someone in need; those who offer hospitality also receive it, and often in unanticipated ways. Both the impetus and immediate goal of hospitality are rooted in the temporal, in the hope for healing in the present. A vision of future healing, of eschatological wholeness, however, frames the practice.[56]

Hospitality has long animated Christian life. Scripture witnesses to the importance of both the divine and the human provisions of hospitality and portrays hospitality as gracious, lifesaving, life giving, and abundant, with both physical and spiritual dimensions.[57] "Images of God as gracious and generous host"—providing manna, shelter, and protection—"pervade the biblical" record.[58] God appeared as host but also, as the Genesis 18 account of God's appearance to Abraham by the Oaks of Mamre shows, as a worthy guest. With Old Testament accounts as a backdrop, Christ's life and ministry anchor the witness of Christian hospitality.[59] Jesus both offered and received hospitality, cementing the practice as one of giving and receiving. Following the witness of Jesus, the apostle Paul "urged fellow Christians to welcome one another as Christ had welcomed them," and "early Christian writers claimed that transcending social and ethnic differences by sharing meals, homes, and worship with persons of different backgrounds was a proof of the truth of the Christian faith." Hospitality in the early church encompassed "physical, social, and spiritual dimensions of human existence and relationships." It both met physical needs and "recognized" the "worth and common humanity" of all encountered.[60] Early Christian provisions of hospitality were personal and direct, but eventually care for strangers became more distant and anonymous.[61]

Hospitality as a Christian practice is a human endeavor that happens in relationship with God and others. It is an ongoing practice, not an isolated event.[62] Christian practices are integrated with belief and imbedded in a community—they rely on the truth proclamation of the community and form a social endeavor. That social nature proves critical for the practice of Christian hospitality to combat stigma generated by social norms.[63] To be sure, congregations offer hospitality imperfectly. But, even though human efforts rarely lead to perfect execution, practices prove viable and useful in the life of communities.[64]

Practice—Christian practice—calls for ongoing participation and consideration of activity and aims. The Christian practice of hospitality seeks to enfold both guest and host into the life of the Triune God, and it does so through acts of welcome, compassion, incorporation, and patience. The discussion of each of these four elements of hospitality below includes a sense of what hospitality requires and what it counters and examples of the shape it takes in congregations attentive to suffering caused by mental illness. These categories offer a glimpse of a reshaping of Christian practice.

WELCOME

> For I was hungry and you gave me food, I was thirsty and you gave
> me something to drink, I was a stranger and you welcomed me.
>
> —Matthew 25:35

Welcome forms the first element of the practice of hospitality. Welcome assumes that there are hosts and guests, both insiders and outsiders. It requires that those who host, those on the inside, signal to outsiders that they are free to join, and not only free, but desired and wanted guests. Hosts exert the primary effort of welcome, but hospitality also requires the willingness of the outsider to embrace the invitation to enter. The willingness to respond to an invitation of welcome requires a leap of faith or a bit of risk taking on the part of the one who has been invited.[65]

The practice of welcome, as part of Christian hospitality, is rooted in recognition of God's welcome and a sense that "God values all creatures whether or not we consider them useful" or "like us."[66] The act of welcome involves hope that outsiders will receive the invitation, but welcome does not require reciprocity.[67] Nor does welcome require assimilation or a need for guests to take on the characteristics of their hosts. Though contact risks deepened stigmatization, outsiders are welcomed to be present, to be included, just as they are. For outsiders and insiders to come together through welcome requires openness to what is strange and different on the part of both host and guest. Often, this means the host must initiate contact (or signal availability) across boundaries, whether physical or social.[68] Welcoming involves risks on the part of the host too, perhaps of having to set limits for involvement for sufferers who in the past have proven a danger to themselves or others, but caution, and not inaction, should prevail. The act of welcome counters experiences of exclusion and debunks notions that the church is an "out of bounds place" where the stigmatized may not enter. Welcome also counters past experiences of rejection and limitation. Finally, welcome counters isolation, signaling to the "other" that as fellow children of God, they are worthy of welcome.

In light of mental illnesses, acts of welcome take the form of extending invitations to those, outside of the church, who suffer. Congregations might host meetings of mental illness advocacy organizations and support groups like the National Alliance on Mental Illness. Welcome also includes opening spaces for those already part of the church community to be present more visibly with their joys and their concerns, including suffering stemming from mental illness, perhaps in the form of spiritual care provided in group settings or in one-on-one conversations. Because stigma carries risks for sufferers and causes reluctance to share experiences of suffering broadly, welcome need not require those who suffer to make their ailments known throughout the full congregation.

COMPASSION

> You shall also love the stranger, for you were strangers in the land of Egypt.
>
> —Deuteronomy 10:19

Welcome brings together insiders and outsiders, hosts and guests, but a more complete practice of hospitality also includes compassion. As God in Christ

entered the world to suffer (and rejoice) with and for humanity, congregations suffer (and rejoice) with one another. Compassion "is a visceral response
to the suffering of another" that "moves us to want to do something in
response." Christian compassion, though, need not (and perhaps should not)
have the cessation of suffering as its lone goal.[69] Rather, compassion calls for
the creation of safe space—physical and emotional—for the brave and honest
telling of stories of pain, suffering, and joy. When believers enter into the
suffering of another, "by suffering-with (*mit-leiden*) the alienated other, the
healer establishes a community that transcends the form of community from
which the sufferer became alienated in the illness experience."[70] In doing so,
compassion dissolves the classifications of "us" and "them." In place is the
formation of a "we" who encounter life side by side.

That willingness to listen, to try to understand the experience of pain
and suffering with another, requires a commitment that the other is worth
listening to and a sense that all are part of the same story, God's story. Goffman argued that "normals" (those not stigmatized) sometimes "believe the
person with a stigma is not quite human."[71] Similarly, Swinton observes that
"in the minds of the media and the general public, people with mental health
problems frequently 'cease being persons.' Instead they become identified by
their pathologies—'schizophrenics,' or 'manic depressives,' . . . terms that
substitute their primary identity as human beings made in God's image and
passionately loved by God, for a socially constructed way of being" that then
shapes their self-understanding and relationships.[72] Such views are acknowledged but set aside when compassionate listening takes place.

Compassion also requires a theological understanding of humanity that
accommodates finiteness. Through the work of Enlightenment thinkers like
Descartes (cogito, ergo sum—"I think, therefore I am"), Locke, Hume, and
Kant, "to be human came to be identified with the ability to doubt, to think,
and then to will."[73] Such views left those living with mental disease or disability, those whose brains seemed to function deficiently, suspected to be less
than fully human. An alternate anthropology, rooted in a sense of shared and
interdependent created-ness, proves more faithful by resisting cultural proc-
lamations of the value of humanity rooted only in productive achievement.
Compassion requires that primary human identities are centered in God's
baptismal covenant through Christ, not in medically driven definitions of
health, economic productivity, or cultural normativity.

For those living with mental illnesses and facing stigma, the work of
compassion combats silence, shame, and the necessity of remaining hidden.
Compassion helps displace a sense of defective humanity and restores to the
community the voices of those who suffer. By providing an environment for

sufferers to voice their pain as part of the full community's suffering, compassion also combats the fear of exposure.

Attentive to the realities of suffering, compassion includes the provision of casseroles during periods of acute illness—of the tending to physical needs in times of hardship. Compassion also takes the shape of friendship or formal caregiving ministries such as Stephen Ministry.[74] Similarly, outside of the congregation, compassion involves offering spiritual care in hospitals that treat those with mental illnesses. In any setting, compassion includes the incorporation of practices of communal lament for suffering.[75] Finally, healing services or other liturgical practices that recognize sickness and provide assurance of healing in public settings demonstrate compassion.[76]

INCORPORATION

> So then you are no longer strangers and aliens, but you are citizens
> with the saints and also members of the household of God.
>
> —Ephesians 2:19

Welcoming others and offering compassion are first steps in the practice of hospitality. Those considered strangers, however, must not simply be brought into the fellowship of believers; hospitality calls for them to be incorporated as full members. To the extent that welcome and compassion offer solidarity *for* the one who suffers, incorporation involves solidarity *with* and full mutuality between guest and host. In that sense, incorporation moves beyond mere inclusion or tolerance, each of which signal joint physical presence but not necessarily mutual participation. The incorporation Christian hospitality offers is mindful that guest and host are incorporated not just into human fellowship but also in the ongoing narrative and life of the people of God.

Incorporation reinforces the dissolution of divisions between "us" and "them," focusing instead on the whole community as one. Incorporation also requires awareness that both guest and host are changed by their encounter.[77] At the same time that the afflicted find relief from their suffering and stigmatization, others find freedom in being able to more fully acknowledge their own limitations and finiteness.

By grounding identity in membership among the people of God, incorporation counters the loss of identity and yearning for belonging that can accompany mental illness. Incorporation mitigates the church's propensity to exist as a "civil place" where some only seem welcome. At the same time, incorporation requires confidence that diversity will not dissolve the community. To be sure, incorporation as part of hospitality requires risk taking. Both hosts and guest must be willing to subordinate their differences as they live and work side by side as members of the body of Christ. Because Christian unity is grounded in the Triune God, that divine mutuality offers a model for human community.

Congregationally, incorporation takes many forms. Participating in one of the oldest traditions of Christian hospitality, eating together, literally brings individuals to the table to share in sustenance and fellowship.[78] Shared meals reach across the social boundaries established by stigma and, with ongoing practice, begin to dissolve those forces that both deepen suffering and inhibit caregiving. Liturgically, baptism and Eucharist signal the enfolding of believers into God's creation.[79] Worship services name all who gather—not just those whose suffering is known—as new creations in Christ. Finally, incorporation includes making room for those who suffer in the broader life and ministry of the congregation as teachers, caregivers, and leaders, even when mental illness makes those who suffer able to participate only sporadically.

PATIENCE

> Do not neglect to show hospitality to strangers, for by doing
> that some have entertained angels without knowing it.
>
> —Hebrews 13:2

Finally, in addition to welcome, compassion, and incorporation, Christian hospitality requires patience. Given the chronic nature of mental illness and the elusiveness of cures, patience proves especially important.[80] Patience demands the courage to live in a tragic world and relies on fortitude that is sustained only in a community that understands that temporal suffering and tragedy do not have the final word. Patience amidst suffering proves possible with an eschatological view and a sense that while the life, death, and resurrection of Christ ushered in the kingdom of God, it has yet to arrive fully. Amidst pain, patience allows communities to bear and absorb the suffering of one another, providing meaning in the face of meaninglessness through human and divine relationship.

Patience requires tolerance for unpredictability. It also calls for a sense of God's abundance amidst the world's alarm about scarce resources.[81] The gift of companionship proves unlimited. While complete healing may be only fully realized eschatologically, healing is experienced and witnessed to in the body of Christ. While prompted to pray for cures to be brought by God, Christians are also called to play a more active role in reliving the distress of those who suffer.[82]

The long view of patience counters despair and an absence of hope and meaning amidst suffering. Patience also counters the idolatrous view of medical technologies as the only solutions to suffering. While medicine and the forces of stigma seem to be in a hurry to categorize and classify conditions, diseases, and humans, Christian hospitality allows the gracious gift of time for guests and hosts to live into their roles of beloved followers of Christ instead of as merely the sick or stigmatized.

Christian patience involves determining, as a full community, how to let a sufferer return to worship, again and again, despite illness and frightening behavior. Patience involves the provision of casseroles for individuals and families, even after a fifth, or tenth, hospitalization. Despite the persistence of mental illness and notwithstanding the ongoing power of social stigma, Christian patience claims the luxury of time to continue to work to align practices and beliefs and to witness to the healing power of God in Christ.[83]

Hospitality transforms both individual lives and Christian communities. Christine Pohl reflects that a community that embodies

> hospitality to strangers "is a sign of contradiction, a place where joy and pain, crises and peace are closely interwoven." Friendships forged in hospitality contradict contemporary messages about who is valuable and "good to be with," who can "give life to others."[84]

Such communities offer the "gift of hope" that "nourishes, challenges, and transforms guests, hosts, and, sometimes, the larger community."[85] In the face of mental illnesses, such communities are ones that counter the forces of stigma and enfold those who suffer into the life of the community and into the life of God in Christ.[86]

THE SHAPE OF LIFE TOGETHER

Suffering stemming from mental illness calls Christian congregations into discussion of the shape of their life together in light of a loving and redeeming God. Churchgoers claim both solidarity with and solidarity for the suffering and the stigmatized, and hospitality—through acts of welcome, incorporation, patience, and compassion—opens that possibility. Through the sustained, face-to-face provision of hospitality, believers challenge their complicity in social interactions shaped by stigma, and they witness to alternatives. They also provide care beyond what the medical establishment offers. Hospitality makes companionship, comfort, and healing possible, and even small attempts at the practice of hospitality witness to the claim that all of humanity is good and worthy of the love of God and the love of the Christian community.

Mental illnesses present challenges, but they are not the only sort of suffering worth attending to. Through an ongoing investigation of the problems of mental illness and the transformations possible through the practice of hospitality, Christian communities may be more aware of both the invisibility of, and their responses to, distress of many types. Suffering not only demands redress, but it also enables the possibility of new thinking, thinking that sparks believers to respond in creative ways to overcome stigma and fear and become more faithful participants in the kingdom of God.

Notes

INTRODUCTION

1   "Mental Illness: Facts and Numbers," National Alliance on Mental Illness, http://www
    .nami.org/factsheets/mentalillness_factsheet.pdf (accessed July 16, 2014).
2   "Facts and Figures," American Foundation for Suicide Prevention, https://www.afsp
    .org/understanding-suicide/facts-and-figures (accessed October 27, 2014).
3   Donald Capps, *Fragile Connections: Memoirs of Mental Illness for Pastoral Care Profession-
    als* (Atlanta: Chalice, 2005), 6.
4   "20 to 25% of the homeless population in the United States suffers from some form of
    severe mental illness. In comparison, only 6% of Americans are severely mentally ill. . . .
    In a 2008 survey performed by the U.S. Conference of Mayors, 25 cities were asked for
    the three largest causes of homelessness in their communities. Mental illness was the third
    largest cause of homelessness for single adults (mentioned by 48% of cities). For home-
    less families, mental illness was mentioned by 12% of cities as one of the top 3 causes of
    homelessness." "Mental Illness and Homelessness," National Coalition for the Homeless,
    http://www.nationalhomeless.org/factsheets/Mental_Illness.pdf (accessed July 16, 2014).
    See also "Current Statistics on the Prevalence and Characteristics of People Experienc-
    ing Homelessness in the United States," Substance Abuse and Mental Health Services
    Administration, http://homeless.samhsa.gov/ResourceFiles/hrc_factsheet.pdf (accessed
    July 16, 2014).
5   Some have argued that Christianity is, at its core, a religion of healing. Amanda Por-
    terfield, e.g., argued, "Healing has persisted over time and across cultural spaces as a
    defining element of Christianity and a major contributor to Christianity's endurance,
    expansion, and success." Porterfield, *Healing in the History of Christianity* (New York:
    Oxford University Press, 2005), 19. Christian attention to healing, she asserted, involved
    both "relief of suffering and enhanced ability to cope with chronic ailments" (4). Histo-
    rians of religion have explored the history of physical healing in Christianity, with some
    attention to the history of pastoral care, but they have undertaken virtually no investi-
    gation of the history of specific Christian responses to mental illness. Mental maladies

appeared in Porterfield's account only briefly, in discussion of the premodern era (85–86, 102–3). See also brief coverage in Ronald L. Numbers and Darrel W. Amundsen, *Caring and Curing: Health and Medicine in the Western Religious Traditions*, 2nd ed. (Baltimore: Johns Hopkins University Press, 1998).

6   Wave III of the *Baylor Religion Survey* showed that those who "strongly believe that they have a warm relationship with God [reported] 31% fewer mental issues" and that those who "strongly believe that God knows when they need support [reported] 19% fewer mental health issues" than those without such beliefs. F. Carson Mencken, Paul Froese, and Lindsay Morrow, "Mental Health and Spirituality," in *The Values and Beliefs of the American Public: Wave III Baylor Religion Survey* (Baylor University, 2011), 12. For additional research on religion and mental health, see Harold G. Koenig, *Faith and Mental Health: Religious Resources for Healing* (Philadelphia: Templeton Foundation, 2005), 43–160.

7   Kathryn Greene-McCreight, *Darkness Is My Only Companion: A Christian Response to Mental Illness* (Grand Rapids: Brazos, 2006), 13.

8   Greene-McCreight, *Darkness*, 4–5.

9   Historians have addressed mental illness in America from the perspective of medical, institutional, legislative, and social narratives. Most significant are the historian Gerald N. Grob's detailed accounts, especially *The Mad among Us: A History of the Care of America's Mentally Ill* (New York: Free Press, 1994). Others attended briefly to the historical intersection of faith and mental illness as part of more general investigations of mental health in America. The psychiatrist Dr. Harold Koenig's *Faith and Mental Health: Religious Resources for Healing* (2005), e.g., included a chapter-length account of historical vignettes about ecclesial care for the mentally ill in Europe and the United States. The theologian Rosemary Radford Ruether's *Many Forms of Madness: A Family's Struggle with Mental Illness and the Mental Health System* (2010) offered similar, cursory historical detail as she shared details of her son's thirty-year struggle with schizophrenia. Other texts deployed firsthand reflections about mental maladies to offer theological reflections and recommend productive connections between religion and mental health. A representative sample includes Stewart D. Govig's *Souls Are Made of Endurance: Surviving Mental Illness in the Family* (1994); Kathryn Greene-McCreight's *Darkness Is My Only Companion: A Christian Response to Mental Illness* (2006); Nancy Kehoe's *Wrestling with Our Inner Angels* (2009); and Amy Simpson's *Troubled Minds: Mental Illness and the Church's Mission* (Downers Grove, Ill.: IVP Books, 2013).

10 The historian Ann Taves described such differences in terms of "experiencing religion" or "explaining experience." Labels, she found, "reflect[ed] the . . . historical and explanatory commitments" of those making assessments: "Psychiatrists most commonly refer to dissociation (or more distantly hysteria); anthropologists to trance, spirit possession, and altered states of consciousness; and religionists to vision, inspiration, mysticism, and ecstasy." Taves, *Fits, Trances, & Visions: Experiencing Religion and Explaining Experience from Wesley to James* (Princeton: Princeton University Press, 1999), 7.

11 Attentive to how historical figures discussed mental dysfunction, I sought mention of "conditions that disrupt a person's thinking, feeling, mood, ability to relate to others and daily functioning." Using current medical terminology, the range of ailments I incorporated include those cohering with modern diagnoses of "major depression, schizophrenia, bipolar disorder, obsessive compulsive disorder (OCD), panic disorder, post traumatic stress disorder (PTSD) and borderline personality disorder." I also took note

of less severe instances of mental distress, assuming that diagnoses and cures applied to both chronic and episodic mental distress. Where possible, I have differentiated between mental illness and mental disability and excluded the latter (which is characterized by permanent cognitive deficits). "What Is Mental Illness: Mental Illness Facts," National Alliance on Mental Illness, http://www.nami.org/template.cfm?section=about_mental _illness (accessed March 27, 2012). While I acknowledge medical diagnoses for illness throughout my historical work, diagnoses included ambiguity and fluidity over time.

12   White, middle-class Protestants form the primary subject of my account. By the 1950s and 1960s, those Christians were known as mainline Protestants, but that label is anachronistic before the middle of the twentieth century. The Protestants that form the basis for my account were those Protestant leaders and flocks that enjoyed culture-shaping authority and offered the dominant public voice of Protestantism through the middle of the twentieth century. Within this group, I focus on the work and thought of clerical and lay leaders, believers that had the resources to take action in the face of mental illness but also to communicate with a wider American public. When sources provided access, I also attend to the voices of Protestants not in leadership positions.

13   The theologian Kathryn Tanner advocated for this sort of "historically funded constructive theology" that "looks to the Christian past not for models for simple imitation" but for how to expand "one's sense of the possibilities for present Christian expression and action." Tanner, "Christian Claims: How My Mind Has Changed," *Christian Century*, February 23, 2010, 43. H. Richard Niebuhr offered a similar sentiment: "This may seem to be an effort to present theology in the guise of history, yet the theology has grown out of the history as much as the history has grown out of the theology." Niebuhr, *The Kingdom of God in America* (Middletown, Conn.: Wesleyan University Press, 1988), xxiii.

CHAPTER 1

1   Cotton Mather, *The Angel of Bethesda*, ed. Gordon W. Jones (Barre, Mass.: American Antiquarian Society, 1972), 10, 326n20. Quotation is a translation of text provided in notes to Capsula I. Jones notes that Hendrick de Roy authored the quotation. De Roy was also known as Henricus Regius and was a Dutch philosopher and physician. Mather wrote that the translation from the Dutch was made by a Lorrichini, a text Jones was unable to identify. Jones transcribed Mather's writing with the capitalization, punctuation, and spelling used by Mather. I have retained those elements to display Mather's intended emphasis.

2   Cotton Mather, *Diary of Cotton Mather: Volume I, 1681–1708* (Boston: Massachusetts Historical Society Collections, 1911), 447.

3   Mather, *Diary of Cotton Mather: Volume I*, 448.

4   Mather, *Diary of Cotton Mather: Volume I*, 448. Kenneth Silverman notes that breast cancer and an infection may have contributed to Abigail's illness and death. Silverman, *The Life and Times of Cotton Mather* (New York: Harper & Row, 1984), 179.

5   For a representative series of laments about the illness and deaths of family members and fellow townspeople, see Cotton Mather, *Diary of Cotton Mather: Volume II, 1709–1724* (New York: F. Ungar, 1957), 639–53. For "sanctimonious" reference, see Perry Miller, *The New England Mind: From Colony to Province* (Cambridge, Mass.: Harvard University Press, 1953), 350. Harry S. Stout noted that Mather was vilified "at the hands of historians." Despite Mather's erudition and public service, "for two centuries, Mather survived in history annals as the Puritan hypocrite historians loved to hate." Stout credits work

after 1975—by David Levin, Richard Lovelace, Kenneth Silverman, and others—with
offering more "balanced" studies that "concede shortcoming in Mather's character (nota-
bly his inflated ego and willful participation in the Salem witchcraft trials), but subordinate these to the unsurpassed contributions he made to Puritanism and his Native New
England." Stout, "The Life and Times of Cotton Mather," *Reformed Journal* 35, no. 8
(1985): 24. Richard F. Lovelace discussed interpretations of Mather, noting that Mather
"retains a dark image in the popular mind," although, among scholars, "Mather's portrait
has brightened a little with the revival of sympathetic and objective Puritan scholarship"
in the twentieth century. See Lovelace, *The American Pietism of Cotton Mather: Origins
of American Evangelicalism* (Grand Rapids: Christian University Press, 1979), 1. There,
Lovelace notes the role of historian Perry Miller's work in shaping negative projections.
Miller, e.g., named Mather "the most intransigent and impervious mind of his period,
not to say the most nauseous human being." Miller, however, also admits that in other
respects, Mather "is the most sensitive and perceptive, the clearest and most resolute."
Miller, *The New England Mind: The Seventeenth Century* (Cambridge, Mass.: Harvard
University Press, 1954), 476. For additional Mather historiography, see Brett Malcolm
Grainger, "Vital Nature and Vital Piety: Johann Arndt and the Evangelical Vitalism of
Cotton Mather," *Church History* 81, no. 4 (2012): 852–54. As will be noted below, scholars
debate the extent of Mather's participation in the witchcraft trials.

6   Gordon W. Jones, "Introduction: Part I," in Mather, *Angel of Bethesda*, xv. Silverman
     noted the "prodigious Proxysms" his wife experienced and the hardship they caused
     Mather. Silverman characterized her as "vain, jealous, manipulative, and perhaps psy-
     chopathic." Silverman, *Life and Times*, 309. Lovelace, *American Pietism*, 25.

7   Jones, "Introduction: Part I," in Mather, *Angel of Bethesda*, xiv. Silverman, *Life and Times*,
     15–17, 33. Silverman credits Mather's prodigious publication record to his attempt to
     prove that, despite a stammer, he could produce worthy written material.

8   Mather, *Angel of Bethesda*, 326. See note 1 above for quotation source information.

9   The historian Winton U. Solberg observed, "Mather welcomed science as a handmaid
     of theology, a new instrument for discovering the mind of God." Solberg, "Science and
     Religion in Early America: Cotton Mather's 'Christian Philosopher,'" *Church History* 56,
     no. 1 (1987): 75. Puritans, historian Perry Miller showed, assumed a "unity of knowledge"
     in which "sense and reason" were "God's [works] as well as grace." Miller, *New England
     Mind: The Seventeenth Century*, 201. The "fusion" of faith and reason, Miller argued,
     required effort on the part of New England clergymen who needed to explain both
     God's sovereignty and the order inherent in nature. Throughout his writings, Mather
     worked hard to justify both that sovereignty and order (208). Such fusion proved harder
     to maintain in later centuries, but Miller observed that seventeenth-century Puritans like
     Mather "did not see the dangers ahead, the possibility that . . . descriptions of faith in the
     terms of reason . . . could give rise to a naturalistic morality and a belief that education
     would achieve everything usually ascribed to grace, because they were convinced that
     theology would remain forever the norm of reason" (202). While for Mather theological
     and scientific thought were one, the same would not hold true a century later, a shift that
     influenced the loss of clerical authority over matters of health and healing.

10   For Puritans, "nature was seen as the revelation of God's will in action." Miller, *New
     England Mind: The Seventeenth Century*, 214. See also discussion of Mather's exploration
     of nature to learn of the divine, in George Harrison Orians, ed., *Days of Humiliation:*

Times of Affliction and Disaster; Nine Sermons for Restoring Favor with an Angry God (1696–1727) (Gainsville, Fla.: Scholars' Facsimiles & Reprints, 1970), xxii.

11 Biographer Kenneth Silverman asserted, "Esteem, prestige, position, and respect belonged to Cotton Mather by birth, for his flesh and name united two of the most honored families in early New England, the Cottons and the Mathers." Silverman, *Life and Times*, 3.

12 Basic biographical details are drawn from "Cotton Mather," in Robert Dean Linder et al., eds., *Dictionary of Christianity in America* (Downers Grove, Ill.: InterVarsity, 1990), 715–16; Stout, "Life and Times," 23; Lovelace, *American Pietism*, 14. Mather was the son of Increase Mather (1639–1723), grandson of John Cotton (1584–1652), and grandson of Richard Mather (1596–1669). Mather had access to more volumes than nearly any other colonial American. In addition to proximity to Harvard's library, the Mather's collection is estimated as one of the largest, if not the largest, in the colonies. Otho T. Beall and Richard H. Shryock, *Cotton Mather, First Significant Figure in American Medicine* (Baltimore: Johns Hopkins University Press, 1954), 60nn22, 23. "Although much of his library was dispersed," 849 titles survived. Thomas E. Keys, "The Colonial Library and the Development of Sectional Differences in the American Colonies," *Library Quarterly* 8, no. 3 (1938): 375.

13 Cotton Mather, *Essays to Do Good; Addressed to All Christians, Whether in Public or Private Capacities*, 2nd ed. (London: Williams and Smith, Burtton, Conder, R. Ogle, and C. Taylor, 1808). For a sample of sources for this volume, see Athanasius (100), Calvin (167), Eusebius (156), Hippocrates (107), Justin Martyr (97), Luther (39, 126), Melanchthon (75), Socrates (151), Tertullian (43), legal theory (135), and church histories (86).

14 "Truth faith involved inward, overt, and obedient preparation, appropriation, humility, dedication, gratitude—and a commitment to walk in God's way according to his Law." Sydney E. Ahlstrom, *A Religious History of the American People*, 2nd ed. (New Haven, Conn.: Yale University Press, 2004), 132.

15 See the following sources for discussion of covenant theology in Puritan thought: "Covenant Theology," in Linder et al., *Dictionary of Christianity in America*, 322–24; Ahlstrom, *Religious History*, 30–132; Miller, *New England Mind: From Colony to Province*, 21–24. Covenant theology emerged before Puritan settlement in the American colonies but took on a distinctive shape in a region founded, in part, on Puritan principles. Cotton Mather died just before the revivals of the Great Awakenings, thus his ministry fell near the end of the Puritan reign in New England. For a discussion of the interplay between Mather and emerging religious traditions (including his conversation with European pietists/ pietism), see Lovelace's *American Pietism*.

16 Silverman, *Life and Times*, 406. Beall and Shryock note that many of the chapters of *The Angel of Bethesda* appeared in Mather's earlier writings and sermons, thus indicating some public distribution of Mather's thought even without the publication of the text during his lifetime. Beall and Shryock, *Cotton Mather*, 62. A diary entry from 1693 points to Mather's early thoughts about developing the volume. See Mather, *Diary of Cotton Mather: Volume I*, 163.

17 Nancy Tomes noted that debate over medical versus spiritual origins of mental illness had bubbled for centuries: "The conception of madness as disease dated back to classical medicine and the Hippocratic texts. Throughout the medieval period, a tradition of medical rationalism continued to dispute the widespread popular belief that mental disorder had a supernatural or demonic origin." The debate gained traction outside of the

medical profession in significant ways during the eighteenth century. Tomes, *A Generous Confidence: Thomas Story Kirkbride and the Art of Asylum-Keeping, 1840–1883* (New York: Cambridge University Press, 1984), 24. For additional sources for the history of insanity (for Mather's era and earlier), see Mary Ann Jimenez, *Changing Faces of Madness: Early American Attitudes and Treatment of the Insane* (Hanover, N.H.: University Press of New England, 1987), 1–8.

18 He also pledged to "apply [himself] both to Heaven and Earth, to bring on the Publication of it." Mather, *Diary of Cotton Mather: Volume II*, 698–99.

19 Silverman named *The Angel of Bethesda* Mather's "single most important achievement in science." Silverman, *Life and Times*, 406.

20 Mather, *Angel of Bethesda*, 281–85.

21 With a few exceptions, *The Angel of Bethesda* presented Mather's summary of existing medical knowledge rather than original work. A "summary of the medical practice, beliefs, and theory of the seventeenth century" filled the text. Gordon W. Jones, "Introduction: Part II," in Mather, *Angel of Bethesda*, xviii.

22 Madness and "distraction" appeared as the most common labels for mental maladies in colonial writings, and both appeared in Mather's writings.

23 Mather, *Angel of Bethesda*, 129. He attributed madness to inflamed "animal spirits" in the brain.

24 Mather, *Angel of Bethesda*, 129. Mather also cited a paucity or disturbance of "Animal Spirits" as the cause of "Dizziness, but there, at fault is a giddy, or over ambitious soul." In addition, he listed obstruction of the "Animal Spirits" at fault for nightmares (148–49, 153).

Mather cited his contemporary, Italian physician Gjuro Baglivi, about the connection between mental and physical health: "Baglivi is not the only physician who has made the observation, 'That many of our diseases, either arise from a weight of cares lying on the minds of men, or are thereby increased. Some diseases that seem incurable, are eerily cured by agreeable conversation. Disorders of the mind first bring diseases on the stomach; and so the whole mass of blood gradually becomes infected: and as long as the mental cause continues, the diseases may indeed change their forms, but they rarely quit the patients.' Tranquility of mind will do wonderful things towards the relief of bodily maladies." Mather, *Essays to Do Good*, 111.

25 Mather, *Angel of Bethesda*, 133.

26 Mather, *Angel of Bethesda*, 133.

27 Mather, *Angel of Bethesda*, 133.

28 Mather, *Angel of Bethesda*, 130.

29 The role of gender in predisposing individuals to certain types of mental maladies made only scant appearance in Mather's account. For example, women might suffer "*Madness of an Uterine Original*," or hysteria. Mather, *Angel of Bethesda*, 132.

30 Mather, *Angel of Bethesda*, 130–31. Of these two differences, the second faded in descriptions of mental maladies in the coming century. Presumptions about the curability of mental illness and a renewed emphasis on human productivity brought about by the market economy (which demanded productive workers) meant that madness came to be understood as an exception, rather an a universal reality. With the rise of scientific medicine, biological causes for illness moved to the forefront, but suspicions of sin, particularly individual sin, causing illness persisted.

31   Mather, *Diary of Cotton Mather: Volume I*, 490. Mather noted that he had taken an almost parental role with the servant—"unto whom I had been so much a Father." In a November 1702 entry, Mather noted, "My godly Maid . . . lay horribly full of the Small-pox, distracted, and hardly escaping her life" (447). See also p. 451: "My poor Servant, who knew and lov'd my Family, and would have been a tender Nurse to my Children, continued so distracted after getting up from the Small-pox, that I was under a Necessity of dismissing her out of my Family." Mather's household was cared for by a variety of white, black, and Indian servants. Though not an abolitionist, his writing urged humane treatment of slaves. For a discussion of Mather and slavery, see Silverman, *Life and Times*, 263–64.

32   Mather, *Diary of Cotton Mather: Volume I*, 452. Mather seems to have a selfish motive in mind here as he reflects. If such a "Disorder of the Mind" would have befallen his wife, he worried that it would have "rendered [his] Condition insupportable."

33   The historian Virginia Bernhard affirmed the difficulty his wife's behavior caused Mather. Bernhard, however, cast doubt on Mather's and later historical assertions of his wife's chronic madness: "Claims that Lydia Mather never recovered her sanity after falling ill in 1719 cannot be substantiated. In fact, given the existing evidence, it is impossible to determine whether [she] ever suffered from mental illness at all." Bernhard speculated Mather interpreted Lydia's anger (over finances and other matters) as madness. Regardless, Mather's diary revealed that he worried about exposing his wife's mental illness: "I have lived a Year in continual Anguish of Expectation, that my poor Wife, by exposing her Madness, would bring a Ruine on my Ministry." He does not comment further, but the confession displays the presence of social stigma associated with mental maladies in the colonial era. Bernhard, "Cotton Mather's 'Most Unhappy Wife': Reflections on the Uses of Historical Evidence," *New England Quarterly* 60, no. 3 (1987): 348, 342.

34   For accounts of Lydia's behavior, see Mather, *Diary of Cotton Mather: Volume II*, 583–84, 715, 723, 735, 742, 743, 745, 749, and 752. Often, Mather recorded his observations and fears either in a separate notebook or in Latin and Greek, a technique he seemed to use when he hoped to keep his thoughts private. Latin entries: see pp. 715, 723, 735, 742, and 745.

35   Mather, *Diary of Cotton Mather: Volume II*, 723.

36   Routine illness afflicted colonists, but epidemics posed dangerous, if periodic, threats. A smallpox epidemic in 1721, e.g., "infected half of the inhabitants of Boston." Cristobal Silva, *Miraculous Plagues: An Epidemiology of Early New England Narrative* (New York: Oxford University Press, 2011), 14. On the 1713 epidemic that struck the Mathers, see Margaret Kendrick Hostetter, "What We Don't See," *New England Journal of Medicine* 366, no. 14 (2012): 1329.

37   Oscar Reiss asserted that the geographically dispersed and generally poor colonial population made it difficult for physicians to establish financially viable medical practices in the colonies. Reiss, *Medicine in Colonial America* (Lanham, Md.: University Press of America, 2000), chap. 1.

38   Beall and Shryock, *Cotton Mather*, 29. Reiss, *Medicine in Colonial America*, 26. Apprenticeship involved several years of assisting an experienced physician before launching a solo practice.

39   As part of that training, the school acquired bodies for studies in anatomy.

40   Reiss, *Medicine in Colonial America*, 20.

41   Mather, *Angel of Bethesda*, 186–91.

42 Mather, *Angel of Bethesda*, 189. Capsula XL. "A Pause made upon, The Uncertainties of the *PHYSICIANS.*"

43 In contrast, Beall and Shryock noted, "The majority of physicians of Mather's day" had "abandoned theological explanations of illness." Beall and Shryock, *Cotton Mather*, 79.

44 Confident in the power of prayer, Mather urged physicians to pray for their patients: "When we consider how much the lives of men are in the hands of God; what a dependence we have on the God of our health for our cure when we have lost it; what strong and remarkable proofs we have had of angels, by their communications or operations, contributing to the cure of the diseases with which mortals have been oppressed; and the marvellous efficacy of prayer for the recovery of the sick brother who has not sinned a 'sin unto death:'—what better thing can be recommended to a physician who desires to do good than this—to be a man of prayer. In your daily and secret prayer, carry every one of your patients, as you would your own children, to the glorious Lord our healer, for his healing mercies; place them, as far as your prayers will do it, under the beams of the Sun of Righteousness." Mather, *Essays to Do Good*, 109–10.

45 Reiss, *Medicine in Colonial America*, 298. Clergy were not of one mind about inoculation. Some believed the illness to be the work of God, and thus to prevent it was "an unrighteous act." Others felt inoculation was given by God to humans, that God "through his mercy" showed humanity how to help itself (305). This paragraph and the next draw on Beall and Shryock, *Cotton Mather*, 95–113.

46 For commentary about the controversy, see Mather, *Diary of Cotton Mather: Volume II*, 624–25n1. For Mather's account of the 1721 smallpox outbreak, see pp. 618–62.

47 Beall and Shryock, *Cotton Mather*, 104.

48 Miller, *New England Mind: From Colony to Province*, 20.

49 For discussion of jeremiads that predicted epidemics and theological opposition to inoculation, see Miller, *New England Mind: From Colony to Province*, 346–49.

50 The debate spilled over into "newspaper and pamphlet warfare." Beall and Shryock, *Cotton Mather*, 106.

51 A message tied to the grenade (which failed to detonate) read, "COTTON MATHER, You Dog, Dam you; I'll inoculate you with this, with a Pox to you." Silverman, *Life and Times*, 350.
        Mather's suspicions of the devil's involvement deepened his sense "that the souls of the colonists were in jeopardy." Margaret Humphreys Warner, "Vindicating the Minister's Medical Role: Cotton Mather's Concept of the *Nishmath-Chajim* and the Spiritualization of Medicine," *Journal of the History of Medicine* 36, no. 3 (1981): 281.

52 Margaret Warner asserted that the expansion of authority by Mather was a calculated effort to offset the societal "status loss" he and other clergy experienced. "In sermon after sermon the clergy, including Mather, opposed creeping secularization and disrespect for the ministry. . . . Mather sought to study the invisible world scientifically, so that the slumbering souls of his congregation . . . would be convinced of the truths of Christianity and of the existence of the spirit world." Only ministers held the expertise to bridge the scientific and the spiritual worlds. Warner, "Vindicating the Minister's Medical Role," 280.

53 The relative status of professions proves complex. "At least since the late Middle Ages, Western societies had commonly recognized medicine, along with divinity and law, as one of the prototypical professions." Clergy, however, claimed authority from God. Medical professionals earned authority as the result of treatment successes. In Puritan America, a world where God's sovereignty was an infrequently challenged assumption,

clerical authority could trump medical authority. Ronald L. Numbers traces the unsteady authority of American physicians through the late nineteenth century. See Numbers, "The Fall and Rise of the American Medical Profession," in *The Professions in American History*, ed. Nathan O. Hatch (Notre Dame, Ind.: University of Notre Dame Press, 1988), 51. For an accompanying discussion of the history of clerical authority in America, see Martin E. Marty's chapter in the same volume. Marty cites the work of Donald Scott in describing the broad authority claimed by clergy in colonial America, a "theocentric culture." See Marty, "The Clergy," in Hatch, *Professions in American History*, 78–79.

54   Ahlstrom, *Religious History*, 280.

55   Reiss, *Medicine in Colonial America*, 22.

56   Reiss, *Medicine in Colonial America*, 23. King's College in NYC, later Columbia University, granted its first M.D. degree one year earlier, in 1770. The King's College medical school stopped operations during the British occupation of the Revolutionary War. Within three decades, the training plan changed, eliminating the bachelor's degree and strengthening the requirements for an M.D. See chap. 2 for discussion of the professionalization of medicine in early America.

57   Reiss, *Medicine in Colonial America*, 28.

58   Reiss, *Medicine in Colonial America*, 59.

59   Mather, in Beall and Shryock, *Cotton Mather*, 35.

60   Mather, *Angel of Bethesda*, 7.

61   Mather, *Angel of Bethesda*, 8–9.

62   Mather, *Angel of Bethesda*, 272.

63   Mather, *Angel of Bethesda*, 5.

64   Mather, *Angel of Bethesda*, 5. The historian Perry Miller noted that for Puritans the "seeming contradictions between the creator's goodness and the creation's visible evils necessitated no denial of either; they merely reinforced the distinction between God's revealed and secret wills. . . . No matter how exasperating, no matter how disastrous, because all experience is given of God, it must have some reason behind it." Miller, *New England Mind: The Seventeenth Century*, 39.

65   Mather, *Angel of Bethesda*, 5. Miller described the Puritan understanding of original sin: Adam, the "spokesman for all men," broke the covenant with God and thus "the guilt was 'imputed' " to all humans as a "legal responsibility. . . . The debt of Adam is laid at their door." Miller, *New England Mind: The Seventeenth Century*, 400–401.

66   Mather, *Angel of Bethesda*, 271.

67   Mather, *Angel of Bethesda*, 6.

68   Miller, *New England Mind: The Seventeenth Century*, 407.

69   Mather, *Angel of Bethesda*, 6. Scripture, the primary source of authority for understanding the causes of illness for Mather, was displaced by scientific and medical knowledge in the following centuries.

70   Norman Dain, "Madness and the Stigma of Sin in American Christianity," in *Stigma and Mental Illness*, ed. Paul Jay Fink and Allan Tasman (Washington, D.C.: American Psychiatric, 1992), 75.

71   Silverman, *Life and Times*, 381–82. For the corresponding diary entry, see Mather, *Diary of Cotton Mather: Volume II*, 715.

72   "Kibroth Hattaavh" appears in the Old Testament book of Numbers (11:34) as "*the graves of craving*" or "*graves of lust.*" Not satisfied with the provision of manna, the exiled Israelites complained to God for meat. God provided abundant meat (quail) but grew angry

and sent a plague that afflicted greedy Israelites. Those who "had the craving" for meat died and were buried in Kibroth Hattaavh.

73   Mather, *Angel of Bethesda*, 116–20.

74   Mather, *Angel of Bethesda*, 8.

75   Mather, *Diary of Cotton Mather: Volume II*, 105.

76   In *The Angel of Bethesda*, Mather deployed his concept of the *nishmath-chajim* (from the Hebrew "breath of life"), "a vital spirit that formed a bridge between man's physical and spiritual components"—it linked the rational spirit and the physical body. He assumed illness to be rooted in imbalances in the *nishmath-chajim*. Warner, "Vindicating the Minister's Medical Role," 278, 285, 287. Mather was convinced of the connection between physical/mental and spiritual health, and the concept of "*nishmath-chajim* enabled Mather to make the minister central to the healing process" (283). For deeper discussion of Mather's use of *nishmath-chajim*, see Grainger, "Vital Nature," 854, 869–71. Grainger argued that Mather's use of this concept helped him reconcile "natural philosophy, Puritan covenant theology," and other intellectual traditions.

77   Given this sense, illness was purposeful in the life of faith and in a way that would not be the same after the revivals of the First and Second Great Awakenings. The stress during those revivals on New Birth, the confidence to mark conversion at a point in time, reconfigured and perhaps even diminished the purposeful role for chronic sickness, like mental illness, in the lives of faithful Americans.

78   The historian David D. Hall declared, "The people of seventeenth-century New England lived in an enchanted universe. Theirs was a world of wonders." Hall, *Worlds of Wonder, Days of Judgment: Popular Religious Belief in Early New England* (New York: Knopf, 1989), 71. With the rise of science, the tight connections to the supernatural loosened in the eighteenth and nineteenth centuries, but those notions held fast in the colonial period, and suspicion of supernatural origins of mental disease remained in modern America. See Mary Ann Jimenez, "Madness in Early American History: Insanity in Massachusetts from 1700 to 1830," *Journal of Social History* 20, no. 1 (1986): 30.

79   Such signs were "demonstrations of God's power to suspect or interrupt the laws of nature." Hall, *Worlds of Wonder*, 71. Hall demonstrated that interpretation of such "abnormalities" simultaneously drew on explanations from theology, astrology, natural history, and Greek meteorology (p. 76 and following). Mather, however, urged that not every natural abnormality displayed divine punishment. He proved more likely to infer divine punishment in significant natural events such as hurricanes than in more isolated abnormalities. See Orians, *Days of Humiliation*, xxiii–xxiv.

80   Silverman offers a representative example of the hysteria surrounding accusations of witchcraft. In June of 1692, Bridge Bishop, the "thrice-married owner of an unlicensed tavern," was found guilty of witchcraft and hung. In the next two weeks, seven hundred additional people were accused and more than one hundred were imprisoned. In that episode, Mather and other ministers cautioned against the use of "spectral evidence." Silverman, *Life and Times*, 99–100, 103–4.

81   Lovelace, *American Pietism*, 17. Grainger argues Mather worked to "discriminate between 'good' and 'bad' varieties of occult practice." Grainger, "Vital Nature," 857.

82   Jones noted, "In 1688 [Mather] took charge of two Boston girls who could produce the most amazing parapsychological phenomena seen in his region. . . . He treated the girls as ill, and cured them." Jones, "Introduction: Part II," in Mather, *Angel of Bethesda*, xiii. Silverman noted that, while "in the popular imagining of the American past" Mather

and the Salem witchcraft trials are "nearly synonymous," "the exact connection between the two remains obscure." Silverman, *Life and Times*, 87.

83 Jones, "Introduction: Part II," in Mather, *Angel of Bethesda*, xiii. For a discussion of witchcraft in Puritan thought, see also Miller, *New England Mind: The Seventeenth Century*, 321. Miller places witchcraft in the Puritan discussion of "providence": seemingly unnatural phenomena like witchcraft, comets, and earthquakes "might have come about by purely natural means, none of them are miracles; yet all illustrate the constant and unceasing government of God by showing Him, not rudely interrupting, but, as it were insinuating Himself into nature—working not in defiance of natural law, but through skillful manipulation of it." All realities fall under the purview of the divine.

84 Beall and Shryock, *Cotton Mather*, 71 (referencing Mather's *Magnalia*, see https://archive.org/details/magnaliachristia00math).

85 Mather, cited in Jimenez, *Changing Faces of Madness*, 12.

86 Mather, cited in Jimenez, *Changing Faces of Madness*, 13 (*Balneum Diaboli*, "the Devil's Bath").

87 In such situations, he recommended prayer and fasting as treatments. Mather, *Angel of Bethesda*, 135, 130.

88 For a discussion of different colonial-era perceptions of madness and witchcraft, see Jimenez, *Changing Faces of Madness*, 42–43. There, she notes, "Witches were seen as people with a great potential for doing harm; they were blamed for all kinds of things, personal and communitywide, that may have gone wrong in early New England. Not so the mad. Rather than epitomizing potential harm or evil, the distracted residents of Massachusetts Bay Colony became a serious problem only when they actually engaged in harmful or destructive behavior."

89 Jimenez, "Madness in Early American History," 30. Mather rarely attributed mental illness to heredity but did so in the case of his third wife's illness, speculating that she suffered from " 'a Distraction which may be somewhat Hereditary' or perhaps demonic possession." Mather, in Dain, "Madness," in Fink and Tasman, *Stigma and Mental Illness*, 75.

90 Not yet diagnosed as medical conditions, "mental illness posed social and economic rather than medical problems." Grob, *Mad among Us*, 6. This section draws on Grob's account.

91 Grob, *Mad among Us*, 7. Jimenez observed, "Guardianship laws were based on the fear that the insane would squander their estate and end up a town charge." Jimenez, "Madness in Early American History," 28.

92 Jimenez, "Madness in Early American History," 26.

93 Jimenez, "Madness in Early American History," 26.

94 The Pennsylvania Hospital opened in 1751 but first admitted patients in 1752. Reiss, *Medicine in Colonial America*, 134.

95 Reiss, *Medicine in Colonial America*, 138.

96 Like other early facilities, the Virginia Eastern Asylum (its later name) "served a caring rather than a medical function evident by the choice of a layperson—not a physician—as its principle officer." Grob, *Mad among Us*, 20.

97 Mather, *Essays to Do Good*, 16–17.

98 Mather, *Angel of Bethesda*, 133.

99 Mather, *Diary of Cotton Mather: Volume II*, 211. For others Mather noted in need of help, see distracted youth (448), a friend under "some Degree of Alienation of Mind" (453), a

"noted Neighbor" fallen into an "uncomfortable Distraction" (551), a church member "fallen into a crazy Melancholy" (581), and "a poor Man in the Flock" (617).

100 In response to the distraction of an aged neighbor "of some Consideration," Mather procured "a Number of the pious Neighbors to meet and pray together with him." Mather, *Diary of Cotton Mather: Volume II*, 576.

101 Mather, *Angel of Bethesda*, 130, 131. In his diary, Mather recorded the following ejaculatory prayer to be offered in the sight of "One crazy and sickly": "Lord, lett the Sun of Righteousness arise to that person with Healing in His Wings; In the Lord, lett him have Righteousness and Strength." Mather, *Diary of Cotton Mather: Volume I*, 82.

102 Mather, *Diary of Cotton Mather: Volume II*, 141.

103 Mather, *Diary of Cotton Mather: Volume I*, 160–61. This episode occurred during the time of the witchcraft trials in Salem.

104 Jimenez, "Madness in Early American History," 31.

105 These four humors corresponded to the presumed four elements of the universe: fire, water, earth, and air. Reiss, *Medicine in Colonial America*, 145.

106 Beall and Shryock, *Cotton Mather*, 25. The use of pharmaceuticals was rare in colonial America, and "only two specific drugs were known in 1700, cinchona bark against malaria and mercury against syphilis," and the latter was known to be dangerous enough to limit its use (26).

107 Mather, *Angel of Bethesda*, 131–32.

108 Mather, *Angel of Bethesda*, 136. See also notes, p. 355.

109 Mather, *Angel of Bethesda*, 134.

110 Mather, *Angel of Bethesda*, 133, 135.

111 Mather, *Angel of Bethesda*, 135.

112 Mather, *Angel of Bethesda*, 326. Quotation is a translation of text provided in notes to Capsula I. Jones noted Hendrick de Roy as the author. Mather indicated that the translation from the Dutch was made by Lorrichini, a text Jones was unable to identify.

CHAPTER 2

1 Benjamin Rush, *Medical Inquiries and Observations upon the Diseases of the Mind*, 4th ed. (1812; Philadelphia: John Grigg, 1830), 241.

2 *The Autobiography of Benjamin Rush: His "Travels through Life" together with His Commonplace Book for 1789–1813*, ed. George Washington Corner (Princeton: Princeton University Press for the American Philosophical Society, 1948), 220–21. Despite Rush's explicit focus on mental disorders in his later years, and his attention to them in his journal, they receive no mention in his autobiography. For additional information on Glendinning's insanity, including his suicide attempt in 1784, see John H. Wigger, *American Saint: Francis Asbury and the Methodists* (New York: Oxford University Press, 2009), 203–6; and Christine Leigh Heyrman, *Southern Cross: The Beginnings of the Bible Belt* (New York: Knopf, 1997), 28–33, 36–37, 279n39; and others. Glendinning's strange behavior, violent agitation, and "spewing curses and babbling blasphemies" earned him "exile" by fellow Methodist clergy from Virginia to a remote plantation in North Carolina.

3 *Autobiography of Benjamin Rush*, 269. Laudanum, a preparation of opium, was used to treat a variety of ailments.

4 For "insisting on humane treatment," see Alyn Brodsky, *Benjamin Rush: Patriot and Physician* (New York: Truman Talley Books, 2004), 5.

5   The intellectual revolution of the Enlightenment "flourished in America" during Rush's
     era (c. 1750–1800). The movement stressed reason, not revelation, as the "way to truth"
     and included an "optimistic belief in human ability to make progress." See "Enlighten-
     ment Protestantism," in Linder et al., *Dictionary of Christianity in America*, 393. Addi-
     tional discussion of Enlightenment influence on Rush and conceptions of mental illness
     appears below.

6   In 1768, after medical study in Edinburgh, Rush lived for a time with Franklin's family in
     London, where Franklin served as agent to several American colonies. The elder states-
     man provided Rush with letters of introduction when he left London for Paris in Febru-
     ary 1769. *Autobiography of Benjamin Rush*, 55, 66. Rush consulted with Paine during the
     writing of Paine's *Common Sense*. See *Autobiography of Benjamin Rush*, 113–14.

7   *Autobiography of Benjamin Rush*, 161. Based on his own experiences, Rush entreated his
     sons "to take no public or active part in the disputes of their country beyond a vote at an
     election." His son Richard disregarded this advice and served as a statesman and diplo-
     mat (162).

8   *Autobiography of Benjamin Rush*, 10. Rarely willing to remain silent on an issue he cared
     about, Rush created loyal friends and enemies in the political and medical realms.

9   Adams, in Carl Binger, *Revolutionary Doctor: Benjamin Rush, 1746–1813* (New York:
     Norton, 1966), 296.

10   Brodsky claimed, "Rush set the record among Philadelphia physicians for attending
     worship, even keeping pews in several churches simultaneously so that he might visit
     the nearest one should he desire communion with his Maker during rounds." Brodsky,
     Benjamin Rush, 346.

11   Rush's father was a member of the Episcopal Church; his mother was reared Presbyte-
     rian. Religion also animated decisions of Rush's ancestors. In the seventeenth century,
     John Rush, Benjamin's great-great-great-grandfather, left England for Pennsylvania to
     practice his Quaker beliefs without persecution. He, his wife, their eight children, and
     several grandchildren arrived in 1683, just a year after the launch of William Penn's
     colony. Rush's family eventually fell away from the Society of Friends, a group he grew
     to detest for their pacifist opposition to fighting during the American Revolution. *Auto-
     biography of Benjamin Rush*, 23–25.

12   Brodsky, *Benjamin Rush*, 16. For more on the First Great Awakening, see "Great Awak-
     ening," in Linder et al., *Dictionary of Christianity in America*, 494–96.

13   Brodsky, *Benjamin Rush*, 16. Rush was baptized at Christ Church (Episcopal) in Phila-
     delphia by Rev. Eneas Ross, the father-in-law of Betsy Ross, the purported maker of the
     first U.S. flag. *Autobiography of Benjamin Rush*, 162n11.

14   Finley later became the fifth president of the College of New Jersey (later Princeton).
     Linder et al., *Dictionary of Christianity in America*, 438–39.

15   Brodsky, *Benjamin Rush*, 20.

16   *Autobiography of Benjamin Rush*, 226.

17   *Autobiography of Benjamin Rush*, 339. Here Rush observed, "Thus to the Catholics and
     Moravians he has committed the Godhead of the Savior, hence they worship and pray to
     him; to the Episcopal, Presbyterian, and Baptist Church the decrees of God and partial
     redemption, or the salvation of the first fruits, which they ignorantly suppose to include
     all who shall be saved. To the Lutherans and Methodists he has committed the doctrine
     of universal redemption, to the Quakers the Godhead and influence of the Holy Spirit,
     to the Unitarians, the humanity of our Savior, or the doctrine of 'god manifested in the

flesh.' . . . Let the different Sects of Christians not only bear with each other, but love each other for this kind display of God's goodness whereby all the truths of their Religion are so protected that none of them can ever become feeble or lost. When united they make a great whole, and that whole is the salvation of all men" (339–40). Rush also found providential the roughly simultaneous lives of Martin Luther and John Calvin, John Wesley and George Whitefield (345).

18   After "submitting" to confirmation at the Episcopal St. Peter's Church with his wife in 1788, he "declined after a year or two" to commune in the church and had his children baptized Presbyterian. Rush's church attendance remained steady throughout his adulthood. He reported "constant" attendance while living in Edinburgh. *Autobiography of Benjamin Rush*, 47. Rush proved informed of the larger Protestant landscape. While in London after medical school, he befriended the evangelist George Whitefield, who he first heard preach in America. While he never met John Wesley, Rush heard him preach twice in Edinburgh. He called these two ministers "the two largest and brightest orbs that appeared in the hemisphere of the Church in the 18th Century" (56). Rush never formally aligned with the emerging Universalist Church, but he participated in its convention held in Philadelphia in 1790 and edited the convention's "articles of religion and plan of worship" (164n14) and June 5, 1790, entry in *Commonplace Book* (185).

19   Mark A. Noll, "The Rise and Long Life of Protestant Enlightenment in America," in *Knowledge and Belief in America: Enlightenment Traditions and Modern Religious Thought*, ed. William M. Shea and Peter A. Huff (Cambridge: Cambridge University Press, 1995), 88. Noll commends three definitions of the Enlightenment in America. Henry F. May's: "The Enlightenment consists of all those who believe two propositions: first, that the present age is more enlightened than the past; and second, that we understand nature and man best through the use of our natural faculties." D. H. Meyer's: "There was, above all, a new faith in science . . . a heightened interest in the natural world, including significantly, human nature . . . a growing impatience with mystery and 'metaphysics' [and] new hope for man." Henry Steel Commanger's: "Recognition of a cosmic system governed by the laws of Nature and Nature's God; faith in Reason . . . commitment to 'the illimitable freedom of the human mind,' . . . to the perfectability of Man . . . and confidence that Providence and Nature had decreed happiness for mankind" (88–89n1).

20   As Henry F. May argued, "Americans perceived several Enlightenments." While they rejected the skeptical (Voltaire, Hume) and revolutionary (Rousseau, Paine) strands of the Enlightenment, and put some faith in the moderate strand (Newton, Locke), they embraced wholeheartedly the didactic Enlightenment (the Common Sense Realism, shaped largely by Scottish thinkers). See Noll's summary of May's classification: Noll, "Rise and Long Life," in Shea and Huff, *Knowledge and Belief*, 93–95. For discussion of the intellectual and personal connections between the colonies and Scotland, see idem, 98–108.

21   Noll, "Rise and Long Life," in Shea and Huff, *Knowledge and Belief*, 96.

22   In their discussion of the Puritan intellectual tradition, Charles Hollinger and David A. Capper name a "synthesis" formed by study of "Christian and biblical scholarship" and "Renaissance humanism" that combined to "achieve the highest cultural goal of the religious intellectual—a justification of the ways of God to man and woman." God and not humanity proved central to the Puritan intellectual effort. Capper and Hollinger, eds., *The American Intellectual Tradition: Volume I, 1630–1865* (New York: Oxford University Press, 2006), 3.

23   For revelation and "experiential reason," see Capper and Hollinger, *American Intellectual Tradition*, 91. For discussion of the inherent goodness of humanity, see Linder et al., *Dictionary of Christianity in America*, 394.

24   See Brodsky, *Benjamin Rush*, 47–50.

25   *Autobiography of Benjamin Rush*, 163.

26   Brodsky, *Benjamin Rush*, 269. Until the late nineteenth century, Universalists professed generally orthodox Trinitarian beliefs alongside the view that humans did not possess the power to frustrate God's will to save. Rush's beliefs remained firmly Trinitarian, and thus not Unitarian. See, e.g., Rush's July 18, 1792, entry in his *Commonplace Book*. There he lamented, "how few Sects honor Father, Son, and Holy Ghost in Religion as they should do." *Autobiography of Benjamin Rush*, 224.

27   *Autobiography of Benjamin Rush*, 163, 344. See also Catherine A. Brekus' discussion of the continued Evangelical Protestant embrace of "the reality of hell." Brekus, *Sarah Osborn's World: The Rise of Evangelical Christianity in Early America* (New Haven, Conn.: Yale University Press, 2013), 9. Brekus' biography of Sarah Osborn offers detailed discussion of how eighteenth-century American Protestants simultaneously rejected and embraced elements of Enlightenment thought. For discussion of the "surprising cross-fertilization of Protestantism and the Enlightenment," see idem, 171, 7–12.

28   *Autobiography of Benjamin Rush*, 164. Brodsky noted Rush's peripatetic church affiliation: "He moved back and forth no less than four times between the Episcopalian, Presbyterian, and Unitarian faiths." Brodsky, *Benjamin Rush*, 346.

29   The influence of faith and intellectual traditions worked in both directions. Rush's Calvinist heritage likely tempered the influence of Enlightenment principles on his study and practice of medicine. During his instruction at West Nottingham and Princeton, e.g., he learned to "account for all things by invoking God, the first cause," a view he never abandoned. Because finding God's hand amidst scientific phenomena presented no problem for the faithful medical man, he accepted Newtonian and Cartesian modes of scientific thought but also valued experientially based, theological reasoning. Rush adopted the empirical medical approaches of his Scottish teachers and came to embrace the idea of "secondary causes to explain natural events," but his approach to religion remained unchanged. "To keep science consistent with Christianity," Rush claimed, "the Newtonian universe was designed by God." Lynn Gamwell and Nancy Tomes, *Madness in America: Cultural and Medical Perceptions of Mental Illness before 1914* (Ithaca, N.Y.: Cornell University Press, 1995), 20.

30   Brodsky, *Benjamin Rush*, 270. Rush also understood religion as serving political ends. He advocated for sectarian schools, in part because "[a] Christian cannot fail of being a republican" (Rush, in idem, 290).

31   *Autobiography of Benjamin Rush*, 165.

32   Scotland proved a popular place for eighteenth-century Americans to study. For a discussion of the intellectual connections between the colonies and Scotland (and the Scottish Enlightenment), see Hideo Tanaka, "The Scottish Enlightenment and Its Influence on the American Enlightenment," *Kyoto Economic Review* 79, no. 1 (2010). Rush came fully to support republican forms of government while in Europe. An earlier opponent of the 1765 Stamp Act, Rush reflected of his time abroad, "Never before had I heard the authority of Kings called into question." *Autobiography of Benjamin Rush*, 46. Rush also gained exposure to men who would later bear "an active part in the events of the first years of the French Revolution" (68). Rush's thesis for the degree of doctor of medicine (written

in Latin) addressed the digestion of food in the stomach. Binger, *Revolutionary Doctor*, 40.

33 *Autobiography of Benjamin Rush*, 37. See also Rush, in Brodsky, *Benjamin Rush*, 26n24.

34 Brodsky, *Benjamin Rush*, 40.

35 Rush identified with Jeremiah's life of strife and controversy and sensed that he, like Jeremiah, was "called upon by God to set the crooked straight." Binger, *Revolutionary Doctor*, 298.

36 *Autobiography of Benjamin Rush*, 88.

37 *Autobiography of Benjamin Rush*, 104.

38 Rush, however, believed that each religious sect was best equipped to train its own youth and, in his educational reforms, called for separate schools by sects.

39 Binger, *Revolutionary Doctor*, 95–96.

40 *Autobiography of Benjamin Rush*, 82–83. Rush admitted that while the publication helped sway public opinion, it also resulted in lost business from those who presumed he had "meddled with a controversy that was foreign to [his] business." Despite later opposition to slavery, Rush did own a slave, William Grubber, whom he "bought and liberated" after ten years of service. He noted Grubber's death on June 17, 1799 (246).

41 *Autobiography of Benjamin Rush*, 90. Rush supported Richard Allen and Absalom Jones in the formation of the nation's first African American churches in Philadelphia. Allen wrote, "Dr. Rush did much for us in public by his influence. I hope the name of Dr. Benjamin Rush and Mr. Robert Ralston will never be forgotten among us. They were the two first gentlemen who espoused the cause of the oppressed, and aided us in building the house of the Lord for the poor Africans to worship in." Richard Allen, *The Life, Experience, and Gospel Labours of the Rt. Rev. Richard Allen.* . . . (Philadelphia: Martin & Boden, Printers, 1833), 14. Rush's *Commonplace Book* recorded his participation with emerging African American churches. *Autobiography of Benjamin Rush*, 202, 228, 250.

42 Rush's public activities demonstrate the rational religion of Enlightenment Protestantism that asserted that "people everywhere experience a sense of obligation or ethical demands toward neighbors." Linder et al., *Dictionary of Christianity in America*, 393.

43 *Autobiography of Benjamin Rush*, 238.

44 In these endeavors, Rush serves as a prime example of how leaders in the new nation combined Protestantism, classical Republicanism, and Scottish Common Sense into a "discourse of virtue" that prompted action. Revolutionary-era Americans proved "confident that the exercise of reason would enable them to fulfill their divinely ordained historical mission." James T. Kloppenberg, "Knowledge and Belief in American Public Life," in Shea and Huff, *Knowledge and Belief*, 33, 34–35.

45 Reiss, *Medicine in Colonial America*, 53.

46 Jimenez, *Changing Faces of Madness*, 66.

47 *Autobiography of Benjamin Rush*, 78–79, 83–84.

48 *Autobiography of Benjamin Rush*, 84, 106.

49 *Autobiography of Benjamin Rush*, 83–84.

50 Political forays interspersed, and sometimes interrupted, Rush's medical career. At times—such as when he tended to the sick and wounded in the Pennsylvania militia and served as a surgeon general (and later physician general) in the Revolutionary War—Rush combined his passions.

51 "Break bone fever" referred to the mosquito-transmitted dengue fever, an ailment that included severe joint pain.

52 *Autobiography of Benjamin Rush*, 85–86.
53 *Autobiography of Benjamin Rush*, 86.
54 Brodsky, *Benjamin Rush*, 84.
55 Reiss, *Medicine in Colonial America*, 23.
56 Brodsky asserted that many believed "every outstanding American physician down to the Civil War was either a pupil of Rush or of a Rush pupil." This figure does not account for the many physicians who continued to train via informal apprenticeship or those that claimed medical expertness for other reasons. Brodsky, *Benjamin Rush*, 5. See also idem, 345. Between 1779 and 1812, 872 students registered in Rush's medical classes. In addition, he shepherded between six and thirty private apprentices at any one time. Binger, *Revolutionary Doctor*, 84.
57 Rush, in Brodsky, *Benjamin Rush*, 94, 252. From an article published in the *Pennsylvania Journal*.
58 Brodsky, *Benjamin Rush*, 96–97.
59 Brodsky, *Benjamin Rush*, 178–81. Flannel clothing helped soldiers avoid illness, but not for the reasons Rush presumed. Rush thought flannel (versus linen) would prevent fevers. Instead, flannel proved too thick for illness-carrying mosquitoes to penetrate. In addition, his prescriptions aimed at cleanliness (to remedy excess sweat) likely helped stem the spread of a variety of insect-borne illnesses. Binger, *Revolutionary Doctor*, 124–25.
60 Brodsky, *Benjamin Rush*, 91. Lacking knowledge of the central nervous system, Rush and his contemporaries assumed that the nervous and the vascular systems were synonymous.
61 Bloodletting often proved extreme, with sometimes four-fifths of the body's blood removed. Reiss, *Medicine in Colonial America*, 169; Brodsky, *Benjamin Rush*, 332. Rush's medical approach developed from his study with William Cullen in Edinburgh. *Autobiography of Benjamin Rush*, 361–66. For additional details about Rush's treatment plans—including remedies that induced "vigorous vomiting and purging of the bowels"—during the 1793 epidemic, see Wigger, *American Saint*, 227, 229.
62 Some Philadelphia "Quakers saw [the outbreak] . . . as divine vengeance for their sons having forsaken the sect's drab traditional garb for the lace and ruffles and bejeweled shoe . . . as well as forsaking traditional values." That view presumed a connection between sin and illness. Brodsky, *Benjamin Rush*, 323, 332.
63 Wigger, *American Saint*, 229.
64 Rush argued "that the disease, like so many others, like malaria, was indigenous, and not endemic like, say, the plague, and was therefore avertable through proper hygiene and maintenance of salubrious environmental conditions." Brodsky, *Benjamin Rush*, 5.
65 Brodsky, *Benjamin Rush*, 333.
66 *Autobiography of Benjamin Rush*, 96.
67 Benjamin Rush, Letter from Rush to Board of Managers of Pennsylvania Hospital: September 24, 1810, in "Letters of Benjamin Rush on the Treatment of Insanity at the Pennsylvania Hospital," *American Journal of Insanity* 58, no. 1 (1901): 196.
68 Rush, in Norman Dain, *Concepts of Insanity in the United States, 1789–1865* (New Brunswick, N.J.: Rutgers University Press, 1964), 16.
69 *Autobiography of Benjamin Rush*, 240.
70 To this, Rush notes, "Dr. [Benjamin] Franklin bequeathed £1000 for that very purpose," demonstrating Rush's doubt in the strength of the charge, although not necessarily the man's insanity. *Autobiography of Benjamin Rush*, 188n49.
71 *Autobiography of Benjamin Rush*, 350.

72 *Autobiography of Benjamin Rush*, 219. Here he also reported, "As yet I have heard of not one instance of Insanity" because of dire economic conditions. On September 4, 1801, Rush noted, "Amos Taylor died this day of suicide by rope. He had been unsuccessful in speculation" (255).
73 *Autobiography of Benjamin Rush*, 231.
74 *Autobiography of Benjamin Rush*, 252.
75 *Autobiography of Benjamin Rush*, 266. Alongside other ailments, Rush also wondered whether madness was "known among them" (265).
76 *Autobiography of Benjamin Rush*, 242.
77 *Autobiography of Benjamin Rush*, 288. For additional background on John Rush and his illness, see idem, 369–70; Binger, *Revolutionary Doctor*, 282–83; and Brodsky, *Benjamin Rush*, 105, 348, 364.
78 Perhaps hoping to comfort his friend, Jefferson "told Rush that he knew of many persons who recovered from insanity and that he had always believed it was one of those diseases for which a cure was highly probable; he related the history of one of his relatives who was restored to sanity and became a successful teacher." Dain, *Concepts of Insanity*, 33–34.
79 The historian Mary Ann Jimenez named the period in which Rush worked "a watershed in the history of insanity" because of the reconceptualization of causes of mental maladies that occurred. Jimenez, *Changing Faces of Madness*, 65. Jimenez's account focused on Massachusetts, but opinions in the rest of the colonies followed this pattern by the early nineteenth century.
80 Rush, *Medical Inquiries*, vi.
81 Brodsky, *Benjamin Rush*, 344. The book went through five editions between 1812 and 1835. See also Dain, *Concepts of Insanity*, 22.
82 Dain, *Concepts of Insanity*, 20.
83 Jimenez, *Changing Faces of Madness*, 65.
84 Grob, *Mad among Us*, 11.
85 This discussion of the role of the passions relies heavily on Jimenez, *Changing Faces of Madness*, 68–71. For Jimenez's sources, see also idem, 163–64nn13, 14.
86 Jimenez, *Changing Faces of Madness*, 68.
87 Kathleen M. Grange, "Pinel and Eighteenth-Century Psychiatry," *Bulletin of the History of Medicine* 35 (1961): 446.
88 Grange, "Pinel and Eighteenth-Century Psychiatry," 447. Grange cites a passage of medical advice from 1745 declaring the separate realms of body and soul: "The Operations of the Mind, and those of the Body, are not confusedly to be considered together, since what disturbs the Mind, is principally owing to the distractions and disorders of the Soul; whereas the Diseases of the Body almost always depend upon the figure and motion of the solid Parts, and the various dispositions of the Fluids contained in the Vessels" (448).
89 Dain demonstrates that physicians of the era, including Rush, offered a mix of views, often fluctuating between materialistic and nonmaterialistic explanations. Dain, *Concepts of Insanity*, 16. This displays the transitional nature of thought during the period and accounts for the variety of physical and psychological remedies that were deployed.
90 Here, Jimenez draws from three medical dissertations written by medical school students in the Unites States between 1794 and 1796. Those works, including one by Edward Cutbush that Rush cited, were the first written American treatments of insanity since Mather's *The Angel of Bethesda*. Jimenez, *Changing Faces of Madness*, 68–69.
91 Grob, *Mad among Us*, 11.

92   Jimenez, *Changing Faces of Madness*, 29.

93   *Autobiography of Benjamin Rush*, 185.

94   Jimenez, "Madness in Early American History," 32. Jimenez argues, "The Divine element [in explaining mental illness] was still present, but God was now a passive figure, not the active punisher or tester of men."

95   *Autobiography of Benjamin Rush*, 353. See also Binger, *Revolutionary Doctor*, 213, 206.

96   *Autobiography of Benjamin Rush*, 339.

97   Wigger, *American Saint*, 205.

98   Wigger, *American Saint*, 480n3.

99   Binger, *Revolutionary Doctor*, 181. Dain, *Concepts of Insanity*, 63.

100 *Autobiography of Benjamin Rush*, 350.

101 Phillips, cited in Jimenez, "Madness in Early American History," 32.

102 Wigger, *American Saint*, 203. Glendinning tried to "cut his throat with a razor, but couldn't bring himself to do it."

103 Edward Cutbush, *An Inaugural Dissertation on Insanity* . . . (Philadelphia: Zachariah Poulson, 1794), 14. Dain, *Concepts of Insanity*, 6. That definition included a symptomology coupled with the assertion that those symptoms fell outside of established social norms and showed the influence of social perceptions on illness.

104 Rush, *Medical Inquiries*, 28–33.

105 Rush, *Medical Inquiries*, 35–40.

106 Trained in chemistry, Rush fell into the category of the less predisposed.

107 Rush, *Medical Inquiries*, 56–66.

108 Rush, *Medical Inquiries*, 57.

109 Rush, *Medical Inquiries*, 59.

110 Rush, *Medical Inquiries*, 135–36

111 Rush, *Medical Inquiries*, 135–36.

112 Rush, *Medical Inquiries*, 158–59.

113 Jimenez, *Changing Faces of Madness*, 72.

114 Gerald N. Grob, *Mental Institutions in America: Social Policy to 1875* (New York: Free Press, 1973), 2.

115 "In place of political power, they sought to influence society at large through private, voluntary, and nonsectarian organizations that embodied positive social purposes. . . . Quakers attempted to retain moral leadership through example, remonstrance, and persuasion." Grob, *Mental Institutions in America*, 17.

116 Benjamin Franklin, *Some Account of the Pennsylvania Hospital: From its First Rise to the Beginning of the Fifth Month, Called May, 1754* (Philadelphia: Office of the United States Gazette, 1754), 4–5. The nation's second hospital, it was chartered in New York City in 1771. Hospital plans included cells for the insane. Though a fire and then the Revolutionary War slowed the hospital's completion, it finally opened in 1791. The nation's first hospital devoted to the insane—located in Williamsburg, Virginia—received approval in 1769 and admitted its first patient four years later. Grob, *Mad among Us*, 19–20.

     Also referred to as Bedlam, Bethlehem Hospital was founded in 1247 and rebuilt in 1547 and 1676. Albert Deutsch, *The Mentally Ill in America: A History of Their Care and Treatment from Colonial Times* (New York: Columbia University Press, 1949), 20.

117 Reiss, *Medicine in Colonial America*, 137.

118 Gamwell and Tomes, *Madness in America*, 32. Public visits to the Pennsylvania Hospital show the presumed "bestial nature of the insane." At times the hospital charged

admission for the ability to gaze upon its patients in hope of discouraging such visits, but public viewings continued through the 1830s (35).

119 Binger, *Revolutionary Doctor*, 250.

120 Rush's earliest advocacy for humane care predated Pinel's writings. However, the first work by the French reformer was available before Rush's *Medical Inquiries and Observations upon the Diseases of the Mind*. Whether Rush knew of Pinel's volume when writing that work remains unclear because he did not cite outside sources or inspirations for his recommendations in his volume. Regardless, Rush's and Pinel's/Tuke's suggestions for humane approaches to treatment bear significant affinities. Dain, *Concepts of Insanity*, 15. Nancy Tomes suggested Rush was unaware of Tuke's and Pinel's work until the 1800s. On that point, and for a broader discussion of Tuke and Pinel, see Tomes, "Notes and Documents: The Domesticated Madman; Changing Concepts of Insanity at the Pennsylvania Hospital, 1780–1830," *Pennsylvania Magazine of History and Biography* 106, no. 2 (1982): 275.

121 Dain, *Concepts of Insanity*, 5. Grob, *Mad among Us*, 26. Moral treatment, Pinel and Tuke asserted, would "assist patients in developing internal means of self-restraint and self-control" and aid healing. Grob, *Mad among Us*, 28.

122 Grob, *Mad among Us*, 26–27.

123 Koenig, *Faith and Mental Health*, 24.

124 Tuke, in David Gollaher, *Voice for the Mad: The Life of Dorothea Dix* (New York: Free Press, 1995), 110.

125 The staff treated patients as "brothers capable of living a moral, ordered existence if treated with kindness, dignity, and respect in a comfortable setting." Koenig, *Faith and Mental Health*, 24.

126 Reiss, *Medicine in Colonial America*, 125–27.

127 Grob, *Mad among Us*, 65–66.

128 Dain, *Concepts of Insanity*, 25.

129 This action hints at the presence of stigma associated with mental illnesses. Bethlehem Hospital in London became famous as a tourist destination and for many years charged visitors admission to view patients.

130 Rush, *Medical Inquiries*, 235–38.

131 "Balance, order, and harmony" were central tenets of the moderate Enlightenment. Jimenez, *Changing Faces of Madness*, 68. Here, Jimenez draws from Henry May's account of four phases of the Enlightenment. See idem, 164n15. Rush argued, e.g., "Depleting the stomach with emetics transferred the morbid excitement of the brain to the stomach and restored sanity." Dain, *Concepts of Insanity*, 18.

132 Rush, in Dain, *Concepts of Insanity*, 19n47. By "lessening muscular action or reducing motor activity, the tranquilizer [chair] was supposed to control the rush of blood toward the brain and presumably reduce the force and frequency of the pulse, thereby inducing a calming effect." Brodsky, *Benjamin Rush*, 361.

133 Brodsky, *Benjamin Rush*, 361–62.

134 Dain, *Concepts of Insanity*, 15.

135 This example is taken directly from Dain, *Concepts of Insanity*, 20.

136 Rush, *Medical Inquiries*, 104.

137 Rush, *Medical Inquiries*, 113.

138 Rush, *Medical Inquiries*, 116.

139 Binger, *Revolutionary Doctor*, 177.

140 *Autobiography of Benjamin Rush*, 216.
141 *Autobiography of Benjamin Rush*, 262.
142 Dain, *Concepts of Insanity*, 15.
143 Rush, Letter from Rush to Board of Managers of Pennsylvania Hospital: November 11, 1789, in "Letters of Benjamin Rush," 193–94.
144 From April 30, 1798: "Mr Coates will please to recollect the following Propositions to be laid before the Managers for the benefit of the Asylum for Mad people, viz: 1st Two Warm and two cold Bath rooms in the lowest floor—all to be Connected; also a pump in the Area to supply the Baths with Water, 2d Certain Employments to be devised for such of the deranged people as are Capable of Working, spinning, sewing, churning &c. might be contrived for the women: Turning a Wheel, particularly grinding Indian Corn in a Hand Mill, for food for the Horse or Cows of the Hospital, cutting Straw, weaving, digging, in the Garden, sawing or planing boards . . . would be useful for the Men. Benj Rush." Rush, Letter from Rush to Board of Managers of Pennsylvania Hospital: April 30, 1798, in "Letters of Benjamin Rush," 194.
145 Brodsky, *Benjamin Rush*, 357.
146 Rush noted that separate buildings should be built for the admission of severely ill patients "in order to prevent the injuries done by the noises" from causing other patients to miss sleep or experience "distress from sympathy with their sufferings." Male and female patients should be kept on separate floors. "Certain kinds of labour, exercise and amusements" should be "contrived" for patients in order to "exercise their bodies and minds" and speed recovery. Labors should include the ordinary work of the hospital. For those whose social status ranks them "above the obligations or necessity of labor," the recommended exercise and amusements include swinging, seesaw, riding a hobbyhorse, chess, checkers, listening to music, and short excursions into town. Patients should be attended to by "intelligent" staff members of their own gender. Visitors should be restricted to those approved by the attending physician in order to prevent the types of exposure and embarrassment that prevented those who suffered from receiving treatment. Comfortable accommodations, including "a number of feather beds and hair mattresses, with an arm chair," should be provided to patients whose conditions warrant and who are able to pay sufficiently for boarding at the hospital. Instead of unhealthy, malodorous chamber pots, patients should be provided with "a close stool with a pan half filled with water in order to absorb the foetor from their evacuations." Rush, Letter from Rush to Board of Managers of Pennsylvania Hospital: September 24, 1810, in "Letters of Benjamin Rush," 194–96.
147 Rush, *Medical Inquiries*, 7.
148 *Autobiography of Benjamin Rush*, 88.
149 *Autobiography of Benjamin Rush*, 148.
150 *Autobiography of Benjamin Rush*, 297.
151 Rush, *Medical Inquiries*, 241.

CHAPTER 3

1 Dorothea Lynde Dix, *Memorial to the Legislature of Massachusetts 1843*, Old South Leaflets (Boston: Directors of the Old South Work, 1902), 490.
2 This paragraph and the next rely on David Gollaher, *Voice for the Mad: The Life of Dorothea Dix* (New York: Free Press, 1995), 125–27. Dix's earliest biographer, Francis Tiffany,

discusses Dix's earliest awareness of conditions at the East Cambridge jail. Tiffany, *Life of Dorothea Lynde Dix*, 13th ed. (1891; Boston: Houghton Mifflin, 1918), 73–74.

3   Frederick Buechner, *Wishful Thinking: A Theological ABC* (New York: Harper & Row, 1973), 119. "The place God calls you to is the place where your deep gladness and the world's deep hunger meet."

4   Women shaped and led much nineteenth-century benevolence work. For an exploration of how gender and class shaped antebellum benevolence efforts, see Lori D. Ginzberg, *Women and the Work of Benevolence: Morality, Politics, and Class in the Nineteenth-Century United States* (New Haven, Conn.: Yale University Press, 1990). As will be noted below, Dix—as a single woman working effectively on a broad public scale—defied traditional gender norms that shaped many other benevolence efforts. Female antislavery societies, e.g., mirrored and sometimes spun off from male societies. No such male-dominated counterpart existed in the work to ameliorate conditions for mentally ill Americans.

5   The historian E. Brooks Holifield distinguished between authority stemming from office, profession, and calling. His categories described "the legitimate use of power" generated by "charisma of office," "rational authority," and "charisma of person" (via divine gift). While Holifield's account focused on Protestant clergy, his categorization helps characterize Dix and her predecessors. In his attention to mental maladies, Mather used the authority of his office, Rush invoked the rational authority of his profession and medical training, and Dix claimed the charismatic authority of her calling as a Christian. See Holifield, *God's Ambassadors: A History of the Christian Clergy in America* (Grand Rapids: Eerdmans, 2007), 2 and following. The physician Karl Menninger (chapter 5, below) also claimed rational authority. Anton Boisen (chapter 4, below) claimed elements of all three types of authority.

6   S. R. I. Bennett, *Woman's Work among the Lowly: Memorial Volume of the First Forty Years of the American Female Guardian Society and Home for the Friendless* (New York: American Female Guardian Society, 1880), 256.

7   For an assessment of Dix's leadership of Civil War nurses, see Ginzberg, *Women and the Work of Benevolence*, 145–46; and Tiffany, *Life of Dorothea Lynde Dix*, 336–43.

8   Dix also harnessed authority as a Christian to transgress gender social norms (of speaking publically, moving outside of the domestic sphere) but did so in a way that differed from her abolitionist and equality-seeking contemporaries. She thought, e.g., that the abolition and the suffrage movements were a waste of time.

9   Thomas J. Brown, *Dorothea Dix: New England Reformer* (Cambridge, Mass.: Harvard Unversity Press, 1998), 2. As evidence of his wealth, in 1789 Elijah Dix had the second-highest tax assessment in Worcester, Massachusetts.

10   Brown, *Dorothea Dix*, 350, cf. n. 16. Some sources, including Gollaher's biography, indicate that Elijah Dix was murdered. Brown disputed this claim, citing circumstantial evidence.

11   Gollaher, *Voice for the Mad*, 17.

12   Unitarianism encouraged a "gradual, self-disciplined cultivation of piety and rectitude." Brown, *Dorothea Dix*, 7.

13   Gollaher shared this assessment but noted that corporeal punishment and harsh discipline characterized the parenting style of early nineteenth-century Evangelicals and so may not have been unusual. Brown refuted accounts of abuse. Gollaher, *Voice for the Mad*, 20.

14   Dix adopted a "lasting image of herself as an orphan prematurely deprived of parental attention and burdened with the grave responsibilities of adulthood." Brown, *Dorothea Dix*, 8.

15   Brown, *Dorothea Dix*, 68.

16   Dix found in the natural sciences "a demonstration of the divine order of the world." Brown, *Dorothea Dix*, 19–20.

17   Dix hoped study would provide a "means to unriddling the mystery of God's calling for her life." Gollaher, *Voice for the Mad*, 44.

18   Gollaher, *Voice for the Mad*, 40.

19   Dix, in Brown, *Dorothea Dix*, 19.

20   In a letter to Dix's earliest biographer, Francis Tiffany, Mary C. Eustis, one of William Ellery Channing's daughters, described Dix as "strict and inflexible" as a teacher. Eustis also noted her later indebtedness to Dix's "iron will from which it was hopeless to appeal." Tiffany, *Life of Dorothea Lynde Dix*, 34.

21   Gollaher, *Voice for the Mad*, 29.

22   "Her main goal was always to instill habits of discipline, perseverance, and seriousness of purpose." Brown, *Dorothea Dix*, 19.

23   Gollaher, *Voice for the Mad*, 93. Brown, *Dorothea Dix*, 18.

24   Gollaher, *Voice for the Mad*, 47. Dix's thirty-year scientific correspondence through the mail with Benjamin Silliman, a leading geologist, suggested the breadth of her intellectual interest and capability. For discussion of *Conversations on Common Things*, see Brown, *Dorothea Dix*, 21.

25   Teaching allowed Dix to "keep her mind alive and even exercise a measure of ambition." Gollaher, *Voice for the Mad*, 84.

26   Elizabeth Peabody, e.g., an "intellectual Unitarian" and fellow teacher, remarked, "Dix's students were educated 'more nearly to . . . the true principles of education' than any other children she knew." Gollaher, *Voice for the Mad*, 84.

27   Brown, *Dorothea Dix*, 1.

28   For a discussion of nineteenth-century "spinsterhood," see Zsuzsa Berend, " 'The Best or None!' Spinsterhood in Nineteenth-Century New England," *Journal of Social History* 33, no. 4 (2000).

29   In a letter to H. A. Buttolph, Dix remarked, "I find traveling *alone* perfectly easy" (emphasis in original). Neither language barriers nor the lack of letters of introduction deterred her desire to find and study European asylums. Tiffany, *Life of Dorothea Lynde Dix*, 295.

30   Gollaher argued that for Dix, "life had a purpose that revolved around discovering and carrying out the will of God." Gollaher, *Voice for the Mad*, 34.

31   Grob, *Mad among Us*, 23.

32   E. Brooks Holifield, *A History of Pastoral Care in America: From Salvation to Self-Realization* (Nashville: Abingdon, 1983), 112. Holifield, through an exploration of the "private interchange" between clergy and "parishioners seeking counsel," documented the theory and practice of pastoral care used by centuries of ministers in the United States. Undoubtedly, mental illnesses prompted some parishioners to seek clergy counsel. In doing so, Holifield narrated changes in the relationships among theology, psychology, and "changing social and economic patterns in America." He also argued that attitudes toward the "self" in American religion—understandings that shaped pastoral care—shifted from an ideal of self-denial to self-love to self-culture to self-mastery to

self-realization. Holifield's account of the "cure of souls," however, attended to a large set of causes for clerical and lay interaction and did not focus on mental distress (11–12).

33 Holifield, *History of Pastoral Care*, 113. Portions of this section rely on Holifield's discussion of "Social Order" in antebellum America.

34 Grob, *Mad among Us*, 24.

35 Grob, *Mad among Us*, 30.

36 Populism "instinctively associated virtue with ordinary people rather than with elites." The historian Nathan O. Hatch named the post-Revolutionary shift and diversification in American Protestantism the "democratization of Christianity." Hatch, *The Democratization of American Christianity* (New Haven, Conn.: Yale University Press, 1989), 9–11. Dix adopted Unitarianism, a tradition not central to Hatch's presentation. (Hatch explored the Christian Movement, Methodism, Afro-American Christianity, Baptist traditions, and Mormonism.) The impulses and animating spirit Hatch outlined, however, shaped Protestantism more broadly than the traditions that form his focus.

37 The revivals in the young nation "empowered ordinary people by taking their deepest impulses at face value rather than subjecting them to the scrutiny of orthodox doctrine and the frowns of respectable clergyman." And "religious outsiders, flushed with confidence about their prospects, had little sense of their limitations." Hatch, *Democratization of American Christianity*, 10.

38 Dix was "exhorted to be contrite, repent of her sins, and desperately throw herself on the mercy of God. Only at this point, having purged her soul of sin and committing it purely to the divine will, could she receive sanctification." She rejected the "unbridled emotionalism and abandonment of self-control" of her father's revival Methodism. Gollaher, *Voice for the Mad*, 22.

39 Strands of liberal Protestantism first appeared in the eighteenth century and were advocated by those like Rev. Charles Chauncy, who emphasized the "truths of religion and the morality duties" of humanity rather than a pietistic religion of the heart. Such individuals also downplayed specific conversion experiences and instead affirmed that "the Christian life was a continuous rational process of self-dedication." Historian Sydney E. Ahlstrom placed Unitarianism as the first formalized liberal tradition in America. For additional discussion of the emergence of liberalism and Unitarianism, see Ahlstrom, *Religious History*, 390–402.

40 Three characteristics defined that modernist Protestant impulse according to the historian William R. Hutchison. First, it included "the conscious, intended adaptation of religious ideas to modern culture." It also assumed "God [was] immanent in human cultural development and revealed through it," instead of solely through scripture or tradition. Finally, there was the belief that "human society [was] moving toward realization (even though it may never attain the reality) of the Kingdom of God." Hutchison, *The Modernist Impulse in American Protestantism* (Durham, N.C.: Duke University Press, 1992), 2. Hutchison's main task was to explore the origins of twentieth-century Protestant liberalism in the United States. He pinned the origins of that movement in the first decades of the nineteenth century.

41 Hutchison defined the "spirit of the age" as a "tutelary authority perceived as a projection of individual reason, yet increasingly spoken of as something palatable and identifiable in itself." Hutchison, *Modernist Impulse*, 16–17.

42 Channing, cited in Hutchison, *Modernist Impulse*, 17.

43   Discourse should be "given over to an attempt to define the leading intellectual and social imperatives of the age." Hutchison, *Modernist Impulse*, 17.

44   Hutchison, *Modernist Impulse*, 17.

45   Hutchison, *Modernist Impulse*, 19.

46   Channing, in Ahlstrom, *Religious History*, 399.

47   Dix set the first hour of her day aside for religious devotions, and while she "rarely" spoke "of her personal religious feelings except in confidential hours, religion was the very breath of her life." Dix was "passionately fond" of hymns. Tiffany, *Life of Dorothea Lynde Dix*, 181.

48   "Sinful human nature was a constant drag on her soul." Gollaher, *Voice for the Mad*, 49.

49   Gollaher, *Voice for the Mad*, 50.

50   Gollaher, *Voice for the Mad*, 35.

51   Brown, *Dorothea Dix*, 41.

52   Gollaher, *Voice for the Mad*, 39.

53   Dix came to believe "salvation depended solely on 'purity of life, and devout affections'" and found little value in "speculative opinions, abstract principles, and creeds." Brown, *Dorothea Dix*, 10.

54   Gollaher, *Voice for the Mad*, 39.

55   Dix, in Gollaher, *Voice for the Mad*, 52.

56   Gollaher, *Voice for the Mad*, 56.

57   Dix, in Gollaher, *Voice for the Mad*, 64. After worshipping at Federal Street, Dix became part of Channing's religious, social, and family circles.

58   Channing held the "belief that the Gospel applied to social problems and his confidence in the redemptive power of moral education influenced Dorothea's ideas about religious reform more than any other factor before she was forty." Gollaher, *Voice for the Mad*, 79. While not every early nineteenth-century Unitarian rejected historical Christian doctrines, Channing did. He, e.g., rejected orthodox Protestant conceptions of the Trinity. See idem, 55.

59   Gollaher, *Voice for the Mad*, 65. In addition to weekday classes, Dix taught Sunday school classes at Channing's church. For a time in the 1820s, she served as a tutor and governess for the Channing family. As part of those duties, she accompanied them on summer trips and other travels, including a several month stay in St. Croix. The trip seemed well timed for Dix, who decided to accept the family's invitation, in part, to recover from exhaustion.
        Letters from Dix's time in St. Croix reveal a contradiction in her care for humanity. Dix expressed outrage over drinking and sexual relationships between whites and blacks on the island but none about the harsh conditions resulting from slavery and an unrestricted slave trade. For Dix's commentary on slavery during her time in St. Croix with the Channing family, see letters from Dix to friends, in Tiffany, *Life of Dorothea Lynde Dix*, 30–32.

60   Biographer Francis Tiffany concluded that she "had drunk in with passionate faith Dr. Channing's fervid insistence on the presence in human nature, even under its most degraded types, of germs, at least, of endless spiritual development." Tiffany, *Life of Dorothea Lynde Dix*, 58. Social outreach by the members of Federal Street Church, and other congregations, can be viewed, on one hand, as faithful Christians working to ameliorate poverty and poor living conditions. It might also be understood as an effort on the part of Boston's wealthy to make the lives, lifestyles, and education of their "inferiors" conform

to their expectations. Likely, both motivations existed, even if subconsciously. Suspicions of this darker side of social reform efforts remained unspoken for decades, but, as we will see, critique of "good deeds" eventually surfaced, particularly in response to mental hygiene efforts of the early twentieth century. See discussion of social control at the close of this chapter.

61 Brown, *Dorothea Dix*, 39.

62 Protestantism continued to exert wide influence "despite forces from the Enlightenment, Revolution, and denominational rivalries that might have undermined Christianity's cultural impact." George M. Marsden, *Religion and American Culture* (San Diego: Harcourt Brace Janovich, 1990), 48.

63 Quoted in Grob, *Mad among Us*, 30. See also Lillian Foster, *Andrew Johnson, President of the United States: His Life and Speeches*, ed. Andrew Johnson, Sabin Americana collection (New York: Richardson, 1866), 104.

64 Alongside a "millennial vision of a perfected society, evangelical Protestantism was transformed into an active social force" with a "generalized faith that institutions could be improved and that individuals could be perfected." Grob, *Mad among Us*, 30.

65 These and "a host of other voluntary organizations were formed in an effort to bring the salutary effects of Christian faith to citizens in Antebellum America." See "Second Great Awakening," in Linder et al., *Dictionary of Christianity in America*, 1068.

66 Gollaher, *Voice for the Mad*, 37, quoting Dix's journal.

67 Gollaher, *Voice for the Mad*, 37.

68 Gollaher, *Voice for the Mad*, 37, quoting Dix's journal.

69 Dix regarded "her religion as a diffuse movement to improve individual spiritual direction rather than a sharply defined denomination." Brown, *Dorothea Dix*, 40.

70 Richard H. Shryock, *Medicine in America: Historical Essays* (Baltimore: Johns Hopkins University Press, 1966), 12.

71 See Tomes, *Generous Confidence*, 68.

72 Hydropathy practitioners used water—internally and externally—to bring cures. Grahamism and Thomsonianism focused on dietary and botanical remedies, respectively. For additional details on these approaches and homeopathy, see Dain, *Concepts of Insanity*, 160–62. See also William G. Rothstein, *American Physicians in the Nineteenth Century: From Sects to Science* (Baltimore: Johns Hopkins University Press, 1985), chaps. 7 and 8.

73 Rosemary Stevens, *American Medicine and the Public Interest* (Berkeley: University of California Press, 1998), 21.

74 "Popular distrust of medical treatments was based . . . on more than a dislike of unpleasant or dangerous remedies. . . . Medicine seemed to have fallen behind the other sciences." Shryock, *Medicine in America*, 170–71.

75 Stevens, *American Medicine*, 26.

76 Dr. Nathaniel Chapman, a University of Pennsylvania physician, asserted that, while European doctors might have had more schooling, "in penetration, and promptness of remedial resources . . . we are perhaps unrivaled" and that "it may be safely said . . . that in no country is medicine . . . better understood or more successfully practiced than in the United States." Shryock, *Medicine in America*, 203.

77 "By 1845 there were at least eight states which gave their populations no guidance as to medical standards, and in many others, graduates of chartered medical colleges could ignore the remaining licensing provisions." Stevens, *American Medicine*, 27.

78 Stevens, *American Medicine*, 28.

79   The humorial approach assumed that illness stemmed from an imbalance in the four major fluids or humors of the human body: cold, dry, hot, and moist. See my chapter 1 above for additional discussion.

80   Technological advances also changed nineteenth-century medicine. Stethoscopes appeared by the 1820s; anesthesia and antiseptics, later in the century. The use of immunizations continued, and by the end of the century, germ theory, which had been debated since Cotton Mather's time, began to be put into practice. Finally, the emergence of the field of statistics meant that medical professionals could track and share details about illness and treatment effectiveness. With the exception of statistical analysis, few of those innovations benefited those suffering from mental maladies. Increasingly squalid conditions in cities generated a formal interest in public health, and hygiene appeared. From 1810 to 1857, e.g., the death rate in New York City grew from twenty-one to thirty-seven out of one thousand. Cities established boards of education that offered advice to residents and city leaders, particularly in times of epidemics. Independent public hygiene efforts combined with more targeted treatments and led to amelioration of the devastating effect of diseases. By the end of the nineteenth century, public health efforts focused on prevention of disease as much as treatment. Disagreement appeared, however, between contagionists, who advised limited contact between sick and others, and sanitarians, who argued that cleaning up the city environment would prevent the most illness. Shryock, *Medicine in America*, 128.

81   "The gloomy ruminations reflected in her letters and journals [from this time] show a woman increasingly depressed by her failure to settle on a suitable vocation, to work out an acceptable relation with society, to decipher God's calling and lead a life worth living." Gollaher, *Voice for the Mad*, 83.

82   Dix, in Gollaher, *Voice for the Mad*, 105.

83   Dix, in Gollaher, *Voice for the Mad*, 94.

84   Such trips formed conventional therapy among the well-to-do of nineteenth-century America, although an extended trip abroad, such as Dix's, was unusual for a woman. Gollaher, *Voice for the Mad*, 116.

85   Channing, in Gollaher, *Voice for the Mad*, 96.

86   Disturbing to Dix was the prevailing assumption that "heredity determined one's proclivity to contract any disease, from tuberculosis to lunacy." To a friend she confessed being haunted by a " 'hidden disposition' that threatened 'to overcome and destroy' her best qualities." Thinking of her parents, she lamented that "she could place little hope 'upon a fabric the basis of which is insecure.' " Gollaher, *Voice for the Mad*, 108.

87   See chapter 2 above for a discussion of the work of William Tuke and moral treatment and its origins. "Moral treatment," rather than working to inculcate morality, referred to the humane methods of care provided. It involved the absence of harsh physical restraints and a focus on psychological (frequent recreation, occupational therapies) rather than medical approaches to treatment.

88   Grob asserted, "Faith in reason and science and in the ability of humanity to alleviate problems and change its environment slowly began to influence theories of insanity and prevailing practices." Grob, *Mad among Us*, 25.

89   Grob, *Mad among Us*, 18.

90   Brodsky, *Benjamin Rush*, 357.

91   Charles E. Rosenberg, cited in Grob, *Mad among Us*, 18.

92 Standards of care improved only in the postbellum era as hospitals emerged as "centers for specialized varieties of disease and treatments" and the location for medical research and the training of medical students. Gert H. Brieger, ed., *Medical America in the Nineteenth Century: Readings from the Literature* (Baltimore: Johns Hopkins University Press, 1972), 233–34.

93 Quaker commitment to pacifism, "faith in the perfectibility" of humanity, and an understanding that all possessed an "inner light" and were thus "partly divine and worthy of humane treatment" shaped the Friends' optimistic and gentle care of the insane. While Quakers at the Friends Asylum emphasized moral treatment, records show that they also deployed physical treatments (restraints, bleeding, purging) when thought necessary. Dain, *Concepts of Insanity*, 30–31. Two other early institutions with church ties appeared. The McLean Asylum for the Insane (chartered in 1812, opened in 1818, renamed in 1826) stemmed from religious philanthropic rivalries in Boston. The Hartford Retreat (Connecticut, 1824) grew out of the revivals of the Second Great Awakening in that state. See Grob, *Mad among Us*, 31–35.

94 Dain, *Concepts of Insanity*, 32; Grob, *Mad among Us*, 37–39.

95 Both Grob and Dain mark this transition year. See Dain, *Concepts of Insanity*, 5; and Grob, *Mad among Us*, 39.

96 See chapter 2 above for a fuller discussion of the work of Tuke and Pinel.

97 The three forces outlined in this paragraph are taken from Grob's analysis. Grob, *Mad among Us*, 29–31.

98 Cited in Grob, *Mad among Us*, 33–34.

99 Grob, *Mad among Us*, 31. The movement of care out of homes and communities implied that more traditional modes of dealing with mental maladies began to fail in early nineteenth-century society. It also signaled growing trust in medical treatments.

100 Grob declared that the shift from private to public institutions was driven jointly by optimism and fear: optimism about the ability of institutions to solve problems, and fear about the burden and threat that pauperism and sickness posed to the productivity of society. See Grob, *Mad among Us*, 40.

101 Grob, *Mad among Us*, 32. Clergy also campaigned to raise funds for the construction of the Hartford Retreat and the McLean Asylum.

102 Grob, *Mad among Us*, 32.

103 Evidence demonstrated that both laity and clergy also hoped to heal mental maladies in order to "save their souls, for persons bereft of their reason could not receive Christian dispensation." See Dain, *Concepts of Insanity*, 37, 51.

104 Dain, *Concepts of Insanity*, 36.

105 Grob, *Mad among Us*, 44.

106 Mann, in Grob, *Mad among Us*, 44 (emphasis in original).

107 Worcester State Lunatic Hospital "shone as a model of Christian charity and civic responsibility for the helpless." Gollaher, *Voice for the Mad*, 4.

108 Grob, *Mad among Us*, 45. Later study revealed the inaccuracy of reported high cure rates. See my chap. 4 below.

109 Dix, *Memorial to the Legislature*, 492 (emphasis in original).

110 She drew "pictures of real individual men and women" and asked her hearers to "sympathize with them and to acknowledge their dignity." In doing so, she "transported the insane out of the realm of impersonal phenomena." Gollaher, *Voice for the Mad*, 152.

111 Dix, *Memorial to the Legislature*, 510.

112 For description of the memorial's impact as a "bombshell," see Tiffany, *Life of Dorothea Lynde Dix*, 83. The Worcester hospital held a number of names during its operation, including Worcester Insane Asylum, Worcester State Lunatic Hospital, and Worcester State Hospital.

113 Dix, *Memorial to the Legislature*, 490. Dix later spoke directly to state legislatures. Her "Massachusetts Memorial" was presented by Samuel Gridley Howe on January 19, 1843. Dix presented her *Memorial* "as an amalgamation of humanitarianism, colored with religious imagery, and stark facts." Gollaher, *Voice for the Mad*, 143. In the Bible, 2 Corinthians 11:25 states, "Three times I was beaten with rods. Once I received a stoning. Three times I was shipwrecked; for a night and a day I was adrift at sea" (NRSV).

114 Dix, *Memorial to the Legislature*, 490 (emphasis in original).

115 Grob, *Mad among Us*, 47.

116 Dix, *Memorial to the Legislature*, 490 (emphasis in original). In later work, Dix spread blame more broadly, denouncing "the inhumanity of jailers and almshouse keepers." Tiffany, *Life of Dorothea Lynde Dix*, 103.

117 Gollaher, *Voice for the Mad*, 3. That approach also allowed Dix to keep asylum physicians as allies. She needed their permission and assistance in bringing change.

118 Gollaher, *Voice for the Mad*, 153.

119 Dix asked, "Could we in fancy place ourselves in the situation of some of these poor wretches, bereft of reason, deserted of friends, hopeless, troubles without, and more dreary troubles within, overwhelming the wreck of the mind as 'a wide breaking in of the waters,'—how should we, as the terrible illusion was cast off, not only offer the thank-offering of prayer, that so mighty a destruction had not overwhelmed our mental nature, but as an offering more acceptable devote ourselves to alleviate that state from which we are so mercifully spared?" Dix, *Memorial to the Legislature*, 511.

120 The most influential included the following: Friends Asylum at Frankfort, Pennsylvania (1817); Massachusetts General Hospital's McLean Asylum, Somerville, Massachusetts (1818); New York Hospital's Bloomingdale Asylum, New York City (1821); Hartford Retreat, Hartford, Connecticut (1824); Worcester State Hospital, Worcester, Massachusetts (1833); Maine Insane Asylum, Augusta, Maine (1840). Tomes, *Generous Confidence*, 74.

The terms psychologist and psychiatrist did not come into general use until the twentieth century. Dain, *Concepts of Insanity*, 55. Early nineteenth-century physicians with an interest in the mentally ill often called themselves alienists. I use the terms "asylum physician" and "alienist" interchangeably. Grob, *Mad among Us*, 36.

121 Pennsylvania Hospital for the Insane (1841); New York State Lunatic Asylum, Utica, New York (1843); Butler Hospital for the Insane, Providence, Rhode Island (1845). Tomes, *Generous Confidence*, 74.

122 Grob, *Mad among Us*, 56. Samuel B. Woodward—a liberal Congregationalist, the first superintendent at the asylum in Worcester, Massachusetts—"rejected the mere pursuit of worldly goods and insisted that human beings had a duty 'to contribute to the happiness and welfare of all the creation of God . . . and to exhibit in our lives and conversation the influence of the principles of Christianity, and the love of God in our hears the governing motive of our conduct' " (57).

123 This predates the formation of the American Medical Association by three years. In the same year, publication of the *American Journal of Insanity* (later the *American Journal of Psychiatry*) began.

124 This section draws from Tomes, *Generous Confidence*, 74–75.
125 In this period, asylum superintendents were the nation's experts on mental illness. "No systematic, consistent instruction in psychiatry was available [at medical schools] from [Benjamin] Rush's death in 1813 until 1867, and psychiatry probably received little attention in regular medical lectures." That segmentation left doctors specializing in the care of mental diseases isolated from the rest of the medical community. Dain, *Concepts of Insanity*, 149–50.
126 Dain, *Concepts of Insanity*, 57–66.
127 Dain, *Concepts of Insanity*, 57, 61.
128 Pliny Earle, in Dain, *Concepts of Insanity*, 64–65.
129 Dain, *Concepts of Insanity*, 64.
130 Dain, *Concepts of Insanity*, 66.
131 Before considering institutionalization for their patients, "local doctors . . . attempted to treat mental illness by traditional methods. . . . Long after most hospitals had discarded venesection, superintendents complained about new patients who were exhausted from excessive bleeding by their local physicians." Dain, *Concepts of Insanity*, 152.
132 Grob, *Mad among Us*, 59–60.
133 Dain, *Concepts of Insanity*, 111. Eventually, heredity and incurability were linked in nineteenth-century psychiatric thought. See idem, 12.
134 Jarvis, in Grob, *Mad among Us*, 61–62.
135 For a discussion of causes of, and assumptions about, disease prevalence, see Dain, *Concepts of Insanity*, 90–104.
136 Nineteenth-century medical professionals awakened "to the needs of the insane and the possibility of their cure," but "only the most educated and religiously liberal persons of the urban classes followed the progress of physicians" and understood mental illness as primarily a medical problem. Grob, *Mad among Us*, 55.
       Asylum medicine offered a secure profession in the first half of the nineteenth century—not only could physicians help shape an emerging field, but "compensation and benefits were both secure and above average." In a time when the "supply of orthodox physicians far exceeded demand," asylum specialists enjoyed a secure client base and strong control over their patients, staffs, and practices. Living expenses for physicians and their families were often covered by asylums. Paid by the state, alienists did not need to worry about collecting fees from patients (56, 57).
137 Dain, *Concepts of Insanity*, 28.
138 Relatives were "reluctant to talk or write freely about it; to them insanity was the mark of the devil or a deplorable strain in their heredity." Dain, *Concepts of Insanity*, 37.
139 Dain, *Concepts of Insanity*, 43.
140 Buchan (1729–1805) first published *Domestic Medicine* in 1769. It became the "foremost 'home' medical book" in both England and New England. Its influence persisted for several generations, with American printings in Philadelphia (1774); Hartford and Boston (pre-1800); Charleston (1807); Exeter, New Hampshire (1828); and elsewhere averaging one edition per year for one hundred years. Adam G. N. Moore, "Dr. Buchan and American Family Medicine," Boston Medical Library, https://www.countway.harvard.edu/bml/william_buchan.htm (accessed May 17, 2011). "According to Buchan, melancholy and mania were caused by: hereditary predisposition; intense thinking, especially about one subject; violent passions or affections such as love, fear, joy, and 'over-weening pride';

excessive venery; 'narcotic or stupifactive poisons'; a sedentary life; solitude; suppression of evacuation; and acute fevers or other diseases." Dain, *Concepts of Insanity*, 38.

141 Dain, *Concepts of Insanity*, 39.

142 Wesley published an earlier version of the text anonymously in 1745 as *A Collection of Receits for the Use of the Poor*. Expanded as *Primitive Physic* in 1773. See "Primitive physic, or, an easy and natural method of curing most diseases" (1846), available online at https://archive.org/details/primitivephysico00wesl (accessed November 6, 2014). See also Numbers and Amundsen, *Caring and Curing*, 320–22.

143 Dain, *Concepts of Insanity*, 40.

144 Dain, *Concepts of Insanity*, 44–45. News reports from trials revealed characteristics of those considered insane: irrationality, inability to distinguish right from wrong, lack of a sense of guilt for crime, violent temperament. "The courts assumed that the moral faculty was almost always intact; unless totally insane, a person knew right from wrong.... Physicians like Rush, who acknowledged the possibility that the moral faculty could be deranged while the reason remained unaffected, appeared to leave the courts without any moral basis for punishing crime" (49).

145 Dix, *Memorial to the Legislature*, 505. The provision of humane, moral treatment did not require knowledge of causes

146 Dix, *Memorial to the Legislature*, 493.

147 Dix, *Memorial to the Legislature*, 505 (emphasis in original).

148 Brown, *Dorothea Dix*, 143.

149 Dix, *Memorial to the Legislature*, 513. This citation refers to the parable of the talents in Matthew 25:23: "His master said to him, 'Well done, good and trustworthy slave; you have been trustworthy in a few things, I will put you in charge of many things; enter into the joy of your master' " (NRSV).

150 Dix, *Memorial to the Legislature*, 519.

151 Her writing also hinted that she thought religion could bring healing by imparting morality. She "firmly maintained her Unitarian conviction that 'sober thought, steady self-discipline, and close meditation, are [the] agents of conversion and parents of godliness.' " Brown, *Dorothea Dix*, 253.

152 Gollaher, *Voice for the Mad*, 155, 154.

153 Howe and Mann, in Gollaher, *Voice for the Mad*, 156.

154 Gollaher, *Voice for the Mad*, 5.

155 Gollaher, *Voice for the Mad*, 163.

156 Brown, *Dorothea Dix*, 146.

157 Grob, *Mad among Us*, 47; Brown, *Dorothea Dix*, 181.

158 Tiffany, one of the early biographers of Dix, cited in David L. Lightner, *Asylum, Prison, and Poorhouse: The Writings and Reform Work of Dorothea Dix in Illinois* (Carbondale: Southern Illinois University Press, 1999), 3.

159 Tiffany, *Life of Dorothea Lynde Dix*, 115. This quotation is cited in Ginzberg, *Women and the Work of Benevolence*, 76. There, Ginzberg offers Dix's conversations with men as a display of women's efforts to influence male voting.

160 Tiffany, *Life of Dorothea Lynde Dix*, 100–102.

161 Brown, *Dorothea Dix*, 144. For Dix's lack of a home, see Tiffany, *Life of Dorothea Lynde Dix*, 364.

162 Dix, *Memorial to the Legislature*, 513.

163 Dix, *Memorial to the Legislature*, 498.

164 Grob, *Mad among Us*, 48.

165 The historian Nancy Tomes demonstrated that "rising expectations of domestic life, as well as greater faith in the asylum's efficacy predisposed nineteenth-century families to commit insane relatives more readily, and for a broader range of reasons, than did their eighteenth-century ancestors." Tomes, *Generous Confidence*, 13.

166 "Although they shunned institutional care for any other ailment, affluent families were obviously willing or, perhaps more accurately, driven to seek hospital treatment for insanity." Tomes, *Generous Confidence*, 73.

167 Tomes notes that American superintendents, more so than their European counterparts, were willing to combine moral treatments with medical interventions. Tomes, "Notes and Documents," 276–77. In a separate work, Tomes explored this change in the career of Thomas Kirkbride, the inaugural (and long-serving) superintendent of the Pennsylvania Hospital for the Insane. Citing reflections from his journal during his year of training at the Friends Asylum in Frankford, she documented his sense that "medical and moral means were 'parts of the same system' and gave 'full benefit' only when practiced together." See Tomes, *Generous Confidence*, 66.

168 Gamwell and Tomes, *Madness in America*, 55. Reported cure rates later proved exaggerated. See my chap. 4 below.

169 Tiffany, *Life of Dorothea Lynde Dix*, 161.

170 Brown, *Dorothea Dix*, 148. Ginzberg paints Dix's efforts to bring change on a national level as an exception to other nineteenth-century benevolence work by women that more often took place on a more local level. Ginzberg, *Women and the Work of Benevolence*, 126n57.

171 Brown, *Dorothea Dix*, 153. As part of her federal petition, Dix "reported a high incidence of insanity among politicians and noted the dangers of 'protracted attendance upon excited public assemblies.'"

172 Dix, in Brown, *Dorothea Dix*, 156.

173 Gollaher argued that Dix's success resulted, in part, because she belonged "to a generation that was naively optimistic about mental disorder and social welfare." Gollaher, *Voice for the Mad*, viii.

174 Grob, *Mad among Us*, 50.

175 Gollaher, *Voice for the Mad*, 6.

176 Gollaher, *Voice for the Mad*, 2.

177 Grob, *Mad among Us*, 46.

178 Tiffany, *Life of Dorothea Lynde Dix*, 146.

179 Michel Foucault (*Madness and Civilization: A History of Insanity in the Age of Reason* [New York: Vintage Books, 1988]) offers the classic proposal for this "social control" theory.

180 Foucault, *Madness and Civilization*, 70.

181 Tomes, *Generous Confidence*, 9. Tomes outlined the work of other social control theorists. While each assessment varied slightly, all saw the asylum as "an instrument of class domination" (10).

182 For a discussion of individual and corporate responsibility for illness, see Foucault, *Madness and Civilization*, 246–50. Note that for Pinel and Tuke, the term "moral" in "moral treatment" did not signal inherent connections with morality. See discussion of moral treatment in chapter 2 above.

183 Tiffany, *Life of Dorothea Lynde Dix*, 362, 364.

184 Brown, *Dorothea Dix*, 344. Note of Dix's final days spent at the New Jersey asylum—the first new hospital (versus expansion of an existing facility) she helped launch—appears in Tiffany, *Life of Dorothea Lynde Dix*, 104–5. About her choice of resting places, Tiffany argues, "The asylums were her children, and that, when worn out and incapacitated for [further] service, one of these children should thus take her and care for her . . . seemed . . . the natural order of family love and duty."

185 Dr. Charles H. Nichols, cited in Tiffany, *Life of Dorothea Lynde Dix*, 375.

186 Brown, *Dorothea Dix*, 143. Dix was not interested in public recognition. She rejected efforts of others to write a biography during her lifetime. In a letter to her friend Sarah Hale, who wanted to profile her in a book of "Distinguished Women," she rejected the offer, explaining, "I am not ambitious of nominal distinctions, and notoriety is my special aversion. . . . My reputation and my services belong to my country." Tiffany, *Life of Dorothea Lynde Dix*, v. Part of her rationale was that she had undertaken work that all should have been eager to pursue: "Much of my work has been where neglects and omissions demanded remonstrance and persistent efforts for reforms . . . , implying much wrong on the part of others, who must be at least noticed as blameworthy through either habitual negligence or willful wrong" (vii).

187 Brown, *Dorothea Dix*, 146.

188 The ability for Christians suffering from mental illness to garner authority for care directly from their experience of suffering developed very slowly, with only a few individuals, like Rev. Anton Boisen, embracing that power.

CHAPTER 4

1 Anton T. Boisen, "Concerning the Relationship between Religious Experience and Mental Disorder (1923)," in *Vision from a Little Known Country: A Boisen Reader*, ed. Glenn H. Asquith (Decatur, Ga.: Journal of Pastoral Care, 1992), 17.

2 Anton T. Boisen, *Out of the Depths: An Autobiographical Study of Mental Disorder and Religious Experience* (New York: Harper, 1960), 91.

3 Boisen, *Out of the Depths*, 113.

4 Asquith, "Introduction," in Asquith, *Vision from a Little Known Country*, 2.

5 Anton T. Boisen, *The Exploration of the Inner World: A Study of Mental Disorder and Religious Experience* (New York: Willett, Clark, 1936), 7.

6 Boisen wrote frequently about "religion" and "religious experience." While he used generic language, it is clear that Christianity, and specifically Protestantism, was the norm he assumed when talking about religion. Reflecting Boisen's descriptions, I use the terms interchangeably in this chapter. While he spent little analytic effort on other religions, nowhere does he seem dismissive of non-Christian traditions. See, e.g., a mention of the mystical experiences of Hinduism, in Anton T. Boisen, "The Problem of Sin and Salvation in Light of Psychopathology (1942)," in Asquith, *Vision from a Little Known Country*, 73.

7 Boisen, *Out of the Depths*, 113.

8 Boisen's illness shaped his life's work, but stigma about mental illness meant that he kept the depth of his illness quiet until his 1960 autobiography, *Out of the Depths*. Boisen's early recounting of his first committal, e.g., indicated that despite the severity of his initial delirium, it disappeared as quickly as it arrived. "Only a few days later," he recalled, "I was well again." Boisen, *Exploration of the Inner World*, 4.

9   Boisen "concluded that the gap between professionals had widened in the twentieth cen-
     tury. He set in motion a movement of clinical training and case study that would bring
     together pastors and physicians in a common enterprise that would deal more effec-
     tively with those who may be afflicted emotionally as well as physically." Numbers and
     Amundsen, *Caring and Curing*, 223.

10   Asquith, "Introduction," in Asquith, *Vision from a Little Known Country*, 1.

11   Boisen, *Out of the Depths*, 132.

12   Boisen, *Out of the Depths*, 132.

13   For biographical details, see Asquith, "Introduction," in Asquith, *Vision from a Little
     Known Country*, 3–8. My account relies on Asquith's and Powell's biographical sketches.
     Robert Charles Powell, *Anton T. Boisen, 1876–1965: "Breaking an Opening in the Wall
     between Religion and Medicine,"* AMHC Forum (Buffalo: Association of Mental Health
     Clergy, 1976).

14   "Boisen self-identified as a liberal Protestant and lived out his professional life in the con-
     text of a network of Progressive reformers, social science professionals, and liberal Chris-
     tians. At one point, he declared himself a 'disciple' of liberal clergyman Harry Emerson
     Fosdick. He embraced the fundamental importance of science, believed in the possibility
     of the transformation of human beings through moral striving, and stressed the impor-
     tance of making some kind of contribution to the social good." Susan E. Myers-Shirk,
     Helping the Good Shepherd: Pastoral Counselors in a Psychotherapeutic Culture, 1925–1975
     (Baltimore: Johns Hopkins University Press, 2009), 17.

15   Following his scientific and psychological training, Boisen "made sociological surveys of
     his parishes, and spiritual/psychological inventories of his parishioners," research that led
     to a number of published articles. Powell, *Anton T. Boisen*, 8.

16   Asquith, "Introduction," in Asquith, *Vision from a Little Known Country*, 4.

17   Asquith, "Introduction," in Asquith, *Vision from a Little Known Country*, 5. Despite the
     centrality of the one-sided love affair to his life, Boisen shielded it from public view and
     refrained from writing publically about it until his 1960 autobiography, *Out of the Depths*.

18   Grob, *Mental Institutions in America*, 153. In 1813 Benjamin Rush offered a basic categori-
     zation of mental maladies. Psychiatrists did not publish an updated classification system
     until the early twentieth century.

19   Illness was presumed to stem from "the violation of the natural laws that governed
     human behavior." Grob, *Mental Institutions in America*, 153.

20   Gerald N. Grob, *The Inner World of American Psychiatry, 1890–1940: Selected Corre-
     spondence* (New Brunswick, N.J.: Rutgers University Press, 1985), 3. Views about the
     links between masturbation and insanity offer an example of the presumed connections
     between behavior (and prevailing morality) and mental illness. In 1835 Samuel Wood-
     ward, superintendent of the Worcester State Lunatic Hospital, wrote, "No Cause is more
     influential in producing Insanity, and, in a special manner, perpetuating the disease, than
     Masturbation." Alongside intemperance, Woodward found masturbation the "most
     frequent cause of insanity" and usually incurable "since the vice was almost impossible
     to give up." Jimenez, *Changing Faces of Madness*, 83. Protestants too linked masturba-
     tion and intemperance to insanity. For a discussion of how "the meaning of insanity" is
     "refracted through the moral imperatives" of a particular society, see idem, 88.

21   Physicians working in asylums identified themselves as alienists and often served under
     the title of superintendent. With the professionalization of the field, this group of physi-
     cians came to be known as psychiatrists. I use the terms interchangeably.

22   Brown, *Dorothea Dix*, 327. As discussed in chaps. 2 and 3 above, "moral" treatment, which originated with the work of William Tuke and Philippe Pinel, referred to humane methods of care that avoided harsh punishments and restraints and that instead sought to treat patients as redeemable human beings rather than incurable beasts. "Moral" was a carryover from the French *traitement moral*, which implied "psychologically oriented therapy" but included no moral content. Grob, *Mad among Us*, 27.

23   Pliny Earle, "The Curability of Insanity," *American Journal of Insanity* 33, no. 4 (1877): 498–99. Grob noted that although success rates were "undoubtedly exaggerated, there is some evidence that early nineteenth-century mental hospitals achieved some striking success." He attributed that success to the closely controlled "internal environment" of the earlier hospitals paired with the "charismatic personalities" of the first generation of superintendents. Grob, *Inner World*, 4.

24   Samuel B. Woodward, quoted in Earle, "Curability of Insanity," 497.

25   As noted, this group of superintendents, from thirteen asylums, formed in October 1844.

26   William E. Baxter, *America's Care of the Mentally Ill: A Photographic History*, ed. David W. Hathcox (Washington, D.C.: American Psychiatric, 1994), 30. The plan came to be known as the "Kirkbride Plan," for its creator, psychiatrist Thomas Kirkbride. It served as the authoritative hospital design for six decades.

27   Historian Nancy Tomes used correspondence between patient family members and Thomas S. Kirkbride, the superintendent of the Pennsylvania Hospital for the Insane in West Philadelphia, to assess common views of mental illness. The four-part categorization here is Tomes', and my narration in this section relies on her third chapter in *Generous Confidence*.

28   Families worried when a "great change in natural disposition and bearing" appeared. Tomes, *Generous Confidence*, 102.

29   Tomes, *Generous Confidence*, 94.

30   David Allyn Gorton, *An Essay on the Principles of Mental Hygiene* (Philadelphia: J. B. Lippincott, 1873), xi.

31   The historian Norman Dain isolated three categories of reactions from Christian leaders. The following description relies on his categorization. Dain, *Concepts of Insanity*, 184. From "1825 to 1865 more than seventy articles . . . about insanity and related topics appeared in leading Protestant journals," and religious leaders also addressed insanity in at least two books dedicated to the topic, in one pamphlet, and in four other books. Dain noted that articles were especially frequent in journals sponsored by Quakers and Presbyterians. This section relies on Dain's eighth chapter, "Religious Opinion."

32   Welling, in Benjamin Reiss, *Theaters of Madness: Insane Asylums and Nineteenth-Century American Culture* (Chicago: University of Chicago Press, 2008), 8.

33   Dain, *Concepts of Insanity*, 184–85. For the professional controversy surrounding hiring chaplains, see idem, 255nn5, 9.

34   Dain, *Concepts of Insanity*, 186.

35   Dain, *Concepts of Insanity*, 186.

36   Thomas C. Upham, *Outlines of Imperfect and Disordered Mental Action* (New York: Harper & Brothers, 1855), iii.

37   Other clergy primarily professed interest in theological aspects of insanity and maintained a more important role for religious assessment than medical. Of particular importance for those ministers was defending Christianity against charges that it could cause insanity. Few clergymen thought insanity stemmed from demon possession, but

some—including Rev. Joseph H. Jones, a Presbyterian minister in Philadelphia—granted that possession remained a "theoretical possibility," although he doubted that it caused any of the cases he encountered. While their ruminations were largely theological, even those religious leaders held that medical treatment, not spiritual care, formed the correct response to mental distress. Dain, *Concepts of Insanity*, 87.

38 Clergy could support most asylum practices, but "in dealing with such controversial problems as causation of insanity, moral responsibility, and the origin of religious melancholia and mania, they often sought to counter" what they viewed as incorrectly presumed links between religion and insanity. Dain, *Concepts of Insanity*, 87.

39 Tomes, *Generous Confidence*, 99.

40 Such religious zeal could be "responsible for precipitating the disease in persons who were predisposed." Dain, *Concepts of Insanity*, 187.

41 Abraham Brigham, in Dain, *Concepts of Insanity*, 187–88.

42 Dain, *Concepts of Insanity*, 188.

43 Clergy remained "virtually unanimous that *irreligion* threatened insanity." Dain, *Concepts of Insanity*, 191 (emphasis added). Clergy assumed "a disposition to deny the truths of religion deprived the mind of 'all rational and stable views in regard to the mysteries around and within us, [which] sets it afloat without chart or compass' " (192).

44 Clergy proved reluctant to excuse immoral behavior on the grounds of "moral insanity," preferring to name wrongdoing as sin. "Moral insanity"—a specific diagnosis that came into vogue for a period in the middle of the nineteenth century and that was offered frequently by psychiatrists through the Civil War—declared that illness, and not sin, was at the root of some wrongdoing. That logic allowed criminals—with the aid of physicians—to plead insanity in courts of law. The anthropologist James C. Prichard, who coined the English use of the term "moral insanity," noted that in some cases patients lost "the power of self-government" but not the ability to reason "upon any subject proposed to" them. "Moral insanity" served as a "catchall" for a variety of forms of mental illness, particularly when sufferers failed to follow social moral norms. Earlier, Pinel used the same term in a different way. See Dain, *Concepts of Insanity*, 73–76.

45 Dain, *Concepts of Insanity*, 190. Catalepsy involved the lapse into a catatonic state.

46 Finney, quoted in Dain, *Concepts of Insanity*, 191.

47 For an extended historical exploration of "a class of seemingly involuntary acts alternately explained in religious and secular terms" (including debate among religious communities), see Taves, *Fits, Trances, & Visions*, 3.

48 More liberal clergy tended to agree "with the growing tendency of medicine and . . . psychiatry to view insanity as a physical illness—that is, a disorder whose symptoms and perhaps even sufficient causes were mental but one that was essentially somatic, possibly a dysfunction of the brain." Dain, "Madness and the Stigma of Sin," in Fink and Tasman, *Stigma and Mental Illness*, 78.

49 Dain, "Madness and the Stigma of Sin," in Fink and Tasman, *Stigma and Mental Illness*, 78.

50 Grob, *Mental Institutions in America*, 319.

51 Baxter, *America's Care*, 51. "By 1860 there was virtually no disagreement with the principle that society had a moral obligation toward the mentally ill," and institution building continued through the end of the nineteenth century. Grob, *Mental Institutions in America*, 303.

52   Grob, *Mental Institutions in America*, 4. An equal number of individuals received care at home or in local almshouses. The 1880 census documented nearly 92,000 insane persons out of a total population of 50 million (8). By 1875 more than 60 *public* institutions operated in 32 states. Grob, *Inner World*, 2.

53   Grob, *Inner World*, 2. Initially, alienists argued that chronic and acute patients were best treated in the same institutions. In 1880 the superintendent Thomas S. Kirkbride, e.g., noted, "What is best for the recent [patient] . . . is best for the chronic [patient]."

54   "When states assumed full responsibility for the care and treatment of the mentally ill, for example, local officials saw advantages in redefining insanity to include aged and senile patients, thereby making possible their transfer from almshouses to hospitals and shifting the fiscal burden to the state" and contributing to inpatient population growth at state facilities. Gerald N. Grob, *Mental Illness and American Society, 1875–1940* (Princeton: Princeton University Press, 1983), 74.

55   Grob, *Mad among Us*, 91.

56   Grob, *Mad among Us*, 91.

57   Grob, *Mental Institutions in America*, 300.

58   Brown, *Dorothea Dix*, 324.

59   Stevens, *American Medicine*, 34.

60   Grob, *Mental Institutions in America*, 278–79. Those states were New York, Pennsylvania, Illinois, Rhode Island, and North Carolina.

61   For discussion of how state mental institutions were swept up in larger welfare reform efforts, see chap. 7 of Grob, *Mental Institutions in America*.

62   Grob, *Mental Institutions in America*, 260, 291. Massive immigration in the late nineteenth century also shaped perceptions. Nativism grew sharply in the final decades of the century. Foreign-born citizens were assumed prone to illness, poverty, and degeneracy. As the number of "foreign" patients rose in mental hospitals, ethnic stereotypes affected care. Physicians professed to find "native" populations more receptive to treatments as the result of perceived higher intelligence and better personal habits. The race, class, and gender of patients all affected treatment. Patients were segregated by those factors, and their therapeutic care often differed by their perceived station in life. See Grob, *Mad among Us*, 86–90.

63   The growing welfare system served "to further enmesh mental hospitals in an ambiguous system that alternated between compassion and hostility for dependent groups." Grob, *Mental Institutions in America*, 341.

64   Earle, "Curability of Insanity," 496. The hospital was the Northampton State Hospital.

65   Earle, "Curability of Insanity," 493.

66   Grob, *Mental Illness and American Society*, 14–15. The percentages, as reported by Grob, total 99 percent.

67   "By the mid-nineteenth century . . . medicine had for many Americans degenerated into little more than a trade, open to all who wished to try their hand at healing." Numbers, "Fall and Rise," in Hatch, *Professions in American History*, 51.

68   Numbers, "Fall and Rise," in Hatch, *Professions in American History*, 52. Stevens reported, "In 1800 there were only 4 functioning medical colleges" in the nation. "Between 1810 and 1840, 26 new medical schools were founded; between 1840 and 1876, 47; and in the great wave of immigration at the end of the century (1873–90) 114 new schools were established." Stevens, *American Medicine*, 24.

69   Numbers, "Fall and Rise," in Hatch, *Professions in American History*, 55 (emphasis in original). As part of that diversity, homeopaths, Thomsonians, more orthodox European-trained physicians, and countless other sectarians and charlatans promoted diverse medical systems.

70   Top schools extended training periods to three years, far longer than the many institutes whose coursework spanned weeks or months, and not years. Entrance requirements also increased with more than twenty schools requiring two years of college by 1910. Numbers, "Fall and Rise," in Hatch, *Professions in American History*, 58.

71   Numbers, "Fall and Rise," in Hatch, *Professions in American History*, 58.

72   Though the vast majority of physicians remained generalists serving rural populations through the Civil War, slowly new professional specialties and societies formed. Alienists had declared the first specialized guild, but others followed. Among others: American Ophthalmological Society, 1864; American Otological Society, 1867; American Neurological Association, 1875; American Gynecological Society, 1876; American Dermatological Association, 1876. Stevens, *American Medicine*, 46. General hospitals were part of that expansion—so were the first nonasylum specialty hospitals treating the eyes, the ears, and skin diseases (31). "The specific germ theory of disease and the growing importance of bacteriology gave rise to a faith that understanding the etiology and course of disease was both possible and empirically verifiable, and that effective therapies would surely follow." Grob, *Mad among Us*, 145.

73   Stevens, *American Medicine*, 39.

74   Grob, *Inner World*, 9.

75   Stevens, *American Medicine*, 34.

76   Stevens, *American Medicine*, 10.

77   Grob, *Mental Illness and American Society*, 31.

78   The name change of their professional organization shows the specialty's movement beyond institutions. In "1885 the Association of Medical Superintendents of American Institutions for the Insane (founded in 1844) modified its membership requirements and permitted assistant physicians to become *ex officio* members. Seven years later, it changed its name to the American Medico-Psychological Association (AMPA). Those changes, which culminated in 1921 when the AMPA became the American Psychiatric Association (APA), represented a fundamental shift in focus." Grob, *Inner World*, 7–8. "In 1895 virtually all members [of the American Psychological Association] had been in hospital practice. By 1956 only about 17 percent . . . were employed in state mental hospitals or Veterans Administration facilities; the remainder were either in private practice or are employed in various government and educational institutions, including community clinics" (11).

79   Grob, *Inner World*, 11.

80   Grob, *Inner World*, 56. S. Weir Mitchell's address, cited in Grob, printed as "Address before the Fiftieth Annual Meeting of the American Medico-Psychological Association . . . 1894," *Journal of Nervous and Mental Disease* 21 (1894): 413–37. The American Neurological Association formed in 1875. Those physicians focused on "scientific studies of the nervous system" in hope of "changing treatments of nervous disorders." Their asylum counterparts focused as much on the management of institutions as they did the sources of disease. The two specialties clashed frequently. For additional detail about psychiatry and neurology in the late nineteenth century, see Edward M. Brown, "Neurology's Influence on American Psychiatry: 1865–1915," in *History of Psychiatry and*

Medical Psychology: With an Epilogue on Psychiatry and the Mind-Body Relation, ed. Edwin R. Wallace and John Gach (New York: Springer, 2008).

81 "In a trial that received national publicity, Packard was declared sane" and then spent "nearly two decades campaigning for the passage of personal liberty laws that would protect individuals and particularly married women from wrongful commitment to and retention in asylums." Grob, *Mad among Us*, 84. See also Grob, *Mental Institutions in America*, 263. Committed to Worcester hospital with "brain fever" in 1935 Packard married four years later. Grob reported that sharp religious differences exacerbated an unhappy marriage: "Elizabeth Packard adhered to a liberal theology, while her husband was a devout Calvinistic [*sic*] who accepted the total depravity of humanity. When Packard refused to play the role of an obedient wife and expressed religious ideas bordering on mysticism, her husband had her committed in 1860."

82 Grob, *Mental Institutions in America*, 269.

83 Grob, *Mental Institutions in America*, 305.

84 Grob, *Mental Institutions in America*, 315.

85 Wagner, cited in Grob, *Inner World*, 8.

86 Some "explored the physiological and biological roots of mental disease, some developed a more analytic psychiatry that incorporated Freudian insights; some attempted to integrate psychological and physiological phenomena to illuminate the inner workings of abnormal minds." See chapter 5 in this volume for the divisions in psychiatry and mental hygiene initiatives. Gerald N. Grob, "The Transformation of American Psychiatry: From Institution to Community, 1800–2000," in Wallace and Gach, *History of Psychiatry and Medical Psychology*, 541.

87 With new, more scientific approaches, "proponents of a 'physiological' view of insanity were poised to make a withering onslaught against the 'metaphysical' interpretation" of the founding fathers of the Association of Medical Superintendents and early asylum advocates. Brown, *Dorothea Dix*, 328.

88 Brown, *Dorothea Dix*, 329.

89 Grob, *Mental Illness and American Society*, 31, 5.

90 Grob, *Inner World*, 11. The creation of psychopathic hospitals accompanied the growth of general hospitals. The former appeared after 1890 as alternatives to asylum care. Those "reception" hospitals (and, similarly, psychiatric wards in general hospitals) located in urban areas offered inpatient treatment for acute cases, sometimes as a first step before committal to an asylum. Grob, *Mad among Us*, 147–48. Psychopathic hospitals (versus asylums) developed from Progressive reform efforts around the turn of the twentieth century. They provided outpatient, short-term inpatient, and preventative services in local communities. They were also intended to help reduce the stigma of mental illness attached to asylum patients. Reality fell short of intentions, however, and the facilities served largely as the first step to institutionalization at the larger asylums, and efforts in them focused on processing chronic patients more than treatment and prevention of acute cases. For a thorough assessment of psychopathic hospitals, see David J. Rothman, *Conscience and Convenience: The Asylum and Its Alternatives in Progressive America* (New York: Aldine de Gruyter, 2002), 309–70.

91 See, e.g., Jennifer Graber, *The Furnace of Affliction: Prisons and Religion in Antebellum America* (Chapel Hill: University of North Carolina Press, 2011). Protestant involvement in prison reform offers a contrast to their participation in asylum care. The historian Jen Graber documented Christian influence in nineteenth-century prison reform. Unlike

involvement in asylum building, which Protestants advocated but then turned over to medical authorities, Protestant prison reformers remained integral to shaping the philosophy and daily life in correctional institutions. Asylums and prisons, while often treated by scholars alongside one another because they involuntarily housed citizens, differed in their aims and approaches. Asylums sought to restore patients to health. Prisons hoped to reform and redeem criminals. While some may have suspected mental illness resulted from individual sin, a legal declaration of wrongdoing marked prison inmates. Asylums aimed to alleviate suffering; prisons imposed suffering as part of the reformation process. Heroic treatments and restraint at asylums, however, bore some resemblance to the methods of inflicted suffering at prisons and made public conflation of such institutions understandable. Both aimed to bring a new state of being through pain or isolation, but nineteenth-century Christians shaped life inside of prisons in ways they did not inside asylums.

92   That high anthropology (rooted in a trajectory that began with Immanuel Kant and made its way into Protestant liberalism through Frederick Schleiermacher) placed trust and authority in human experience.

93   The historian Donald B. Meyer argued, "The quest for American identity had assumed that that identity was to be found in purposes, aspirations and achievements, and further, that whatever these purposes were, they were served by energy-packed questing individuals." Meyer, *The Positive Thinkers: Popular Religious Psychology from Mary Baker Eddy to Norman Vincent Peale and Ronald Reagan* (Middletown, Conn.: Wesleyan University Press, 1988), 23.

94   An 1880 statement by the American neurologist E. C. Seguin explains the stigmatized status of those declared mentally ill: "It is fair to say that in the present state of psychiatry in America, to be pronounced insane by physicians, by a judge, or by a jury, means imprisonment for months, for years, or for life. To put it another way, there is a disease which reduces its victims to a level with persons accused of crime, and exposes them to loss of liberty, property and [to] unhappiness." Quoted in Grob, "Transformation of American Psychiatry," in Wallace and Gach, *History of Psychiatry and Medical Psychology,* 540.

95   Boisen, *Exploration of the Inner World,* 1, ix–x.

96   Boisen, *Exploration of the Inner World,* 1.

97   Asquith, "Introduction," in Asquith, *Vision from a Little Known Country,* 5.

98   Boisen, *Exploration of the Inner World,* 2–3.

99   Boisen, *Out of the Depths,* 86.

100 Asquith, "Introduction," in Asquith, *Vision from a Little Known Country,* 6. Boisen published details about his illness only decades later in his autobiography. Of his first hospitalization, he recalled, "Throughout this entire period I was in a violent delirium and spent most of the time reposing in cold-packs or locked up in one of the small rooms on Ward 2, often pounding on the door and singing." Boisen, *Out of the Depths,* 87.

101 The phrase "prophetic delusion" is biographer Robert C. Powell's. Powell, *Anton T. Boisen;* 8. Boisen, *Out of the Depths,* 91.

102 Boisen, cited in Powell, *Anton T. Boisen,* 8. In reference to these words from Boisen, Powell argued, "In view of the extremely productive course Boisen's life took" after his vision, "there is perhaps some justification for agreeing with an assertion he made in a letter written soon after the gross disturbance cleared."

103 Boisen, *Exploration of the Inner World,* 11.

104 Anton T. Boisen, "The Challenge to Our Seminaries (1926)," in Asquith, *Vision from a Little Known Country*, 21.
105 Boisen, "Concerning the Relationship," in Asquith, *Vision from a Little Known Country*, 16.
106 Anton T. Boisen, "Theological Education via the Clinic (1930)," in Asquith, *Vision from a Little Known Country*, 26.
107 Boisen experienced "distinct psychotic episodes" that "came and departed very quickly." "For long periods in between episodes [he] was free from" symptoms. During his first hospitalization, Boisen received the diagnosis of schizophrenia and used that label to describe his symptoms throughout his life. Later assessment of the variety of Boisen's self-reported symptoms led some to assess his illness as a different ailment, bipolar affective disorder. Carol North and William M. Clements, "The Psychiatric Diagnosis of Anton Boisen: From Schizophrenia to Bipolar Affective Disorder," in Asquith, *Vision from a Little Known Country*, 217–27. Boisen recorded his experiences and published them near the end of his life in his autobiography, *Out of the Depths*.
108 Boisen, cited in Powell, *Anton T. Boisen*, 14.
109 Asquith, "Introduction," in Asquith, *Vision from a Little Known Country*, 1.
110 Boisen, "Theological Education," in Asquith, *Vision from a Little Known Country*, 26.
111 Boisen, "Problem of Sin and Salvation," in Asquith, *Vision from a Little Known Country*, 66.
112 Boisen, *Exploration of the Inner World*, 8, 48.
113 Boisen, *Exploration of the Inner World*, 11.
114 Boisen, *Exploration of the Inner World*, 5.
115 Boisen, "Concerning the Relationship," in Asquith, *Vision from a Little Known Country*, 16.
116 Anton T. Boisen, "Theology in the Light of Psychiatric Experience (1941)," in Asquith, *Vision from a Little Known Country*, 57 (emphasis in original).
117 Anton T. Boisen, "Inspiration in the Light of Psychopathology (1961)," in Asquith, *Vision from a Little Known Country*, 122. There Boisen noted that medieval mystics had to learn that some of the "ideas which came surging into their minds could hardly have come from God" and might have come from the devil.
118 In doing so, Boisen "challenged the idea that mentally ill people were depraved" and instead suggested that "the individual who suffered from functional mental illness was actually the most sensitive in moral and ethical matters." Myers-Shirk, *Helping the Good Shepherd*, 17.
119 Boisen observed, "In every mental hospital therefore, we find patients who believe that God has spoken to them, that he has given them some important mission to perform and that they have some important role to act out. Among these there may be some potential George Fox or John Bunyan or some Saul of Tarsus who has it in him to change the course of history. It is therefore a matter of first importance to be able to recognize and give a helping hand to the moulting genius and to have our eyes opened to the significance of such experiences." Boisen, "Inspiration in the Light," in Asquith, *Vision from a Little Known Country*, 114. Boisen draws no connection to his own religious visions.
120 Worcester founded the Emmanuel Movement, an effort to "bring people to health by using psychotherapy in a process of reconciling patients with Christ while at the same time attempting to alleviate their symptoms." Dain, "Madness and the Stigma of Sin," in Fink and Tasman, *Stigma and Mental Illness*, 78.

121 Boisen, cited in Powell, *Anton T. Boisen*, 9. By spiritual pathology, Boisen referred to documenting in patients the types of religious experiences he found outlined in the work of Augustine, George Fox, Paul Bunyan, the apostle Paul, and others. He hoped clergy (and physicians) would attend not only to physical and behavioral symptoms but also to the progression and struggles inherent in spiritual journeys.

122 Powell, *Anton T. Boisen*, 7.

123 Boisen, *Out of the Depths*, 111.

124 Boisen found healing in "religion" but assumed that clergy mediated, enacted, and led congregations and ministered one-on-one to parishioners. Individual healing formed Boisen's ultimate interest, and changing clergy awareness and practice formed the route he pursued to effect change.

125 Boisen, *Exploration of the Inner World*, 6.

126 Boisen, "Theological Education," in Asquith, *Vision from a Little Known Country*, 28.

127 Boisen, "Concerning the Relationship," in Asquith, *Vision from a Little Known Country*, 18.

128 Boisen, "Challenge to Our Seminaries," in Asquith, *Vision from a Little Known Country*, 20–21. There Boisen noted, "According to the Interchurch Survey of 1919, 381 hospitals are supported and are controlled by the Protestant churches of America, only three of these hospitals, so far as I have been able to discover, are especially concerned with the problem of mental disorders, and even in these three the approach is almost wholly medical."

129 Boisen, in Powell, *Anton T. Boisen*, 11n73.

130 Boisen, "Concerning the Relationship," in Asquith, *Vision from a Little Known Country*, 17.

131 Boisen, "Concerning the Relationship," in Asquith, *Vision from a Little Known Country*, 17–18. Similar preventative impulses fed clerical and lay participation in the mental hygiene movement.

132 For a discussion of Boisen's adoption of scientific methods, see Myers-Shirk, *Helping the Good Shepherd*, 18–20.

133 Boisen, "Challenge to Our Seminaries," in Asquith, *Vision from a Little Known Country*, 21.

134 Boisen, "Challenge to Our Seminaries," in Asquith, *Vision from a Little Known Country*, 22.

135 Boisen, in Powell, *Anton T. Boisen*, 20. Boisen frequently used the term "living human documents."

136 Boisen, "Concerning the Relationship," in Asquith, *Vision from a Little Known Country*, 18.

137 Henri J. M. Nouwen, "Anton T. Boisen and Theology through Living Human Documents (1968)," in Asquith, *Vision from a Little Known Country*, 171. Boisen's focus on the centrality, and authority, of human experience betrayed his training in Protestant liberalism. Boisen called for "a new authority, grounded not in tradition but in experience." Boisen, "Challenge to Our Seminaries," in Asquith, *Vision from a Little Known Country*, 23.

138 Alongside work at Worcester, Boisen taught at Chicago Theological Seminary, spending the fall quarter of each year there.

139 Boisen, *Exploration of the Inner World*, 9.

140 Chaplains had served at other institutions, such as prisons, for more than a century, but Boisen forged a new role as a full-time chaplain at a mental hospital. For discussion of prison chaplaincy, see Graber, *Furnace of Affliction*, 48, 61–62, 73–74.

141 Powell, *Anton T. Boisen*, 12.

142 Powell, *Anton T. Boisen*, 9.

143 Powell, *Anton T. Boisen*, 14.

144 Powell, *Anton T. Boisen*, 11n75. Another of Boisen's recurring delusions—"his notion of a 'family of four'—suggested a definite 'plan of collaboration between medical and religious workers' " for the benefit of patients (21). Boisen did not assume, however, that clergy would adopt and use principles of psychotherapy. Medical and religious workers were to cooperate by deploying their individual competencies and sharing insight. Myers-Shirk, *Helping the Good Shepherd*, 39.

145 Boisen, "Challenge to Our Seminaries," in Asquith, *Vision from a Little Known Country*, 22.

146 Popular for many years, the hymnal's fourth and final edition was published in 1950. For Boisen's discussion of his hymnal, see Anton T. Boisen, "The Service of Worship in a Mental Hosptial: Its Therapeutic Significance (1948)," in Asquith, *Vision from a Little Known Country*, 89–96.

147 Students "used those encounters to observe patient behavior and draw conclusions about how religious experience figured in mental illness." Myers-Shirk, *Helping the Good Shepherd*, 16. "In 1925 Dr. Richard C. Cabot, father of medical social work, had written a plea for 'A Clinical Year for Theological Students' at Harvard." In 1930 Cabot, Boisen, and others formalized clinical clerical training efforts with the formation of the Council of Clinical Training. Robert D. Leas and John R. Thomas, "A Brief History," Association for Clinical Pastoral Education, Inc., http://s531162813.onlinehome.us/pdf/History/ACPE%20Brief%20History.pdf (accessed November 7, 2014).

148 Boisen, "Challenge to Our Seminaries," in Asquith, *Vision from a Little Known Country*, 21.

149 Boisen, *Exploration of the Inner World*, 7.

150 Asquith, "Introduction," in Asquith, *Vision from a Little Known Country*, 9.

151 Boisen, *Out of the Depths*, 9.

152 Boisen, *Out of the Depths*, 208.

153 Boisen "did not want to believe that his mental illness was organic or physiological and thus, by the medical standards of the time, incurable. Nor did he wish to believe that he was somehow morally degenerate or corrupt—the other possible explanation for his illness." Myers-Shirk, *Helping the Good Shepherd*, 21.

154 Rev. Dr. Seward Hiltner, a pastoral theologian at Princeton Theological Seminary and ordained Presbyterian clergyman, was one of Boisen's first students at Elgin State Hospital.

155 Powell, *Anton T. Boisen*, 18–20.

156 Asquith, "Introduction," in Asquith, *Vision from a Little Known Country*, 12.

157 Powell, *Anton T. Boisen*, 21.

158 Even Boisen proved vulnerable to stigma. The historian Norman Dain noted an inconsistency in his efforts. The Presbyterian clergyman hoped to help "the 'worthy' insane, those struggling to resolve problems of life and death and of instinctual drives (mainly sexual)." Boisen implied that those were the "kind of people whom religion can help; by implication they would tend to be educated and therefore middle or upper class,"

individuals like Boisen. Absent from the pastor's work were the unworthy, whom he deemed beyond help. Dain noted, "The idea that certain patients either deserved or could benefit better from treatment, religious or psychiatric, than other patients was of course not confined to the religious but was widespread in the psychiatric profession and society at large. . . . The pious individual who became insane might be freed from blame and minimally stigmatized by his or her disorder; the reprobate was likely not to be thus spared." Dain, "Madness and the Stigma of Sin," in Fink and Tasman, *Stigma and Mental Illness*, 79.

CHAPTER 5

1   Karl A. Menninger, *Man against Himself* (New York: Harcourt, Brace, 1938), 449.

2   Karl A. Menninger, "Forward," in *Psychiatry and Religious Faith*, ed. Robert G. Gassert and Bernard H. Hall (New York: Viking, 1964), xiv. David M. Moss, "Karl Menninger: A Centennial Tribute," *Journal of Religion and Health* 32, no. 4 (1993): 254.

3   See the introduction above for a discussion of my use of the term "mainline." My use in *this* chapter follows my earlier practice and captures the group of Protestants that could be named as culturally normative. In this chapter, I attend to what came to be known, by the middle of the twentieth century, as the Protestant mainline. I exclude the groups labeled Evangelical or Fundamentalist. Here, I use the terms "mainline" and "mainstream" to refer to the same group of believers. This chapter characterizes those who read the *Christian Century*, e.g., and not the readership of *Christianity Today*.

4   Menninger, "Forward," *Psychiatry and Religious Faith*, in Gassert and Hall, xiv. Moss, "Karl Menninger," 254.

5   Bart Barnes, "Cancer Stills Psychiatrist Karl Menninger at Age 96," *Houston Chronicle*, July 19, 1990. Besides Albert Schweitzer, Karl was the only living subject represented in the cathedral's stained glass windows.

6   Grob, *Mad among Us*, 198. For a timeline with additional biographical details, see Karl A. Menninger, *The Selected Correspondence of Karl A. Menninger, 1946–1965*, ed. Howard J. Faulkner and Virginia D. Pruitt (Columbia: University of Missouri Press, 1995), ix–xi.

7   Menninger "spoke out every chance he could against individual and social evil," including "the abuse of children, [the care of] prisoners, [treatment of] Native Americans and the environment." James F. Drane, "Karl A. Menninger: Psychiatrist as Moralist," *Christian Century*, August 22, 1990, 758.

8   Flo Menninger taught Sunday school for decades and attracted a large following in Topeka. In 1935 the congregations' Menninger Bible Classes dedicated a memorial rose window in memory of her service and teaching.

9   Lawrence Jacob Friedman, *Menninger: The Family and the Clinic* (New York: Knopf, 1990), 29. Karl Menninger felt the same way about medical insight—that it should be practical for use in daily life.

10   Friedman, *Menninger*, 23, 26. The text of "Rescue the Perishing" demonstrates a sense of Christian discipleship focused on serving one's fellow humans, with help and strength to do so provided by God: "(1) Rescue the perishing, care for the dying, Snatch them in pity from sin and the grave; Weep o'er the erring one, lift up the fallen, Tell them of Jesus, the mighty to save. (Refrain) . . . (4) Rescue the perishing, duty demands it; Strength for thy labor the Lord will provide; Back to the narrow way patiently win them; Tell the poor wand'rer a Savior has died." General Assembly of the Presbyterian Church in the United

States of America, ed., *The Hymnal* (Philadelphia: Presbyterian Board of Publication and Sabbath School Work, 1921), 730.

11   Friedman, *Menninger*, 27–29. See also Paul W. Pruyser, "Religio Medici: Karl A. Menninger, Calvinism and the Presbyterian Church," *Journal of Presbyterian History* 59 (1981): 62. The Student Volunteer Movement, founded by Dwight L. Moody, encouraged students to commit to foreign mission work in hopes of achieving "the evangelization of the world in this generation." See "Student Volunteer Movement for Foreign Missions," in Linder et al., *Dictionary of Christianity in America*, 1143.

12   Lisa Lewis and Roger Verdon, "Menninger, Karl," in *The Encyclopedia of Positive Psychology*, 1st ed., ed. Shane J. Lopez (Malden, Mass.: Wiley-Blackwell, 2009). This quotation of Menninger's is often cited, but without attribution to a specific work.

William Menninger (1899–1966), too, pursued a career shaped by his family's commitment to Christian service. After taking a break in his undergraduate education to enlist in the Student Army Training Corps, Will earned an undergraduate degree from Washburn University in Topeka, Kansas, with a major in zoology and a minor in psychology in 1919. In 1922 he completed a master's degree in zoology at Columbia University, and he earned a doctor of medicine two years later from Cornell University. Initially, "Dr. Will" planned to serve as a medical missionary but was unable to find a "suitable position at a teaching hospital in China." As a result, he joined his father and brother in medical practice in Kansas. For more on Will's career, see W. Walter Menninger, M.D., "Contributions of Dr. William C. Menninger to Military Psychiatry," *Bulletin of the Menninger Clinic* 68, no. 4 (2004): 278.

13   Albert Deutsch, *The Shame of the States* (New York: Harcourt, Brace, 1948), 15.

14   First Presbyterian Church of Topeka, "History of First Presbyterian," http://www.fpctopeka.org/wp-content/uploads/2012/05/History_of_First_Presbyterian.pdf (accessed November 7, 2014). See also Pruyser, "Religio Medici," 70.

15   Pruyser, "Religio Medici," 60. The oldest Menninger worked and worshiped in an increasingly diverse Protestant landscape. His beliefs and practices—not to mention his subscriptions to Christian periodicals—placed them squarely in the Protestant mainline. Those twentieth-century believers were located in denominational clusters including the American Baptist, Congregational (UCC), Disciples, Episcopal, Lutheran (ELCA), northern Methodist, Reformed, and Presbyterian (PCUSA) churches. Descending from early twentieth-century Protestant liberalism, in the face of a rapidly changing world, mainline Protestants viewed God as transcendent and at work in and through history and nature. They understood Christ as a radical incarnation of God, the Bible as the source of faith (although not infallible), and culture as (at least) selectively normative.

Protestants like Menninger shared an "openness, if sometimes cautious, to new ideas in the scientific, social and ethical realms." They tolerated diversity "regarding theological, social, and political opinions among clergy and membership" and viewed social progress as beneficial. Similarly, they understood creation—all of creation—as inherently good and given by God to humanity. Mainline Protestants, however, did find sin and evil in the world. They recognized sin in both individuals and institutions and understood it as contrary to God's ordering of creation. To combat evil and to enact their faith, mainline Protestants willingly and cooperatively engaged the world around them. See Peter W. Williams, *America's Religions: Traditions and Cultures* (New York: Macmillan, 1990), 333–34.

16   Pruyser, "Religio Medici," 63.

17 Pruyser, "Religio Medici," 64.

18 Pruyser, "Religio Medici," 64.

19 Pruyser, "Religio Medici," 64.

20 Pruyser, "Religio Medici," 66.

21 Bernard H. Hall, ed., *A Psychiatrist's World: The Selected Papers of Karl Menninger, M.D.* (New York: Viking, 1959), 777.

22 Karl A. Menninger, "Religio Psychiatri," *Pastoral Psychology* 2, no. 16 (1951): 13.

23 Menninger went on to summarize the work of Alfred B. Haas, professor of practical theology at Drew University, who wrote about "the therapeutic value of hymns" in *Pastoral Psychology*. In that article, Menninger notes that Haas pointed out "that, because of their rich emotional associations, hymns reduce anxiety, alleviate a sense of guilt, strengthen inner resolves, bring comfort, and divert self-preoccupation." Menninger, "Religio Psychiatri," 11–12.

24 Friedman, *Menninger*, 29.

25 Friedman, *Menninger*, 29–30. After his return to Boston, Menninger met his mentor, Dr. E. E. Southard, and worked with the psychoanalyst Smith Ely Jelliffe.

26 Quotation from "Menninger's Long History Began with a Small Idea," previously online at the Menninger Clinic website, http://www.menningerclinic.com.

27 Friedman, *Menninger*, 44.

28 Tim Richardson, "Menninger through the Years," *Topeka-Capital Journal*, http://cjonline.com/indepth/menninger/stories/100100_menninger.shtml (accessed February 14, 2012).

29 Menninger, introduction to Deutsch, *Shame of the States*, 16.

30 Friedman, *Menninger*, xi.

31 J. F. Brown, "The Human Mind," *Psychological Bulletin* 35, no. 1 (1938): 50. Brown also named the text as a "popularization of contemporary psychiatry, conceived with artistry and executed with accuracy and grace" (52). By 1940, in addition to his work at the University of Kansas, Brown served as chief psychologist at the Menninger Clinic.

32 Friedman, *Menninger*, 56. Washburn College became Washburn Municipal University of Topeka in 1941 and Washburn University in 1952. Martha Imparato, "Chapter 2: Washburn University History," http://www.washburn.edu/about/files/washburn-history-chapter.pdf (accessed November 7, 2014).

33 Karl's next two books, *Man against Himself* (1938) and *Love against Hate* (1942), outlined his sense of Sigmund Freud's "most important message—man's tragic intrapsychic struggle." Friedman, *Menninger*, 120. Friedman argued that as a result of his optimism, Karl failed to understand fully the darkness and depth of Freud's "death instinct." With his stress on the power of love, Menninger also departed from Freud's focus on the pervasive influence of "libidinal sexuality." See idem, 121–22. *The Vital Balance* (1963) "argued for the replacement of rigid psychiatric classifications with more dynamic perspectives" (idem, 310). Moving toward more general social advocacy, his *The Crime of Punishment* (1968) explored the nation's criminal system and examined what he saw as the "strange paradox of social danger, social error, and social indifference." There he also challenged the incompetence of the nation's justice system, arguing, "The punishment of incarceration in our penal system is a crime in itself . . . because it is self-defeating and not socially protective." Robert Wallerstein, "Karl A. Menninger, M.D.: A Personal Perspective," *American Imago* 64, no. 2 (2007): 217.

34 Menninger "boasted that his own hospital lacked the expensive physical facilities of his private competitors but that his staff development and treatment programs were better." Friedman, *Menninger*, 41.

35 Friedman, *Menninger*, 142. The Menningers then turned the free clinic over to the city of Topeka, but Karl complained, "In our actual work we labor with a few rich individuals . . . whose personal salvation or lack of salvation will not make very much difference." He had hoped his efforts would reach more broadly.

36 Quotation from "History," previously online at the Menninger Clinic website, http://www.menningerclinic.com.

37 Within a few years of launching, internal estimates indicated "5 percent to 7 percent of all the psychiatrists in the U.S. and Canada were trained at Menninger." Quotation from "History," previously online at the Menninger Clinic website, http://www.menninger clinic.com.

38 Wallerstein, "Karl A. Menninger," 214. The Menningers' facilities earned a loyal following, not only among patients but also with employees. Seventy-five years after father and son began their joint medical practice, the state-of-the-art Menninger Foundation and Clinics employed over one thousand in Topeka and Kansas City. Reflecting on his twenty-five-year career as a psychologist at the Menninger Clinic, Dr. Ira Stamm noted, "The commitment many staff made to [the Menninger Clinic] was akin to a religious or missionary calling. Menninger staff would settle in Topeka, raise their families here and devote their careers to the care of those with mental illness who sought treatment at Menninger." Given their clear vision, the Menninger men easily recruited others to join in their cause. Ira Stamm, "Menninger Has a Distinguished Past but What Is Its Future?" *Topeka-Capital Journal*, http://cjonline.com/indepth/menninger/stories/010602_bus _menninger.shtml (accessed February 14, 2012).

39 Gerald N. Grob, *From Asylum to Community: Mental Health Policy in Modern America* (Princeton: Princeton University Press, 1991), 3.

40 Grob, *Mad among Us*, 165–66.

41 Grob, *Mad among Us*, 124–26.

42 Grob, "Transformation of American Psychiatry," in Wallace and Gach, *History of Psychiatry and Medical Psychology*, 539. State commitment to mental institutions remained strong despite deteriorating conditions. "By 1951 about 8 percent of the current operating budgets of states (a figure that excluded debt servicing and capital outlays) was devoted to mental illness." State averages ranged from 2 percent to nearly 33 percent (New York). Grob, *Mad among Us*, 167.

43 Eventually, paresis and pellagra proved treatable. "The former was the tertiary stage of syphilis in which massive damage to the central nervous system and brain resulted in insanity; the latter, a disease of dietary origins, in many cases caused bizarre and abnormal behavior." See Grob, *Mad among Us*, 144.

44 Albert Q. Maisel, "Bedlam 1946: Most U.S. Mental Hospitals Are a Shame and a Disgrace," *Life*, May 6, 1946, 103.

45 Deutsch, *Shame of the States*, 41–42. Menninger wrote the introduction to Deutsch's volume.

46 Grob, *Mad among Us*, 206.

47 *The Snake Pit* was released as a motion picture of the same name in 1948. Starring Olivia de Havilland, it won one Oscar and was nominated for five more in 1949.

48   Fever therapy developed from the observations of the Austrian psychiatrist Julius Wagner-Jauregg, who found that "mental symptoms occasionally disappeared in patients ill with typhoid fever." By the 1930s, fever therapy (caused by infecting patients with malaria and other viruses) became dominant in the treatment of paresis. Shock therapy—introduced by the Viennese physician Manfred Sakel, and refined by Sakel between 1933 and 1935—involved injecting patients with large enough doses of insulin to induce a hypoglycemic state, which seemed to improve the mental condition of patients. At the same time, Hungarian physician Ladislas von Meduna, having observed that epileptic patients were rarely schizophrenic, began inducing convulsions with camphor and then metrazol. Both forms of shock treatment gained popularity in the United States between 1937 and 1940. See Grob, *Mental Illness and American Society*, 294–99. Even such harsh treatments, with unknown effectiveness, seemed worth using on patients otherwise destined for a lifetime of institutional care and by physicians in search of worthwhile medical innovation. By 1940 electroshock therapy, because it appeared to minimize the risk of injury to patients, began to replace insulin and metrazol shock therapy. Lobotomy involved severing "fibers of the prefrontal areas from the rest of the brain" through the removal of a small piece of skull. The procedure seemed to reduce symptoms but also brought lasting side effects, including the loss of "some spontaneity, some sparkle, [and] some flavor of the personality." For a fuller discussion of the development of, and objections to, prefrontal lobotomy, see idem, 304–5.

49   New drugs included paraldehyde, sulphonal, trional, veronal, chloral hydrate, bromides, hyoscine, and morphine. Grob, *Mental Illness and American Society*, 292. Other novel treatments emerged, including the "focal infection theory of mental illness" in which "patients had allegedly infected teeth removed or underwent tonsillectomies" to improve their mental health. Throughout the twentieth century, Protestants spent little time, at least in the *Christian Century*, discussing pharmaceutical treatments.

50   Grob, *Mental Illness and American Society*, 291.

51   A 1946 study by the Group for the Advancement of Psychiatry found doctor-patient ratios of 1 to 500 and nurse-patient ratios of 1 to 1,320. Grob, *Mad among Us*, 170–71.

52   See my chaps. 3 and 4 above for discussions of "moral" treatment, which names a standard of humane care and not an explicit attempt to inculcate morality. For Karl Menninger's explanation of moral treatment, see Karl A. Menninger, *The Vital Balance: The Life Process in Mental Health and Illness* (New York: Viking, 1964), 67–71.

53   The "passage of years and the extension of experience" only deepened his hopefulness. Friedman, *Menninger*, 46–47, 52. Karl Menninger met with Freud, briefly, during a 1934 trip to Vienna. Despite his devotion to Freud's theories, Menninger thought the Austrian mistreated him by being dismissive and failing to recognize Menninger's grasp and use of Freud's work (110–11). Karl A. Menninger, *The Human Mind (1942)*, 2nd ed. (New York: Knopf, 1942), vii. In 1945 Menninger visited the Buchenwald concentration camp just twelve days after it was liberated, and the horror that he saw tempered his enthusiasm for full-scale adoption of European psychoanalytic theory. Friedman, *Menninger*, 130–31.

54   As Karl's speaking schedule increasingly kept him away from Topeka, managing the day-to-day operations of the clinic transferred to William. A discussion of the details of Karl's theory of the origins of mental illness appears below.

55   The historian Lawrence Friedman found four distinct elements that shaped William's, and thereby the family clinic's, holistic formulation of mental health care. This section draws on his account. See Friedman, *Menninger*, 62–65.

56   The therapeutic philosophy articulated in William Menninger's "Guide to the Order Sheet" "committed everyone to being part of the treatment, including housekeeping staff, aides, cooks, and groundsmen. Treatment was a 24-hour-a-day process that involved every employee," and not just physicians. Roy W. Menninger, "The Legacy of Menninger," *Bulletin of the Menninger Clinic* 66, no. 4 (2002): 354.

57   Friedman, *Menninger*, 62–65.

58   Friedman, *Menninger*, 90.

59   Herbert J. Brinks, *Pine Rest Christian Hospital, 75 years: 1910–1985* (Cutlerville, Mich.: Pine Rest Christian Hospital, 1985), 11.

60   Despite largely falling out of favor, suspicions of demonic influence lingered. With plans for Pine Rest underway, the Dutch Reformed clergyman Jon Keizer concluded that "mental problems . . . frequently resulted from spiritual anxieties—fears of having sinned beyond the power of God's forgiving grace." Such "a weakened state," he held, made "the patient especially vulnerable to the work of Satan." Brinks, *Pine Rest*, 13, 15. Marking some instances of mental distress as religious in nature, and thus the responsibility of the church (and not medicine), was a pronouncement similar to that offered by Anton Boisen.

61   Other religious groups continued or launched similar care efforts. The Christian Sanatorium in Patterson, New Jersey, opened in 1917 after deacons from Reformed and Christian Reformed congregations hoped to "create a facility that would be guided by Christian principles and provide physical, mental, and spiritual care for those with mental afflictions, regardless of ability to pay." Quotation from "Our History," previously online at the Christian Health Care Center website, http://www.christianhealthcare .org. The Seventh-Day Adventist and psychiatrist George T. Harding IV, after years of private practice, opened the Indianola Rest Home for women in 1916. In the 1930s, he launched the Harding Sanitarium. Harding staff members were influenced by Karl Menninger's writings and trained at the Menninger Clinic. See George T. Harding IV, "Adventists and Psychiatry—A Short History of the Beginnings," *Spectrum* 17, no. 3 (1987). American Quakers offered mental health care, as they had for the prior century. They actively advertised their facilities to fellow Friends. Throughout the 1950s and 1960s, e.g., advertisements for the Philadelphia Friends Hospital for the Mentally Ill, the Darlington Sanitarium, and the Marshall Square Sanitarium appeared in the *Friends Journal*.

62   John Maurice Gessell, "State Hospital Scandal," *Christian Century*, October 16, 1946.

63   Elmer M. Ediger, "Roots of the Mennonite Mental Health Story," in *If We Can Love: The Mennonite Mental Health Story*, ed. Vernon H. Neufeld (Newton, Kans.: Faith and Life, 1983), 27 (emphasis in original).

64   Mennonites opened seven additional mental health centers between 1949 and 1967. Planning for the first Mennonite hospital, Brook Lane, began in 1946. It opened in 1949, located on a farm outside of Hagerstown, MD. See Ediger, *Roots of the Mennonite Mental Health Story*, 27. The third Mennonite hospital, Prairie View, opened in Newton, Kansas, in 1954. "They discovered," a correspondent for the *Century* reported, "that mental patients responded to their care, and that Christian love was a prerequisite which had

apparently been lacking in the care and treatment" at other facilities. "Mennonites Aid Mental Therapy," *The Christian Century*, May 5, 1954, 566.

65   "Invite Churches to Aid Mentally Ill," *Christian Century*, April 24, 1946, 517.

66   See, e.g., James Maurice Trimmer, "C.O.'s Bring Reforms in Mental Hospitals," *Christian Century*, September 22, 1943, 1082; O. M. Walton, "Pacifists Protest Beating of Insane: Conscientious Objectors Are Discharged from Ohio Hospital," *Christian Century*, December 8, 1943, 1451.

67   Wartime psychiatrists attended to "high battlefield neuropsychiatric casualty rates." Grob, *Mad among Us*, 193.

68   Wartime needs grew the ranks of psychiatrists and expanded the setting of their work beyond the asylum. In 1940 the American Psychological Association had 2,295 members, two-thirds of whom worked in mental hospitals. In World War II alone, 2,400 physicians served in psychiatric roles. Grob, *Mad among Us*, 193–94, 196.

69   They began to argue that "early identification of symptoms and treatment in community settings could prevent the onset of more serious mental disorders and thus obviate the need for prolonged institutionalization." Undergirding that assumption was a belief that mental health (and illness) existed along a spectrum. Preventative and restorative measures helped reorient ailing individuals toward health. This section relies on Grob, *Mad among Us*, 191–94. Wartime efforts significantly increased demand for psychiatric professions, particularly so because the military used psychiatrists to screen out men deemed unfit for military service. "The military feared in particular that the inadvertent recruitment of homosexual males would have a devastating effect on the armed forces" (192). The condition soldiers suffered was named "combat exhaustion" and not formally diagnosed as mental illness (another indicator of ongoing stigma).

70   The new approach "elevated the significance of the life history and prior experiences of the individual." Grob, *Mad among Us*, 142.

71   In the years after the war, "a shift in psychiatric thinking fostered receptivity toward a psychodynamic and psychoanalytic model that emphasized life experiences and the role of socioenvironmental factors." Grob, *From Asylum to Community*, 4.

72   Menninger, *Vital Balance*, 66.

73   Menninger, "Religio Psychiatri," 14. Freud's psychodynamic theory assumed psychological, not organic, forces shaped human behavior. Psychoanalysis, then, sought to uncover those psychological forces in both conscious and unconscious thought.

74   Grob, *Mad among Us*, 101–2. By 1957 only 17 percent of ten thousand American Psychiatric Association members worked in state asylums or Veterans Administration facilities. A century earlier, membership was restricted to asylum physicians.

75   Grob, *Mental Illness and American Society*, 144–45.

76   Coordinating many mental hygiene efforts was the National Committee for Mental Hygiene, which formed in 1909. Clifford Beers, a former mental patient turned advocate for the insane, founded the organization with the support of the Swiss-born psychiatrist Adolf Myers and psychologist William James. The National Committee for Mental Hygiene hoped to "protect the public's mental health; promote research into and dissemination of material pertaining to the etiology, treatment, and prevention of mental disease; enlist the aid of the federal government; and establish state societies for mental hygiene." Grob, *Mental Illness and American Society*, 153. See Grob's chapter 6 for additional detail about the formation and development of mental hygiene efforts (144–78). Grob argued that "hygienic goals seemed certain to attract broad support from a public increasingly

fearful of the seeming rise in venereal diseases, alcoholism, and a variety of other aberrant behaviors that fostered illness, dependency, and crime." Mental hygiene efforts allowed Americans to address their worries about other citizens. Grob, *Mad among Us*, 154.

77   Menninger, though, rejected hereditarian theories of mental disease. See discussion below.

78   Karl A. Menninger, *The Human Mind (1930)*, 1st ed. (New York: Knopf, 1930), 13n2.

79   Menninger noted that "the distress of a personality struggling with an environment is simply struggle and not a matter of devils and witches, sin and 'orneriness,' or yet of a feeble intellect or feeble will." Karl Menninger, *The Human Mind (1949)*, 3rd ed. (New York: Knopf, 1949), 15.

80   Menninger, *Human Mind (1930)*, 14, 359 (emphasis in original).

81   Theories of mental hygiene changed over time. In the nineteenth century, a "synthesis of Protestantism, Scottish moral philosophy, and Baconian science" linked mental and physical disease to individual behaviors. Prevention efforts "reflected a world view based on an older religious tradition that emphasized natural law, free will, and individual responsibility." While professionals could educate patients about the connections between behavior and disease, individuals held ultimate responsibility for their choices. Grob, *Mental Illness and American Society*, 144. The twentieth-century mental hygiene movement, in contrast, grew from the assumption that disease was "a product of environmental and hereditarian deficiencies" and that "its control and eradication required a fusion of scientific knowledge and administrative activity." Grob, *Mad among Us*, 151. As a result, newer mental hygiene efforts addressed not just mental illness but also feeble-mindedness, alcoholism, juvenile delinquency, crime, prostitution, and dependency, all conditions thought to be influenced by environmental factors and heredity.

82   "Church Offers Courses on Mental Hygiene," *Christian Century*, March 27, 1940, 427.

83   "Great Churches of America: XII. First Community Church, Columbus, Ohio," *Christian Century*, December 20, 1950, 1515.

84   Grob, *Mental Illness and American Society*, 166–67.

85   Grob, *Mental Illness and American Society*, 173.

86   During the war, "revelations about the use of sterilization in Nazi Germany became public." Grob, *Mental Illness and American Society*, 177.

87   This section relies of the work of theological ethicist Amy Laura Hall (*Conceiving Parenthood: American Protestantism and the Spirit of Reproduction* [Grand Rapids: Eerdmans, 2008]).

88   George Huntington Donaldson, cited in Hall, *Conceiving Parenthood*, 260.

89   Hall, *Conceiving Parenthood*, 261–62.

90   Protestants like Donaldson and Osgood interpreted the "scriptural story of salvation in the Old Testament" as "God's refining, purifying, and selecting in order to produce a stronger, heartier stock of humans." Hall, *Conceiving Parenthood*, 265.

91   The language of "mental hygiene" hard largely fallen out of use by the end of the 1950s, but the impulse for church people to aid in prevention efforts continued. In 1959 Herbert H. Stroup, Congregational minister and professor of sociology at Brooklyn College, urged church people to root out "incipient cases" of illness in a quest to sustain "normal existence." Stroup discussed ways Christian resources could be deployed in support of maintaining normality. Different in Stroup's account, however, was the proposal of a more robust theological anthropology to balance church resources with secular tools.

Herbert H. Stroup, "Keeping Sane in a Crazy World," *Christian Century*, September 18, 1959, 1338–40.

92 Hall, *Conceiving Parenthood*, 269.

93 Similarly, the editors of the *Christian Century* argued, "In the light of these current revelations, no Christian minister with a member of his congregation in a mental institution should rest until he knows what the conditions are in that institution and whether or not they call for reform." "Growing Outcry over Mental Hospitals," *Christian Century*, May 15, 1946, 611–12.

94 Gessell, "State Hospital Scandal," 1245–47.

95 Similarly, an April 1946 *Christian Century* editorial advocated support for the same organization and lauded the U.S. House of Representatives for passing the National Mental Health Act. "Invite Churches to Aid Mentally Ill," 518.

96 "Pacifists Give Aid to Mental Hospitals," *Christian Century*, February 24, 1943, 240.

97 "Obsession with the Neurotic," *Christian Century*, May 15, 1946, 613.

98 Charles Leslie Venable, "Launch Campaign for Mentally Ill," *Christian Century*, April 23, 1947, 531.

99 Charles Leslie Venable, "Call for Reform in Institutions: Chicago Ministers Urge Congregations to Work for Improvement in State Hospitals for Mentally Ill," *Christian Century*, June 11, 1947, 748.

100 Justin G. Reese, "Sick Minds Are a Community Problem," *Christian Century*, June 18, 1947, 768.

101 "Church Club Helps Discharged Mental Patients," *Presbyterian Life*, December 15, 1959, 31. Support for public relief agencies and efforts persisted over the next two decades. In 1966, e.g., an article entitled "Mr. Goldwater Talks Sense," in the *Christian Century*, pointed to an "unexpected boost" (and a "shocking rebuke" for the "lunatic fringe of the radical right") from Barry Goldwater, an ultraconservative 1964 presidential candidate. In a speech as the campaign chair of a local Arizona mental health association, Goldwater had called for a "turn-around on our outlook on mental health," expressed dismay at the lack of knowledge of mental illnesses, and called for support for local mental health agencies. *Christian Century* editors were pleasantly surprised by Goldwater's support for such efforts and noted, "So, if the extreme right leaves him [as a result of his stand]— good riddance." Inherent in that commentary about Goldwater was a continued call for support, and an affirmation of the value of local, secular mental health agencies by the mainline. "Mr. Goldwater Talks Sense," *Christian Century*, July 20, 1966, 905.

102 J. R. Nelson, "Bioethics and the Marginalization of Mental Illness," *Journal of the Society of Christian Ethics* 23, no. 2 (2003): 184.

103 Community-based initiatives failed fully to "assume the burdens previously shouldered by state hospitals." "During the 1960s the population of nursing homes rose from about 470,000 to nearly 928,000." Grob, *Mad among Us*, 287–90.

104 Karl A. Menninger, *Whatever Became of Sin?* (New York: Hawthorn Books, 1973), 80–81.

105 Karl A. Menninger, "Psychiatrists Use Dangerous Words," *Saturday Evening Post*, April 25, 1964, 12.

106 Menninger, *Human Mind* (1942), 1.

107 Menninger, *Human Mind* (1942), viii. He also named mental illness a "universal human experience," reflecting a sentiment voiced by Cotton Mather centuries earlier. Menninger, *Vital Balance*, 417.

108 Hall, *Psychiatrist's World*, 796. In that 1953 reflection, Menninger noted that the first type of illness was currently "a more recognized field for psychiatry" and that the other "is coming to be."

109 Hall, *Psychiatrist's World*, 784.

110 Hall, *Psychiatrist's World*, 796 (emphasis original).

111 Menninger, "Religio Psychiatri," 14.

112 L. M. Birkhead, ed., *From Sin to Psychiatry: An Interview on the Way to Mental Health with Dr. Karl A. Menninger*, ed. E. Haldeman-Julius, Little Blue Book, vol. 1585 (Girard, Kans.: Haldeman-Julius, 1931), 10–11.

113 Menninger, *Human Mind (1942)*, viii.

114 Three thinkers influenced that understanding. From the nineteenth-century French physiologist Claude Bernard, he understood that the interaction of one's internal and external environments (milieus) influenced sufferers. From the Swiss psychiatrist Adolf Meyer, Menninger adopted the sense of "mental illness as an unskillful reaction to external stress." Finally, from the creator of psychoanalysis, Sigmund Freud, he embraced notions of "the struggle between creative and destructive forces, between life and death instincts, between love and aggression" that caused mental illness. Menninger held that stress caused "aggressive, hostile and destructive feelings" and that mental illness resulted when those feelings were not "handled effectively." Drane, "Karl A. Menninger," 759.

115 Menninger, cited in Drane, "Karl A. Menninger," 758–59 (emphasis in original).

116 Deutsch, *Shame of the States*, 9–10. Karl Menninger authored the introduction to Deutsch's volume. In 1943 legislation in Illinois officially dropped the terms "lunacy" and "insanity" and substituted "mental illness." Charles Leslie Venable, "Modernize Treatment of Mental Illness," *Christian Century*, August 11, 1943, 926.

117 Jerome G. Manis et al., "Public and Psychiatric Conceptions of Mental Illness," *Journal of Health and Human Behavior* 6, no. 1 (1965): 49.

118 John B. Oman, "Church Help for the Mentally Ill," *Christian Century*, January 23, 1952, 100.

119 Mental patients were not the only ones featured in media portrayals that shaped views of illness. For a period in the early 1960s, coverage indicated that the mental health system—and psychiatrists in particular—had regained prestige lost around the turn of the twentieth century. Between 1957 and 1963, e.g., "Hollywood produced more than twenty films that presented psychiatrists—the purveyors of reason, knowledge, and well-being—in glowing and idealized terms." That praise, however, was short lived. A later batch of films and novels, including *One Flew over the Cuckoo's Nest* (1962) and *Shock Treatment* (1964), displayed psychiatrists as "either malevolent or comedy-like figures." Among the films portraying physicians in a favorable light were *The Three Faces of Eve* (1957), *Splendor in the Grass* (1961), *Pressure Point* (1962), and *Freud* (1962). Despite their reclamation of professional prestige, it seemed psychiatrists could not escape the taint associated with attending to those citizens often relegated to mental institutions and "banished" by fellow Americans. Grob, *Mad among Us*, 173, 268, 275.

120 Jo C. Phelan et al., "Public Conceptions of Mental Illness in 1950 and 1996: What Is Mental Illness and Is It to Be Feared?" *Journal of Health and Social Behavior* 41, no. 2 (2000): 188.

121 Jo C. Phelan et al., "Public Conceptions," 188.

122 Oman, "Church Help for the Mentally Ill," 100.

123 Jim Bryan, "Life's Hard Questions: How Should the Church Handle Mental Illness?"
     Presbyterian Life, September 1, 1968. Similarly, *Christian Century* articles in 1968 and 1969
     cite a 1966 Public Affairs pamphlet that stated twenty-five thousand Americans commit-
     ted suicide in 1966. Both urged reconsideration of traditional church teaching of suicide
     as a sin, and each implored church members to respond. Only the latter article, which
     talked about an overnight ministry, described who might suffer: "night workers, theater
     and night club performers and patrons, tourists . . . drunks . . . hippies . . . or even 'just
     people' trying to walk off problems that won't let them sleep." Elsie Thomas Culver,
     "Suicide: Need for a 'Significant Other,' " *Christian Century*, January 15, 1969, 100. See
     also Donald D. McCall, "Anomie My Enemy," *Christian Century*, July 24, 1968.
124 An exception was a discussion in 1959 about the mental health of former air force major
     Claude Eatherly, who flew the B-29 bomber that dropped the atomic bomb on Hiro-
     shima, Japan, during World War II. After his repeated suicide attempts and a "life of
     delinquency," church leaders wondered if Eatherly needed not just psychiatric care but
     instead "the ministries of religion" to attend, theologically, to his spiritual distress. "Who
     Needs the Psychiatrist?" *Christian Century*, May 6, 1959, 541.
125 Edward Hughes Pruden, "Nerves of Defense Workers Crack: Psychiatrist Condemns
     Capital Strain," *Christian Century*, April 1, 1942, 440.
126 "When the Heroes Come Home," *Christian Century*, May 26, 1943, 629.
127 George Christian Anderson, "Emotional Health of Clergy," *Christian Century*, Novem-
     ber 4, 1953, 1260–61 (emphasis in original). Because church leaders assumed that clergy
     emotional stability might be important to assess, psychological testing for ministerial
     candidates became common practice for mainline denominations in the middle of the
     twentieth century.
128 William H. Hudnut Jr., "Are Ministers Cracking Up?" *Christian Century*, November 7,
     1956, 1288.
129 Hudnut, "Are Ministers Cracking Up?" 1288.
130 Differences between specialties warrant explanation. Formal medical care for mental ill-
     ness grew out of the work of nineteenth-century asylum physicians. The medical doctors
     that were direct descendants of those "alienists" were psychiatrists. M.D. psychiatrists
     attended medical school and then specialized in psychiatry. Neurology, another medi-
     cal specialty, developed in the United States during the Civil War, with an interest "in
     wounds involving nerve tissue." In the nineteenth century, they treated many of the same
     ailments as psychiatrists, but "unlike the founders of institutional psychiatry—many
     of whom were identified with pietistic Protestantism and moral issues—neurologists
     tended to identify themselves with the world of science and especially European scientific
     medicine." With a focus on the brain and the central nervous system, and with a differ-
     ent methodological background, neurologists remained organizationally separate from
     psychiatrists and frequently eschewed work in institutions. See Grob, *Mental Illness and
     American Society*, 50–62. Psychology was a "discipline with its roots in philosophy rather
     than medicine." Doctors of psychology earned Ph.D.s, not medical degrees. In the United
     States, at first, psychology was a research-oriented discipline that studied individuals and
     groups. Eventually, though, "clinical" psychologists began to work outside of universities
     in clinics and schools where they made prescriptive observations about human behavior.
     This led to conflict with psychiatrists, especially as they extended their practice outside
     of mental hospitals. See idem, 260–64. See Grob's ninth chapter, "The Emergence of the
     Mental Health Professions," for additional discussion including overviews of psychiatric

social work and occupational therapy, both of which played a role in twentieth-century mental health care. Psychoanalytic thought and psychoanalysis stemmed from the theories about human behavior of the Austrian neurologist Sigmund Freud, whose work "had relatively little influence on American psychiatry before 1920" (120).

Overlapping convictions—alongside many differences in thought—marked the relationships between these groups in the first five or six decades of the twentieth century. Sometimes they cooperated; often they competed for patients and authority.

131 Grob, *Mental Illness and American Society*, 306. In 1918, with Clifford Beers, Hincks founded the Canadian National Committee for Mental Hygiene.

132 Drane, "Karl A. Menninger," 759. He thought that both religious workers and professionals attending to mental maladies (psychiatrists, psychiatrists' helpers, psychiatric social workers, psychiatric nurses and aides, therapists, and psychologists) were "dedicated to the kind of work in which the importance of the other person is greater than it is natural for that importance to be in a normal person." Hall, *Psychiatrist's World*, 796. Perhaps the earliest joint healing effort was the Emmanuel Movement started in Boston in 1906 by the Episcopal priest Elwood Worcester. Psychiatrists, other medical doctors, and clergy worked together to diagnose and care for patients. The practice of prayer and belief in the "primacy of the mind over the body" shaped the ministry. Numbers and Amundsen, *Caring and Curing*, 256.

133 Menninger, "Religio Psychiatri," 14.

134 Hall, *Psychiatrist's World*, 778.

135 Virgil E. Lowder, "Menninger Relates Religion and Psychiatry," *Christian Century*, April 11, 1951, 475.

136 Lowder, "Menninger Relates Religion," 475. Menninger also identified a morality in psychiatry and assumed that "beliefs which must in the last analysis be described as religious are implicit in the theory and practice of psychiatry." Drane, "Karl A. Menninger," 759.

137 Menninger, "Religio Psychiatri," 14.

138 Hall, *Psychiatrist's World*, 783.

139 Menninger, "Religio Psychiatri," 17. In that explanation, as others, Menninger supported his assertions with a verse from Scripture: "'Passing through the valley of weeping, they make it a place of springs.' (Psalm 84)." His mother's Bible study training had lasting impact.

140 Menninger, in Deutsch, *Shame of the States*, 15.

141 Menninger, *Whatever Became of Sin?* 201.

142 Hall, *Psychiatrist's World*, 778.

143 Menninger, *Vital Balance*, 416.

144 "2,000 Attend Institute on Religion and Psychiatry," *Christian Century*, June 1, 1955, 660.

145 Menninger, *Whatever Became of Sin?* 217–18.

146 Menninger, in Deutsch, *Shame of the States*, 15.

147 "Offer Wisconsin Pastors Aid in Counseling Mentally Ill," *Christian Century*, June 16, 1948, 614. Whether churches or the state made the request is unclear, but, either way, the news item supported the request.

148 Clarence Worthington Kemper, "Ministers Study Psychiatry," *Christian Century*, January 26, 1944, 120.

149 Gessell, "State Hospital Scandal," 1247.

150 "Religion and Mental Health Academy Is Launched," *Christian Century*, April 18, 1956, 477.

151 The groups gathered in celebration of the one hundredth anniversary of Sigmund Freud's birth.

152 "Psychiatry Makes a Move," *Christian Century*, May 9, 1956, 572.

153 John Wright Buckham, "What Has Psychology Done to Us?" *Christian Century*, September 25, 1940, 1171–72.

154 Quotation from "History," previously online at the Menninger Clinic website, http://www.menningerclinic.com.

155 Hiltner, a Presbyterian, was a leader in the field of pastoral counseling and a faculty member at Princeton Theological Seminary for nearly twenty years. He was one of the first students to train with Anton Boisen and went on to publish ten books and hundreds of articles, most dealing with the application of psychology to pastoral care. In the 1930s, he served as executive secretary of the Council for Clinical Training, and later he served as the executive secretary of the Commission on Religion and Health. "Rev. Seward Hiltner, 74, Dies; Taught at Princeton Seminary," *New York Times*, November 28, 1984.

156 A review of the theologian Leslie D. Weatherhead's *Psychology, Religion and Healing* captured that mainline sentiment well. The reviewer noted Weatherhead's reminder that "(1) religion has to do with the whole of man; (2) that the splendid work of doctors in the area of physical methods is in constant need of spiritual assistance in a cooperative fashion; (3) that God works just as thoroughly through the skills of men to bring health and happiness to the minds, bodies, and souls of his children as man will let him." Clyde J. Verheyden, "Healing the Whole Man," *Christian Century*, August 6, 1952, 901.

157 Simon Doniger, ed., *The Minister's Consultation Clinic: Pastoral Psychology in Action* (Great Neck, N.Y.: Channel, 1955). See the volume's table of contents for each section for a list of topics.

158 Karl A. Menninger, "The Minister's Consultation Clinic," *Pastoral Psychology* 7, no. 1 (1956): 5.

159 Friedman, *Menninger*, 263. Because training in pastoral counseling, beyond the knowledge to be gained by the many published books, required financial resources, it likely proved out of reach of all but middle- and upper-class clergy.

160 For detailed discussions of the development of pastoral counseling within the mainline tradition, see Holifield, *History of Pastoral Care*; Myers-Shirk, *Helping the Good Shepherd*; and Warren Anderson Kinghorn, "Medicating the Eschatological Body: Psychiatric Technology for Christian Wayfarers" (Th.D. diss, Duke University, 2011).

161 Robert Edward Luccock, "Seminary in Retrospect," *Christian Century*, April 26, 1950, 524.

162 John Oliver Nelson, "Trends Toward a Relevant Ministry," *Christian Century*, April 26, 1950, 527.

163 William Edward Hulme, "Theology and Counseling," *Christian Century*, February 21, 1951, 239.

164 "Psychiatry and Religion," *Time*, April 16, 1951, 65.

165 William Claire Menninger, "Psychiatry and Religion: Both Aim at the Re-establishment of a Sense of Relatedness, of Self-dignity, of Self-acceptance in Man," *Pastoral Psychology* 1, no. 1 (1950): 14. Voicing concerns in 1947, the Roman Catholic monsignor Fulton J. Sheen declared psychiatry "irreligious." Grob, *Mad among Us*, 271.

166 Menninger, "Religio Psychiatri," 13.

167 Lowder, "Menninger Relates Religion," 475.

168 Other arguments by religious people against psychiatry, psychology, and psychoanalysis, Menninger acknowledged, included assertions that those approaches promoted a dangerous sort of self-knowledge and individual freedom that failed "to relieve the unresolved sense of the guilt of sin." See Menninger, "Religio Psychiatri," 14–16.

169 Harmon Wilkinson, "Conditions in Mental Hospitals," *Christian Century*, April 10, 1946, 466.

170 Willmar L. Thorkelson, "Chaplains Serve State Hospitals: Minnesota Launches New Program for Mentally Ill," *Christian Century*, September 20, 1950, 1114.

171 Ernest M. Fowler, "Appoint Protestant Chaplain for Stockton Hospital," *Christian Century*, January 21, 1953, 83.

172 Charles Leslie Venable, "Hiltner Stresses Role of Church as Healer," *Christian Century*, November 10, 1943, 1316.

173 Oman, "Church Help for the Mentally Ill," 100–101.

174 Seward Hiltner, "Outlook for Mental Health Services," *Christian Century*, October 29, 1975, 970.

175 Robert Drake, "Were You There?" *Christian Century*, October 15, 1986, 902.

176 Drake, "Were You There?" 902.

177 Menninger, *Vital Balance*, 408.

178 Menninger, "Psychiatrists Use Dangerous Words," 12.

179 Menninger, "Psychiatrists Use Dangerous Words," 14.

180 Later research demonstrated that stigma prevented patients from seeking treatment. See, e.g., sources cited in Nelson, "Bioethics and the Marginalization of Mental Illness," 189.

181 Hall, *Psychiatrist's World*, 800–802. There, Menninger seemed to say that Christ called his followers to accept that sort of courtesy stigma. "Jesus said," Menninger reflected, " 'Whosoever shall seek to save his life shall lose it; and whosoever shall lose his life shall preserve it.' And, of course, [Jesus] too has often been called crazy." See the conclusion below for a discussion of Goffman's stigma theory, including "courtesy stigma."

182 Menninger, *Human Mind (1942)*, ix.

183 Menninger, *Human Mind (1942)*, viii.

184 Menninger, *Human Mind (1930)*, ix.

185 For Mennonites, in contrast, whose pacifism already marked them as outsiders, little risk existed, because they already lived outside the cultural norm. They felt freer to hold on to their mission to help those afflicted with mental maladies.

    A Chevrolet advertising campaign in the early 1970s portrayed "baseball, hot dogs, apple pie, and Chevrolet" as quintessentially American.

186 This citation of Scripture is from Menninger, *Human Mind (1930)*, 440.

187 Menninger, *Whatever Became of Sin?* 189.

188 Menninger, "Religio Psychiatri," 18 (emphasis in original).

189 "The Kansas Moralist," *Time*, August 6, 1973, 62.

190 Michael Hooper, "The Legacy of Menninger," *Topeka Capital Journal*, May 4, 2003, http://cjonline.com/stories/050403/our_menninger.shtml.

191 Deutsch, *Shame of the States*, 13.

CONCLUSION

1 Stanley Hauerwas, "Salvation and Health: Why Medicine Needs the Church," in *On Moral Medicine: Theological Perspectives in Medical Ethics*, ed. Stephen E. Lammers and

Allen Verhey, 2nd ed. (Grand Rapids: Eerdmans, 1998), 82. The essay was originally published in 1986.

2 Healing, as the historian Amanda Porterfield demonstrates, has formed "a persistent theme in the history of Christianity, treading its way over time through ritual practice and theological belief, and across space through the sprawling, heterogeneous terrains of Christian community life and missionary activity." Porterfield, *Healing in the History of Christianity* (New York: Oxford University Press, 2005), 4. Porterfield names three aspects of healing in Christian tradition. Healing involved, first, "cures accomplished in the name of Christ and through the agency of" the "Spirit and saints." Often deemed miraculous, cures involved the disappearance of distress and disease. Porterfield argues, however, that Christian healing more commonly involved, second, the "relief of suffering" and, third, an "enhanced ability to cope with chronic ailments" (4).

3 Social context often determined perceived normativity of actions and behaviors. Ian S. Evison noted that broader social ethics and a sense of normative behavior shaped psychiatric diagnoses: "Before the Civil War, psychiatrists discussed whether *drapetomania*, slaves running away from their masters, was a mental disease. . . . During the suffragette campaigns of the late nineteenth century psychiatrists discussed whether the discontent of women was a form of 'nervousness' that might be remedied by a 'rest cure.' . . . During the Vietnam war, psychiatrists discussed how to cure the 'inappropriate' reluctance of soldiers to go into battle. . . . And during recent revisions in the standard diagnostic manual, the DSM-III psychiatrists have classified smoking as an illness and no longer refer to homosexuality as an illness." Ian S. Evison, "Between the Priestly Doctor and the Myth of Mental Illness," in Lammers and Verhey, *On Moral Medicine*, 828.

4 Twentieth-century debates about the permissible use of psychiatry and psychology stemmed from these lines of inquiry. See chap. 5 above for additional discussion.

5 The historian Martin Marty offers a framework for thinking about how theological convictions shape the relationship of faith and healing. Marty names four categories of responses to the question "What precisely do people have in mind when they express the hope or make the claim that their faith has something to do with the understandings of illness and health and the process of healing?" The two theistic options are relevant to the discussion here. Marty first presents a category he labels "God Experiences with Me: Empathy." Assuming a divine agent who experiences illness alongside humans, believers in this group "tend to have accommodated their religious outlooks to modern scientific viewpoints," and they "readily commend themselves to the care of those who advocate and practice the most advanced scientific medical techniques." While reluctant to affirm miraculous cures, they refrain from outright denials and "commend themselves and their fellows to the God whose love they believe to be stronger than death." Their faith provides "courage to cope with tribulation and they often triumph." In many ways, this categorization describes the approach and reactions of mainline Protestants in the twentieth century, as outlined in chap. 5 above. Second, Marty characterizes a group he labels "God Worked a Miracle in Me," or "Monergism." These individuals ascribe "all agency to a God who may withhold physical healing or may impart it to those who follow prescriptions such as praying for cures." God is the "sovereign agent," and humans have no "integral role" in affecting healing. This viewpoint, though, does not necessarily "limit humane sympathy or empathy." Instead, they "relegate to the realm of mystery any final accounting of why God withholds healing and comfort . . . or they may at times blame their own apparent lack of sufficient faith." Martin E. Marty, "Religion and Healing:

The Four Expectations," in *Religion and Healing in America*, ed. Linda L. Barnes and Susan Starr Sered (New York: Oxford University Press, 2005), 490–99.

6   Productive activity did appear, but in isolated pockets. In the late twentieth century, churches and other faith-based organizations provided a range of mental health services. Congregations provided some spiritual and pastoral care, companionship, food, shelter, and support for the afflicted. Networking and advocacy organizations like Pathways to Promise and FaithNet (an initiative of the National Alliance on Mental Illness) offered educational and referral resources. Religiously affiliated organizations—such as the Pine Rest Christian Mental Health Services, the American Association of Pastoral Counselors, and the professionals of the American Association of Christian Counselors—offered a range of medical treatments, social services, and counseling. Though effective, such efforts at the congregational level and beyond were the exception and not the norm. For an overview of these early twentieth-century efforts, see Koenig, *Faith and Mental Health*, 169–72 and chaps. 8–11. For additional information on Pathways to Promise, "an interfaith cooperative" that provides assistance and resources including "liturgical and educational materials, program models, [and] caring ministry with people experiencing a mental illness and their families," see "Pathways to Promise: Ministry and Mental Illness," http://www.pathways2promise.org (accessed April 25, 2012). For more information on NAMI FaithNet, see www.nami.org/namifaithnet/. See also the websites for Pine Rest Christian Mental Health Services (http://www.pinerest.org/) and the American Association of Christian Counselors (http://www.aacc.net/).

7   To be sure, many Christians attended to mental distress as family members and health care professionals. In those endeavors, however, faith and healing often existed in separate realms, at least overtly.

8   Instead of seeking intellectual explanations for suffering or debating the role of medical treatments, I focus on the impulse for a practical, theologically informed response. Rather than ferreting out, e.g., whether individual, corporate, or original sin is to blame for human distress, or focusing on explorations of theodicy (How can a good God have created a world that includes suffering and evil?), in this chapter I assert that an understanding of past action informs ongoing Protestant responses. Others have argued that medicine and psychiatry need the witness of the church and Christian ethics. See, e.g., Hauerwas, "Salvation and Health," in Lammers and Verhey, *On Moral Medicine*, 72–82; and Kinghorn, "Medicating the Eschatological Body." I agree, but my focus differs. I attend to congregational-based practices of Christian hospitality, sensing that until the church can attend faithfully to suffering, it has limited wisdom to offer the world. While the world at large is not the focus of my theological reflection, what the world might gain from the church's faithful practice of hospitality is insight into dismantling social stigma, stigma that prevents care and deepens suffering for many. Because individual encounters with mental distress, medical diagnoses, religious beliefs, and social interactions all shape the experience of mental illness, and each of these elements can generate suffering, I do not define a solely medically based view of illness. Instead of a focus on disease, I consider the broader category of suffering and turn to Christian understandings of health that extend beyond (and sometimes counter) medical assessments of illness.

9   With this suggestion, I draw on theologian Andrew Purves' sense that "practical theology is theology that is concerned with action: first with God's action, the *mission Dei*; and second, with the action or praxis of the church in its life and ministry in faithful communion with the God who acts, the mission of the church." God's acts are first, ours

are second, and "even then," Purves argues, they are "but a participation in the Holy Spirit . . . to the prior act of God." Purves, *Reconstructing Pastoral Theology: A Christological Foundation* (Louisville, Ky.: Westminster John Knox, 2004), xxv.

10 Thinking through suffering in light of Christian practice, I follow the lead of theologians like Stanley Hauerwas, David Kelsey, and John Swinton and attend to questions of God's presence amidst suffering and the faithful responses of believers. Reflecting on suffering and the problem of evil, Hauerwas argues, "Christians have not had a 'solution' to the problem of evil. Rather, they have had a community of care that has made it possible for them to absorb the destructive terror of evil that constantly threatens to destroy all human relations." Stanley Hauerwas, *Naming the Silences: God, Medicine, and the Problem of Suffering* (Grand Rapids: Eerdmans, 1990), 41–42, 39, 53. Considering faith in the light of concrete instances of suffering, Kelsey frames this question as "What earthly difference can Jesus make here?" David H. Kelsey, *Imagining Redemption* (Louisville, Ky.: Westminster John Knox, 2005), 1. Swinton asserts, "We can and always will speculate about why there is evil and suffering in the world and what God's relationship is to it. However, in reality, we can never know the answers to the questions that so deeply trouble us. Indeed, attempting to know the unknowable can actually create fresh suffering and evil." John Swinton, *Raging with Compassion: Pastoral Responses to the Problem of Evil* (Grand Rapids: Eerdmans, 2007), 13. In addition to Swinton and Hauerwas, see, e.g., Edward Farley, *Good and Evil: Interpreting a Human Condition* (Minneapolis: Fortress, 1990); Susan L. Nelson, "Facing Evil: Evil's Many Faces," *Interpretation* 57, no. 4 (2003); Brian Davies, *Thomas Aquinas on God and Evil* (Oxford: Oxford University Press, 2011); and Kenneth Surin, *Theology and the Problem of Evil* (Oxford: Blackwell, 1986).

11 For a discussion of the "usurpation" and "loss of voice" experienced by patients amidst medical treatment, see M. Therese Lysaught, "Patient Suffering and the Anointing of the Sick," in Lammers and Verhey, *On Moral Medicine*, 359.

12 The psychiatrist and theologian Warren Kinghorn, e.g., observed that instead of an "idealized modern science" that names and solves all problems, "contemporary mental health care involves a complicated socio-politico-scientific culture in which the cries of the distressed, the methods of modern scientific inquiry, the economic powerhouse of modern medical and pharmaceutical interests, the self-interests and professional commitments of clinicians, and the wide range of sociocultural attitudes toward madness are inextricably mixed." Kinghorn, "Medicating the Eschatological Body," 129–30.

13 Suffering carries a sense of "surdness," or inability to be fully voiced. It denotes "frustrations for which we can give no satisfying explanation and that we cannot make serve some wider end." To suffer "is to have our identity threatened physically, psychologically, and morally. Thus our suffering even makes us unsure of who we are." Stanley Hauerwas, "Should Suffering Be Eliminated? What the Retarded Have to Teach Us (1984)," in *The Hauerwas Reader*, ed. John Berkman and Michael Cartwright (Durham, N.C.: Duke University Press, 2003), 562, 572.

14 For the goodness of creation, see Genesis 1:31. As the theologian Susan L. Nelson reflects, "The earth, our bodies, and our passions, our dependency upon one another, our strengths and our vulnerabilities, the complexities of life lived in community with all sorts of creation—all of this is good." Nelson, "Facing Evil," 398.

15 The phrase "shadow side" of creation is one that theologian Daniel L. Migliore borrows from Karl Barth. Migliore, *Faith Seeking Understanding: An Introduction to Christian Theology* (Grand Rapids: Eerdmans, 1991), 89. Susan L. Nelson and others distinguish

between suffering and evil. "Evil is an awareness of," she argues, the "disjuncture between the pronouncement that life is God's good creation and the knowledge that suffering and violence are real and threaten not only life and health but also any sense of meaning, order, and blessing. Evil is the experience of suffering, misery and death, *and* the accompanying fear that such suffering undermines any hope of meaning and order in the world of a God who exercises providential care." Nelson, "Facing Evil," 399 (emphasis in original). By differentiating between suffering and evil for the purposes of my reflections here, I do not intend to imply that suffering associated with mental illnesses can never be named evil. The despair of chronic affliction can seem evil. Mental illnesses that prompt violence perpetrated by—or against—the one who ails, e.g., can readily be called evil. Despite, however, frequently overlapping coverage of mental ill-ness and violence in the media, in the vast majority of cases, experiences of mental illness can be categorized as misery more so than evil.

16 Similar to Susan L. Nelson's work, the theologian John Swinton reflects, "If the claim is true that in Christ God has overcome evil and suffering and that even now, the world is not the way it has to be or indeed the way it will be, then the problem of . . . suffering becomes both a mystery and a paradox." Here, and throughout his text, Swinton dis-cusses "suffering and evil." Swinton, *Raging with Compassion*, 1. Although suffering and evil bear commonalities, and often exist simultaneously, my work focuses on instances of human suffering but not necessarily evil.

17 Migliore speaks of the "coexistence and interdependence of all created beings." Migliore, *Faith Seeking Understanding*, 89.

18 Christian communities play a role in witnessing to healing, regardless of the infirmity. The theologian Joel James Shuman argues, "The central issue for Christians is not that illness is fundamentally bad or that God heals the sick (although both of these things are certainly true), but that God cares for and intervenes on behalf of the sick in a variety of ways." Going further, Shuman asserts, "Because God cares for and intervenes on behalf of the sick, Christians must care and intervene as well." Shuman, *The Body of Compas-sion: Ethics, Medicine, and the Church* (Boulder, Colo.: Westview, 1999), xvi.

19 Alongside this hope for reshaping Christian practice, I acknowledge that behaviors often fail to cohere with religious beliefs. Here, my focus is on the ways stigma contributes to religious incongruence. Incongruence of religious belief and practice should not be surprising; it proves as common as suffering—religious *incongruity* is "ubiquitous." The sociologist Mark Chaves notes that we should expect *in*congruence of belief and practice. Chaves, "SSSR Presidential Address Rain Dances in the Dry Season: Overcoming the Religious Congruence Fallacy," *Journal for the Scientific Study of Religion* 49, no. 1 (2010): 2. Chaves uses "religious *congruence*" "in three related senses: (1) individuals' religious ideas constitute a tight, logically connected, integrated network of internally consistent beliefs and values; (2) religious and other practices and actions follow directly from those beliefs and values; and (3) the religious beliefs and values that individuals express in certain, mainly religious, contexts are consistently held and chronically accessible across contexts, situations, and life domains. In short, congruence can mean that religious ideas hang together, that religious beliefs and actions hang together, or that religious beliefs and values indicate stable and chronically accessible dispositions in people." Religious congruence, while rare, is not impossible, and the purpose of reflective, practical theology such as the proposals of this chapter, I argue, is to highlight instances of, and reasons for, incongruence and to seek greater congruity.

20 An American framework that includes a sense of entitlement for what is "better" or "perfect" and a presumption that problems are always solvable exacerbates this phenomena. See discussion of stigma and normality in America in chapter 5 above.

21 Some physical ailments generate stigma, although of a different sort. HIV/AIDS and instances of lung and skin cancer—all ailments with presumed (although not certain) links to willing human action or inaction—serve as examples. Those living with physical *disabilities* face stigma but less frequently face blame for causing—or failing to prevent—their illnesses. In addition, the 1990 Americans with Disabilities Act, and years of advocacy work that preceded it, opened access and reduced significantly the stigma associated with physical disability. Stigma and *mental* disability are more often connected, with parents of those living with mental disabilities often being the targets of stigma, disapproval, and shunning. Because of cognitive limitations, however, those living with mental disabilities are sometimes less disposed than the mentally ill to experience shame and perceive the effects of stigma.

22 The discussion of stigma that follows relies on, and traces, Erving Goffman's account in his *Stigma: Notes on the Management of Spoiled Identity* (Englewood Cliffs, N.J.: Prentice-Hall, 1963). I traced Goffman's framework in a prior publication. See Heather Vacek, "Opening Hearts and Hands to Those in Need: Mental Illness, Stigma, and the Church," *Hinge: A Journal of Christian Thought for the Moravian Church* 10, no. 1 (2012–2013).

23 Goffman, *Stigma*, 2–3 (emphasis added).

24 Goffman, *Stigma*, 4.

25 William F. May discusses how the fear of those not stigmatized—fear of their own limitations—deepens stigma and encourages invisibility on the part of those who suffer. "Not all expedience in our treatment of the distressed springs from gross callousness; rather, we are busily engaged in obscuring from view our own poverty: by hiding from ourselves and hiding our selves. We consign to oblivion the maimed, the disfigured, and the decrepit, because we have already condemned to oblivion a portion of ourselves. To address them in their needs would require us to permit ourselves to be addressed in our needs. . . . The hidden away threaten us with what we have already hidden away from ourselves." May, *The Patient's Ordeal* (Bloomington: Indiana University Press, 1991), 150. Similarly, in a discussion of "emotion of disgust," Richard Allan Beck observes, "Disgust motivates us to avoid and push away reminders of vulnerability and death, in both ourselves and others. What is needed to combat this illusion is a church willing to embrace need, decay, and vulnerability." Beck argues that "the psychology of disgust is at work in the life of the church" and offers an exploration of how it can be acknowledged and its pernicious effects thwarted. Beck, *Unclean: Meditations on Purity, Hospitality, and Morality* (Eugene, Ore.: Cascade Books, 2011), 10, 181. Fear of mental illness—in the self or other—often prompts the sort of disgust Beck discusses.

26 Unlike a broken leg or physical deformity, mental illness often proves invisible in human relationships. In this sense, ex-mental patients (or those masking current illness) can be likened to "expectant unmarried fathers . . . in that their failing [to meet normative social expectations] is not readily visible." Goffman, *Stigma*, 48.

27 I focus here on the negative consequences of stigma, and that emphasis is central in Goffman's account. He does name, however, positive effects ("secondary gains") that are possible for the stigmatized. For example, sufferers might see trials "as a blessing in disguise" bringing valuable lessons about "life and people." Stigma might also allow

sufferers to "re-assess the limitations of normals" and realize that normals lack coping skills gained by the afflicted. Goffman, *Stigma*, 11.

28   Goffman, *Stigma*, 42.

29   With "great rewards in being considered normal, almost all persons who are in a position to pass will do so on some occasion by intent." Goffman, *Stigma*, 74.

30   The sociologist Arthur W. Frank, reflecting about cancer, makes a point germane to mental illness. "Every attempt to hide cancer," he argues, "every euphemism, every concealment, reconfirms that stigma is real and deserved." Frank, *At the Will of the Body: Reflections on Illness* (Boston: Houghton Mifflin, 1991), 97.

31   Goffman, *Stigma*, 81.

32   Goffman's third category of stigma's origins identifies religious beliefs and practices as potential *sources* of stigma. Goffman, *Stigma*, 4.

33   Goffman, *Stigma*, 19.

34   Goffman, *Stigma*, 28.

35   Goffman, *Stigma*, 30.

36   Sympathetic others (sympathetic normals) become wise by first passing "through a heart-changing personal experience" and are often "marginal" individuals. Goffman here does not refer to religious conversion or the choice to affiliate with a community of faith, but a Christian confession of God as loving creator, incarnate in Jesus Christ, seems to fit well as such a "heart-changing" experience that encourages one to become a sympathetic normal. Goffman, *Stigma*, 28.

37   Here, consider Paul's plea in Romans 12:2: "Do not be conformed to this world; but be transformed by the renewing of your minds, so that you may discern what is the will of God—what is good and acceptable and perfect" (NRSV).

38   Reference to Jesus and outcasts, sinners, and tax collectors include Matthew 9:10, 11:19; Mark 2:16; Luke 5:29.

39   Mental illnesses cause suffering whether they stem from physical, emotional, environmental, or moral causes. Here, I refrain from debating the causes of mental illness and instead focus on the suffering it brings. We might think about illness or disease as inflicting two sorts of suffering, primary and secondary. Not only the symptoms of disease (primary) but also the experience of illness (secondary) generate distress. This is the case, as sociologists Freund and others argue, because the "capacity to reflect means that humans typically suffer not merely from disease but also from their experience of illness and the meaning that they and others attach to it." A physical disability such as cerebral palsy might mean, e.g., that one is, in actuality, incapable of "normal" bodily activities, but one might also simply be perceived to be physically and emotionally limited. Such perceptions alter human relationships and inflict a separate sort of secondary suffering. In the case, above, of the young man hospitalized after his congregation called the authorities, his schizophrenia caused hallucinations and odd behavior. Then, as a result, his congregation's fear of behavior they perceived as a danger to the young man, and perhaps themselves, precipitated estrangement. Peter E. S. Freund, Meredith B. McGuire, and Linda S. Podhurst, *Health, Illness, and the Social Body: A Critical Sociology* (Upper Saddle River, N.J.: Prentice Hall, 2003), 126.

40   To be sure, Goffman wrote without Christian practices in mind, but the practice of Christian hospitality seems like the type of "purposeful social action" that he imagined had the power to diffuse stigma and alleviate suffering. Goffman, *Stigma*, 138.

244   *Notes to pages 170–172*

41   The World Health Organization offers a slightly wider description and defines health functionally as "a state of complete physical, mental, and social well-being and not merely the absence of disease and infirmity." "WHO Definition of Health in Preamble to the Constitution of the World Health Organization as adopted by the International Health Conference, New York, 19–22 June, 1946; signed on 22 July 1946 by the representatives of 61 States (Official Records of the World Health Organization, no. 2, p. 100) and entered into force on 7 April 1948," http://www.who.int/about/definition/en/print .html (accessed June 13, 2013). Part of the trouble with such a definition, of course, is that conceptions of "physical, mental and social well-being" prove subjective. Health, as the sociologist Freund argues, is "a social ideal that varies widely from culture to culture or from one historical period to another." Freund, McGuire, and Podhurst, *Health, Illness, and the Social Body*, 126. For a discussion of theories of psychiatric disease, illness, and health, see Kinghorn, "Medicating the Eschatological Body," 91–104.

42   The ethicist Courtney S. Campbell declares that medicine—in its concern for health— summons "theological critique" when health is viewed as "an absolute, the end of the human journey, rather than a value whose meaning is intelligible only within some broader account of human nature and destiny." Campbell, "Religion and Moral Meaning in Bioethics," in Lammers and Verhey, *On Moral Medicine*, 27.

43   To be sure, the opposite holds true—that unhealthiness could be declared, even in the *absence* of disease.

44   John Swinton, *From Bedlam to Shalom: Towards a Practical Theology of Human Nature, Interpersonal Relationships, and Mental Health Care* (New York: P. Lang, 2000), 72.

45   Swinton, *From Bedlam to Shalom*, 155. Here, Swinton draws on the work of Stanley Hauerwas.

46   Michael Warren, *At This Time, in This Place: The Spirit Embodied in the Local Assembly* (Harrisburg, Pa.: Trinity International, 1999), 124.

47   Mary McClintock Fulkerson, *Places of Redemption: Theology for a Worldly Church* (New York: Oxford University Press, 2007), 13–14. Similarly, talking about the early (pre-Enlightenment) church, Hauerwas notes that "suffering was not a metaphysical problem needing a solution, but a practical challenge requiring a response." Hauerwas, *Naming the Silences*, 51.

48   Rather than a comprehensive, systematic theology of mental illness, the practical, theoretical, and theological work of this chapter involves what the theologian David Kelsey names as primary, or pastoral, theology. I refer to it as practical theology, or theological reflection integrated with Christian practice. I ground my reflection in concrete human situations and seek "to throw light on the theological content, rational, and criteria of truly faithful Christian ministry" and practice. This effort involves "critical reflection on the entire range of practices that make up both the common life of communities of Christian faith and the lives of individual persons of faith." Primary and secondary theologies necessarily relate to one another. Kelsey asserts that secondary, or systematic, theology "seeks to throw light on the meaning and truth of beliefs that are inseparable from the practices that make up the life of communities and persons of Christian faith." Secondary theology is systematic in one of three ways: (1) it moves from explanation of simple to "more complex and difficult ideas about God"; (2) it attempts to show connections between elements of beliefs; and (3) "it proposes a coherent scheme of more or less rigorously defined technical concepts by which Christian beliefs can be reformulated to provide an internally coherent network of explanations" that relate to "all aspects of human

experience." Kelsey's text is systematic in the first two ways. Kelsey, *Imagining Redemption*, 87–88. A secondary, systematic, theology of mental illness is an important and much needed addition to the theological literature but beyond the scope of this book. The work of a number of theologians—often theologians of disability—heads in that direction. See, e.g., theologies of disability by Nancy L. Eiesland, *The Disabled God: Toward a Liberatory Theology of Disability* (Nashville: Abingdon, 1994); Hans S. Reinders, *Receiving the Gift of Friendship: Profound Disability, Theological Anthropology, and Ethics* (Grand Rapids: Eerdmans, 2008); and Thomas E. Reynolds, *Vulnerable Communion: A Theology of Disability and Hospitality* (Grand Rapids: Brazos, 2008); and the theological work of John Swinton (particularly *From Bedlam to Shalom*).

49   Theologian John Swinton (in *Resurrecting the Person: Friendship and the Care of People with Mental Health Problems* [Nashville: Abingdon, 2000]) calls congregations to consider how they might offer friendship to those afflicted with mental illness. He outlines practices that congregations might deploy and education they might undertake to receive warmly such individuals into Christian fellowship. In a companion text (*From Bedlam to Shalom*), Swinton presents friendship as a key to "healing" the church's response to cognitive illnesses of all sorts. His focus falls on restoring the humanity of those who suffer from mental health issues by offering them friendship within a community. Hans Reinders' *Receiving the Gift of Friendship* also focuses on the practice of friendship but does so in an effort to broaden theological anthropology in light of profound intellectual disabilities. Reinders rejects any account of what it means to be human that is rooted in an account of agency or rationality, "skills" that the most severely disabled do not, and will not, possess. Writing primarily about physical disability, Nancy Eiesland proposes a reconsideration of the "body practices of the church," including the laying on of hands and the Eucharist. Noting that "for many people with disabilities, the Eucharist is a ritual of exclusion and degradation" (because of "architectural barriers . . . demeaning body aesthetics, unreflective speech, and bodily reactions"), she seeks a "resymbolization" of the sacrament, one shaped by an understanding of God as disabled. She seeks practices that liberate disabled persons from exclusion and a broadened understanding of God for both the bodily disabled and the able. Eiesland, *Disabled God*, 113, 90–93.

50   Hospitality serves "as a framework [that] provides a bridge which connects our theology with daily life and concern." Christine D. Pohl, *Making Room: Recovering Hospitality as a Christian Tradition* (Grand Rapids: Eerdmans, 1999), 8.

51   The Greek word translated as "hospitality," *philoxenia*, means "love of strangers." Pohl names strangers as "those who are disconnected from basic relationships that give persons a secure place in the world" and who "experience detachment and exclusion." Pohl, *Making Room*, 13.

52   Henri J. M. Nouwen argues that hospitality is more than "sweet soft kindness, tea parties, bland conversation and a general atmosphere of coziness." Nouwen, *Reaching Out: The Three Movements of the Spiritual Life* (Garden City, N.Y.: Image Books, 1986), 66. Christine Pohl cites Henri Nouwen's *Reaching Out* and credits Nouwen with "a significant contribution to the recovery of hospitality" in the late twentieth century. See Pohl, *Making Room*, 3. Nouwen names hospitality "a fundamental attitude toward our fellow human being." Nouwen, *Reaching Out*, 67.

53   Pohl, *Making Room*, 15.

54   Letty M. Russell, *Just Hospitality: God's Welcome in a World of Difference*, ed. Kate M. Ott and J. Shannon-Clarkson (Louisville, Ky.: Westminster John Knox, 2009), 2. Russell

names hospitality a "calling and challenge." While I adopt Russell's definition of hospitality, my goal in discussing hospitality differs from hers in one important way. Russell challenges Christians to welcome strangers—individuals made strange by race, class, gender, nationality, and sexuality. She affirms such differences amidst Christian unity, and she hopes individuals are welcomed while able to maintain their distinctness. Not discounting her aims, mine differ slightly. The difference generated by mental illness is another sort of strangeness. Rather than a reality—a difference—to be named "good," mental illness causes suffering. In addition, the resulting stigma is what the practice of hospitality seeks to overcome. I hope that those living with mental illness will be welcomed and cared for and that illness and especially stigma need not be defining features of their created nature.

55 Russell, *Just Hospitality*, 18.

56 As the theologian Amos Yong argues, it is through "hospitable interactions that the church in turn experiences the redemptive work of God in anticipation of the coming Kingdom." Yong, *Hospitality and the Other: Pentecost, Christian Practices, and the Neighbor* (Maryknoll, N.Y.: Orbis Books, 2008), 100. A wide range of assessments of Christian hospitality appeared in the twenty-first century; a sample of the available selection follows. Maria Poggi Johnson's *Making a Welcome* focuses on household hospitality and argues that "hospitality can serve as a useful metaphor for other aspects of life" and can "be a fruitful way to think of one's relationship not only to visitors and strangers, but also to ideas, to people, to God." Johnson, *Making a Welcome: Christian Life and the Practice of Hospitality* (Eugene, Ore.: Cascade Books, 2011), 9. Arthur Sutherland's *I Was a Stranger* "presents hospitality from the point of view of systematic theology," by tracing how it is "founded in Christology, ecclesiology, reconciliation, and eschatology." He does so to distinguish Christian and secular hospitality and to challenge "institutionalized" practices of Christian hospitality that fail to "see the stranger 'as we are going.' " Sutherland, *I Was a Stranger: A Christian Theology of Hospitality* (Nashville: Abingdon, 2006), xvi, 77, 79. Elizabeth Newman's *Untamed Hospitality* focuses on the role of worship as "participation in divine hospitality, a hospitality that cannot be sequestered from our economic, political, and public lives." Newman, *Untamed Hospitality: Welcoming God and Other Strangers* (Grand Rapids: Brazos, 2007), 13. Amy Oden's *God's Welcome* explores human hospitality as an outflowing of "God's welcome into abundant life." Oden, *God's Welcome: Hospitality for a Gospel-Hungry World* (Cleveland: Pilgrim, 2008), 7.

57 For a more thorough discussion of the biblical insight into the history of Christian practices of hospitality, see chaps. 2–3 in Yong, *Hospitality and the Other*. For a discussion of "Luke-Acts and the Trinitarian Shape of Hospitality," see chap. 4 in that same volume.

58 Pohl, *Making Room*, 16.

59 Yong asserts, e.g., "Jesus characterizes the hospitality of God in part as the exemplary recipient of hospitality" throughout his life and ministry. See, e.g., Jesus as a guest of Simon Peter (Luke 4:38–39), Levi (Luke 5:29), Martha (Luke 10:38), and Zacchaeus (Luke 19:5). Yong, *Hospitality and the Other*, 100.

60 Pohl, *Making Room*, 5, 6. The early church, "partly in continuity with Hebrew understandings of hospitality that associated it with God, covenant, and blessing, and partly in contrast to Hellenistic practices which associated it with benefit and reciprocity . . . pressed hospitality outward toward the weakest, those least likely to reciprocate" (17).

61 For Pohl's argument about the loss of a moral dimension to hospitality, see Pohl, *Making Room*, 4. Pohl calls for reclaiming earlier moral urgency in the provision of hospitality.

62 In imagining the contours of hospitality, a more general definition of practice offers a helpful framework. Here, I use the moral philosopher Alasdair C. MacIntyre's definition of a practice as "any coherent and complex form of socially established cooperative human activity through which goods internal to that form of activity are realized in the course of trying to achieve those standards of excellence which are appropriate to, and partially definitive of, that form of activity, with the result that human power to achieve excellence, and human conceptions of the ends and good involved, are systematically extended." In this sense, practice is more than a simple task or activity—it is complex. But it is also coherent—practice, in the MacIntyrian sense, contains a certain internal logic. MacIntyre attests that the performance of practice can be measured against a standard of excellence at any point in time. In the case of the Christian practice of hospitality, Scripture and tradition form the basis of that standard of excellence. Simultaneously, a practice continues to evolve and change as it strives to achieve and then extend the good that results from doing so. Practice, for MacIntyre, moves toward a goal or telos. MacIntyre, *After Virtue: A Study in Moral Theory* (Notre Dame, Ind.: University of Notre Dame Press, 1984), 187. To be sure, alternative definitions of practice exist, and definitions are not always mutually exclusive. See Ted Smith's comparison of MacIntyre's definition with Pierre Bourdieu's conception of practice as "regulated improvisation," in Ted A. Smith and David D. Daniels III, "History, Practice, and Theological Education," in *For Life Abundant: Practical Theology, Theological Education, and Christian Ministry*, ed. Dorothy C. Bass and Craig R. Dykstra (Grand Rapids: Eerdmans, 2008), 217n2.

63 What makes a practice uniquely Christian? We might say that a practice is Christian when it is cooperative activity undertaken by Christians, but this is not sufficient. In addition to Christian participants, the standards of excellence that define both the activity and the goal against which excellence is measured must be rooted in Christian Scripture and tradition. Dorothy C. Bass states this in the following way: "To be called 'Christian,' a practice must pursue a good beyond itself, responding to and embodying the self-giving dynamics of God's own creating, redeeming, and sustaining grace." Bass, "Ways of Life Abundant," in Bass and Dykstra, *For Life Abundant*, 30. Christianity provides a specific understanding of telos—a telos of humanity's communion with God made possible through the birth, life, death, and resurrection of Christ. (This is a broader assertion of the telos noted in my discussion of healing.) Because of sin, humans and human activity exist at a distance from this telos. But, through participation in practice, that distance may be bridged. A social group might define other teloi. In the face of mental illness, a sociological view might seek to eliminate conditions that diminish "life chances" such as educational attainment and professional advancement. Those alternate "ends" are not inherently bad, but they fail to cohere with a Christian notion of telos.

64 "Communities engage in . . . practices forever imperfectly—faltering, forgetting, even falling into gross distortions." As theologian Dorothy Bass recommends, inherent imperfection calls for "theological discernment, repentance, and renewal" as "necessary dimensions" of practices and of "Christian life as a whole." Bass, "Ways of Life Abundant," in Bass and Dykstra, *For Life Abundant*, 29.

65 Goffman observes, "The stigmatized individual may find that he feels unsure of how we normals will identify him and receive him." Goffman, *Stigma*, 13.

66 Migliore, *Faith Seeking Understanding*, 88.

67 "Hospitality is a gift offered without preconditions and expectations, [it is] an emblem of openness to the other." Reynolds, *Vulnerable Communion*, 20.

68   Hauerwas claims, "Only a community that is pledged not to fear the stranger—and ill-
      ness always makes us a stranger to ourselves and others—can welcome the continued
      presence of the ill in our midst." Hauerwas, "Salvation and Health," in Lammers and
      Verhey, *On Moral Medicine*, 82. At times, host and guest hold unequal social power, with
      host often holding more. This invites the host to be aware of the imbalance of power
      (resources, ability to be in communication with outsiders, etc.) and attempt to keep those
      power differentials from deforming practice.

69   See the editors' introduction to chapter 8 in Lammers and Verhey, *On Moral Medicine*,
      325.

70   George Khushf, "Illness, the Problem of Evil, and the Analogical Structure of Healing:
      On the Difference Christianity Makes in Bioethics," in Lammers and Verhey, *On Moral
      Medicine*, 38. Here, bioethicist Khushf draws on Stanley Hauerwas (see 39n5).

71   Goffman, *Stigma*, 5.

72   Swinton, *Resurrecting the Person*, 11, 10.

73   Kelly M. Kapic, "Anthropology," in *Mapping Modern Theology: A Thematic and Historical
      Introduction*, ed. Kelly M. Kapic and Bruce L. McCormack (Grand Rapids: Baker Aca-
      demic, 2012), 123. Kapic's chapter offers a helpful history of theological anthropology
      and the cultural forces shaping those developments.

74   See https://www.stephenministries.org/. Stephen Ministry offers a useful volume for
      discerning when caregivers should refer to mental health professionals. See "When
      and How to Use Mental Health Resources," Stephen Ministries, https://www.stephen
      ministries.org/stephenministry/default.cfm/1578 (accessed July 8, 2014).

75   Hauerwas, *Naming the Silences*, 80. Communal lament might include praying the psalms
      of disorientation, lament psalms where "suffering is simply acknowledged for what it is
      with no explanation" given. "The psalms of lament do not simply reflect our experience;
      they are meant to form our experience of despair. They are meant to name the silences
      that our suffering has created. They bring us into communion with God and one other,
      communion that makes it possible to acknowledge our pain and suffering, to rage that
      we see no point to it, and yet our very acknowledgement of that fact makes us a people
      capable of living life faithfully" (82).

76   For a discussion of suffering and liturgical practices (specifically, the Roman Catholic
      tradition's Sacrament of Anointing the Sick), see Lysaught, "Patient Suffering," in Lam-
      mers and Verhey, *On Moral Medicine*, 360–62.

77   "Our resistance to human vulnerability," the theologian Thomas Reynolds observes,
      "calls for transformation if we are to experience the power of the biblical witness and
      participate more fully in God's inclusive love." Reynolds, *Vulnerable Communion*, 21.

78   Drawing on the work of John Dominic Crossan, the theologian M. Therese Lysaught
      observes, "Jesus' Jewish culture," decisions about "what we eat, where we eat, when we
      eat, and above all, with whom we eat . . . form a miniature map of our social distinctions
      and hierarchies." Lysaught, "Patient Suffering," in Lammers and Verhey, *On Moral Med-
      icine*, 361. Christine Pohl makes a similar point: "Early Christian writers claimed that
      transcending social and ethnic differences by sharing meals, homes, and worship with
      persons of different backgrounds was a proof of the truth of the faith." Pohl, *Making
      Room*, 5.

79   For a discussion of liturgical practices of incorporation (a reshaping of liturgical prac-
      tices, mindful of disabilities), see Eiesland, *Disabled God*, 107–18.

80   "To care for another when we cannot cure," theologians Stanley Hauerwas and Charles Pinchas claim, "is surely one of the many ways we serve one another patiently." God's patience, they argue, is nowhere more "clearly exemplified than in the life of Christ." Hauerwas and Pinchas, "Practicing Patience: How Christians Should Be Sick," in Lammers and Verhey, *On Moral Medicine*, 367, 365.

81   Yong argues that "for Christians, the practices of hospitality . . . embody the Trinitarian character of God's economy of redemption" where there is "never any lack of hospitality to be offered and received." Yong, *Hospitality and the Other*, 126.

82   Patience also requires a particular sort of imagination. In the face of suffering, together, Christians learn to imagine the shape of redemption. "The process of acquiring the capacities," the theologian David Kelsey proposes, "including mastering the concepts, that are needed to perceive the world as created, be-graced, ambiguous, and redeemed is a major part of what is fostered by involvement in the practices that make up persons' lives of faith and the common life of the Christian community." As Kelsey demonstrates, the ability to imagine redemption both enables and sustains patient Christian practice of hospitality. Kelsey, *Imagining Redemption*, 106.

83   Stanley Hauerwas uses the phrase "all the time in the world" in a number of works. See, e.g., Hauerwas, *Prayers Plainly Spoken* (Downers Grove, Ill.: InterVarsity, 1999), 31; and cited in James Samuel Logan, *Good Punishment? Christian Moral Practice and U.S. Imprisonment* (Grand Rapids: Eerdmans, 2008), 162.

84   Here, Pohl draws insight from Jean Vanier and Ken Weinkauf. Pohl, *Making Room*, 10.

85   Pohl, *Making Room*, 10–11.

86   "Because of God's faithfulness," Stanley Hauerwas asserts, "Christians are supposed to be a people who have learned how to be faithful to one another by our willingness to be present, with all our vulnerabilities, to one another . . . in and out of pain." Hauerwas, "Salvation and Health," in Lammers and Verhey, *On Moral Medicine*, 81.

Bibliography

Ahlstrom, Sydney E. *A Religious History of the American People*. 2nd ed. New Haven, Conn.: Yale University Press, 2004.

Albers, Robert H., William Meller, and Steven D. Thurber. *Ministry with Persons with Mental Illness and their Families*. Minneapolis: Fortress, 2012.

Allen, Richard. *The Life, Experience, and Gospel Labours of the Rt. Rev. Richard Allen. To Which is Annexed the Rise and Progress of the African Methodist Episcopal Church in the United States of America. Containing a Narrative of the Yellow Fever in the Year of Our Lord 1793: With an Address to the People of Colour in the United States*. Philadelphia: Martin & Boden, Printers, 1833.

Anderson, George Christian. "Emotional Health of Clergy." *Christian Century*, November 4, 1953, 1260–61.

Asquith, Glenn H., ed. *Vision from a Little Known Country: A Boisen Reader*. Decatur, Ga.: Journal of Pastoral Care, 1992.

Barnes, Bart. "Cancer Stills Psychiatrist Karl Menninger at Age 96." *Houston Chronicle*, July 19, 1990, 3.

Bass, Dorothy C. "Ways of Life Abundant." In *For Life Abundant: Practical Theology, Theological Education, and Christian Ministry*, edited by Dorothy C. Bass and Craig R. Dykstra, 21–40. Grand Rapids: Eerdmans, 2008.

Baxter, William E. *America's Care of the Mentally Ill: A Photographic History*. Edited by David W. Hathcox. Washington, D.C.: American Psychiatric, 1994.

Beall, Otho T., and Richard H. Shryock. *Cotton Mather, First Significant Figure in American Medicine*. Baltimore: Johns Hopkins University Press, 1954.

Beck, Richard Allan. *Unclean: Meditations on Purity, Hospitality, and Morality*. Eugene, Ore.: Cascade Books, 2011.

Bennett, S. R. I. *Woman's Work among the Lowly: Memorial Volume of the First Forty Years of the American Female Guardian Society and Home for the Friendless*. New York: American Female Guardian Society, 1880.

Berend, Zsuzsa. "'The Best or None!' Spinsterhood in Nineteenth-Century New England." *Journal of Social History* 33, no. 4 (2000): 935–57.

Bernhard, Virginia. "Cotton Mather's 'Most Unhappy Wife': Reflections on the Uses of Historical Evidence." *New England Quarterly* 60, no. 3 (1987): 341–62.

Binger, Carl. *Revolutionary Doctor: Benjamin Rush, 1746–1813*. New York: Norton, 1966.

Birkhead, L. M., ed. *From Sin to Psychiatry: An Interview on the Way to Mental Health with Dr. Karl A. Menninger*. Edited by E. Haldeman-Julius. Little Blue Book, vol. 1585. Girard, Kans.: Haldeman-Julius, 1931.

Boisen, Anton T. "The Challenge to Our Seminaries (1926)." In Asquith, *Vision from a Little Known Country*, 19–24.

———. "Concerning the Relationship between Religious Experience and Mental Disorder (1923)." In Asquith, *Vision from a Little Known Country*, 15–18.

———. *The Exploration of the Inner World: A Study of Mental Disorder and Religious Experience*. New York: Willett, Clark, 1936.

———. "Inspiration in the Light of Psychopathology (1961)." In Asquith, *Vision from a Little Known Country*, 113–22.

———. *Out of the Depths: An Autobiographical Study of Mental Disorder and Religious Experience*. New York: Harper, 1960.

———. "The Problem of Sin and Salvation in Light of Psychopathology (1942)." In Asquith, *Vision from a Little Known Country*, 65–75.

———. "The Service of Worship in a Mental Hosptial: Its Therapeutic Significance (1948)." In Asquith, *Vision from a Little Known Country*, 89–96.

———. "Theological Education via the Clinic (1930)." In Asquith, *Vision from a Little Known Country*, 25–32.

———. "Theology in the Light of Psychiatric Experience (1941)." In Asquith, *Vision from a Little Known Country*, 51–64.

Brekus, Catherine A. *Sarah Osborn's World: The Rise of Evangelical Christianity in Early America*. New Haven, Conn.: Yale University Press, 2013.

Brieger, Gert H., ed. *Medical America in the Nineteenth Century: Readings from the Literature*. Baltimore: Johns Hopkins University Press, 1972.

Brinks, Herbert J. *Pine Rest Christian Hospital, 75 years: 1910–1985*. Cutlerville, Mich.: Pine Rest Christian Hospital, 1985.

Brock, Brian, and John Swinton, eds. *Disability in the Christian Tradition: A Reader*. Grand Rapids: Eerdmans, 2012.

Brodsky, Alyn. *Benjamin Rush: Patriot and Physician*. New York: Truman Talley Books, 2004.

Brown, Edward M. "Neurology's Influence on American Psychiatry: 1865–1915." In Wallace and Gach, *History of Psychiatry and Medical Psychology*, 519–32.

Brown, J. F. "The Human Mind." *Psychological Bulletin* 35, no. 1 (1938): 50–52.

Brown, Thomas J. *Dorothea Dix: New England Reformer*. Cambridge, Mass.: Harvard Unversity Press, 1998.

Bryan, Jim. "Life's Hard Questions: How Should the Church Handle Mental Illness?" *Presbyterian Life*, September 1, 1968, 4–5.

Buckham, John Wright. "What Has Psychology Done to Us?" *Christian Century*, September 25, 1940, 1171–72.

Buechner, Frederick. *Wishful Thinking: A Theological ABC*. New York: Harper & Row, 1973.

Campbell, Courtney S. "Religion and Moral Meaning in Bioethics." In Lammers and Verhey, *On Moral Medicine*, 22–30.

Capper, Charles, and David A. Hollinger, eds. *The American Intellectual Tradition: Volume I, 1630–1865*. New York: Oxford University Press, 2006.

Capps, Donald. *Fragile Connections: Memoirs of Mental Illness for Pastoral Care Professionals*. Atlanta: Chalice, 2005.

Chaves, Mark. "SSSR Presidential Address Rain Dances in the Dry Season: Overcoming the Religious Congruence Fallacy." *Journal for the Scientific Study of Religion* 49, no. 1 (2010): 1–14.

Christian Century. "2,000 Attend Institute on Religion and Psychiatry." June 1, 1955, 660.

———. "Church Offers Courses on Mental Hygiene." March 27, 1940, 427.

———. "Great Churches of America: XII. First Community Church, Columbus, Ohio." December 20, 1950, 1513–20.

———. "Growing Outcry over Mental Hospitals." May 15, 1946, 611–12.

———. "Invite Churches to Aid Mentally Ill." April 24, 1946, 517–18.

———. "Mennonites Aid Mental Therapy." May 5, 1954, 566.

———. "Mr. Goldwater Talks Sense." July 20, 1966, 905–6.

———. "Obsession with the Neurotic." May 15, 1946, 613.

———. "Offer Wisconsin Pastors Aid in Counseling Mentally Ill." June 16, 1948, 614.

———. "Pacifists Give Aid to Mental Hospitals." February 24, 1943, 240.

———. "Psychiatry Makes a Move." May 9, 1956, 572.

———. "Religion and Mental Health Academy Is Launched." April 18, 1956, 477.

———. "When the Heroes Come Home." May 26, 1943, 629.

———. "Who Needs the Psychiatrist?" May 6, 1959, 541.

Culver, Elsie Thomas. "Suicide: Need for a 'Significant Other.'" *Christian Century*, January 15, 1969, 100–102.

Cutbush, Edward. *An Inaugural Dissertation on Insanity: Submitted to the examination of the Rev. John Ewing, S.T.P. provost; the trustees and medical professors of the University of Pennsylvania; for the degree of Doctor of Medicine, on the nineteenth day of May, A.D. MDCCXCIV*. Philadelphia: Zachariah Poulson, 1794.

Dain, Norman. *Concepts of Insanity in the United States, 1789–1865*. New Brunswick, N.J.: Rutgers University Press, 1964.

———. "Madness and the Stigma of Sin in American Christianity." In *Stigma and Mental Illness*, edited by Paul Jay Fink and Allan Tasman, 73–84. Washington, D.C.: American Psychiatric, 1992.

Davies, Brian. *Thomas Aquinas on God and Evil*. Oxford: Oxford University Press, 2011.

Deutsch, Albert. *The Mentally Ill in America: A History of Their Care and Treatment from Colonial Times*. New York: Columbia University Press, 1949.

———. *The Shame of the States*. New York: Harcourt, Brace, 1948.

Dix, Dorothea Lynde. *Memorial to the Legislature of Massachusetts 1843*. Old South Leaflets, 489–520. Boston: Directors of the Old South Work, 1902.

Doniger, Simon, ed. *The Minister's Consultation Clinic: Pastoral Psychology in Action*. Great Neck, N.Y.: Channel, 1955.

Drake, Robert. "Were You There?" *Christian Century*, October 15, 1986, 901–2.

Drane, James F. "Karl A. Menninger: Psychiatrist as Moralist." *Christian Century*, August 22, 1990, 758–59.

Dunlap, Susan J. *Counseling Depressed Women*. Louisville: Westminster John Knox, 1997.

Earle, Pliny. "The Curability of Insanity." *American Journal of Insanity* 33, no. 4 (1877): 483–533.

Ediger, Elmer M. "Roots of the Mennonite Mental Health Story." In *If We Can Love: The Mennonite Mental Health Story*, edited by Vernon H. Neufeld, 3–28. Newton, Kans.: Faith and Life, 1983.

Eiesland, Nancy L. *The Disabled God: Toward a Liberatory Theology of Disability*. Nashville: Abingdon, 1994.

Evison, Ian S. "Between the Priestly Doctor and the Myth of Mental Illness." In Lammers and Verhey, *On Moral Medicine*, 828–44.

Farley, Edward. *Good and Evil: Interpreting a Human Condition*. Minneapolis: Fortress, 1990.

Foster, Lillian. *Andrew Johnson, President of the United States: His Life and Speeches*. Edited by Andrew Johnson. Sabin Americana collection. New York: Richardson, 1866.

Foucault, Michel. *Madness and Civilization: A History of Insanity in the Age of Reason*. New York: Vintage Books, 1988.

Fowler, Ernest M. "Appoint Protestant Chaplain for Stockton Hospital." *Christian Century*, January 21, 1953, 83.

Frank, Arthur W. *At the Will of the Body: Reflections on Illness*. Boston: Houghton Mifflin, 1991.

Franklin, Benjamin. *Some Account of the Pennsylvania Hospital: From its First Rise to the Beginning of the Fifth Month, Called May, 1754*. Philadelphia: Office of the United States Gazette, 1754.

Freund, Peter E. S., Meredith B. McGuire, and Linda S. Podhurst. *Health, Illness, and the Social Body: A Critical Sociology*. Upper Saddle River, N.J.: Prentice Hall, 2003.

Friedman, Lawrence Jacob. *Menninger: The Family and the Clinic*. New York: Knopf, 1990.

Fulkerson, Mary McClintock. *Places of Redemption: Theology for a Worldly Church*. New York: Oxford University Press, 2007.

Gamwell, Lynn, and Nancy Tomes. *Madness in America: Cultural and Medical Perceptions of Mental Illness before 1914*. Ithaca, N.Y.: Cornell University Press, 1995.

General Assembly of the Presbyterian Church in the United States of America, ed. *The Hymnal*. Philadelphia: Presbyterian Board of Publication and Sabbath School Work, 1921.

Gessell, John Maurice. "State Hospital Scandal." *Christian Century*, October 16, 1946, 1245–47.

Ginzberg, Lori D. *Women and the Work of Benevolence: Morality, Politics, and Class in the Nineteenth-Century United States*. New Haven, Conn.: Yale University Press, 1990.

Goffman, Erving. *Stigma: Notes on the Management of Spoiled Identity*. Englewood Cliffs, N.J.: Prentice-Hall, 1963.

Gollaher, David. *Voice for the Mad: The Life of Dorothea Dix*. New York: Free Press, 1995.

Gorton, David Allyn. *An Essay on the Principles of Mental Hygiene*. Philadelphia: J. B. Lippincott, 1873.

Graber, Jennifer. *The Furnace of Affliction: Prisons and Religion in Antebellum America*. Chapel Hill: University of North Carolina Press, 2011.

Grainger, Brett Malcolm. "Vital Nature and Vital Piety: Johann Arndt and the Evangelical Vitalism of Cotton Mather." *Church History* 81, no. 4 (2012): 852–72.

Grange, Kathleen M. "Pinel and Eighteenth-Century Psychiatry." *Bulletin of the History of Medicine* 35 (1961): 442–53.

Greene-McCreight, Kathryn. *Darkness Is My Only Companion: A Christian Response to Mental Illness*. Grand Rapids: Brazos, 2006.

Greider, Kathleen J. *Much Madness Is Divinest Sense: Wisdom in Memoirs of Soul-Suffering*. Cleveland: Pilgrim, 2007.

Grob, Gerald N. *From Asylum to Community: Mental Health Policy in Modern America*. Princeton: Princeton University Press, 1991.

———. *The Inner World of American Psychiatry, 1890–1940: Selected Correspondence*. New Brunswick, N.J.: Rutgers University Press, 1985.

———. *The Mad among Us: A History of the Care of America's Mentally Ill*. New York: Free Press, 1994.

———. *Mental Illness and American Society, 1875–1940*. Princeton: Princeton University Press, 1983.

———. *Mental Institutions in America: Social Policy to 1875*. New York: Free Press, 1973.

———. "The Transformation of American Psychiatry: From Institution to Community, 1800–2000." In Wallace and Gach, *History of Psychiatry and Medical Psychology*, 533–54.

Hall, Amy Laura. *Conceiving Parenthood: American Protestantism and the Spirit of Reproduction*. Grand Rapids: Eerdmans, 2008.

Hall, Bernard H., ed. *A Psychiatrist's World: The Selected Papers of Karl Menninger, M.D.* New York: Viking, 1959.

Hall, David D. *Worlds of Wonder, Days of Judgment: Popular Religious Belief in Early New England*. New York: Knopf, 1989.

Harding, George T., IV. "Adventists and Psychiatry—A Short History of the Beginnings." *Spectrum* 17, no. 3 (1987): 2–6.

Hatch, Nathan O. *The Democratization of American Christianity*. New Haven, Conn.: Yale University Press, 1989.

———, ed. *The Professions in American History*. Notre Dame, Ind.: University of Notre Dame Press, 1988.

Hauerwas, Stanley. *Naming the Silences: God, Medicine, and the Problem of Suffering*. Grand Rapids: Eerdmans, 1990.

———. *Prayers Plainly Spoken*. Downers Grove, Ill.: InterVarsity, 1999.

———. "Salvation and Health: Why Medicine Needs the Church." In Lammers and Verhey, *On Moral Medicine*, 72–83.

———. "Should Suffering Be Eliminated? What the Retarded Have to Teach Us (1984)." In *The Hauerwas Reader*, edited by John Berkman and Michael Cartwright, 556–76. Durham, N.C.: Duke University Press, 2003.

Hauerwas, Stanley, and Charles Pinchas. "Practicing Patience: How Christians Should Be Sick." In Lammers and Verhey, *On Moral Medicine*, 364–72.

Heyrman, Christine Leigh. *Southern Cross: The Beginnings of the Bible Belt*. New York: Knopf, 1997.

Hiltner, Seward. "Outlook for Mental Health Services." *Christian Century*, October 29, 1975, 965–71.

Holifield, E. Brooks. *God's Ambassadors: A History of the Christian Clergy in America*. Grand Rapids: Eerdmans, 2007.

———. *A History of Pastoral Care in America: From Salvation to Self-Realization*. Nashville: Abingdon, 1983.

Hooper, Michael. "The Legacy of Menninger." *Topeka Capital Journal*, May 4, 2003. http://cjonline.com/stories/050403/our_menninger.shtml.

Hostetter, Margaret Kendrick. "What We Don't See." *New England Journal of Medicine* 366, no. 14 (2012): 1328–34.

Hudnut, William H., Jr. "Are Ministers Cracking Up?" *Christian Century*, November 7, 1956, 1288–89.

Hulme, William Edward. "Theology and Counseling." *Christian Century*, February 21, 1951, 238–39.

Hutchison, William R. *The Modernist Impulse in American Protestantism*. Durham, N.C.: Duke University Press, 1992.

Jimenez, Mary Ann. *Changing Faces of Madness: Early American Attitudes and Treatment of the Insane*. Hanover, N.H.: University Press of New England, 1987.

———. "Madness in Early American History: Insanity in Massachusetts from 1700 to 1830." *Journal of Social History* 20, no. 1 (1986): 25–44.

Johnson, Maria Poggi. *Making a Welcome: Christian Life and the Practice of Hospitality*. Eugene, Ore.: Cascade Books, 2011.

Jones, Gordon W. "Introduction: Part I." In Mather, *Angel of Bethesda*, xi–xvi.

———. "Introduction: Part II." In Mather, *Angel of Bethesda*, xvii–xxx.

Kapic, Kelly M. "Anthropology." In *Mapping Modern Theology: A Thematic and Historical Introduction*, edited by Kelly M. Kapic and Bruce L. McCormack, 121–48. Grand Rapids: Baker Academic, 2012.

Kelsey, David H. *Imagining Redemption*. Louisville, Ky.: Westminster John Knox, 2005.

Kemper, Clarence Worthington. "Ministers Study Psychiatry." *Christian Century*, January 26, 1944, 120.

Keys, Thomas E. "The Colonial Library and the Development of Sectional Differences in the American Colonies." *Library Quarterly* 8, no. 3 (1938): 373–90.

Khushf, George. "Illness, the Problem of Evil, and the Analogical Structure of Healing: On the Difference Christianity Makes in Bioethics." In Lammers and Verhey, *On Moral Medicine*, 30–41.

Kinghorn, Warren Anderson. "Medicating the Eschatological Body: Psychiatric Technology for Christian Wayfarers." Th.D. diss, Duke University, 2011.

Kloppenberg, James T. "Knowledge and Belief in American Public Life." In *Knowledge and Belief in America: Enlightenment Traditions and Modern Religious Thought*, edited by William M. Shea and Peter A. Huff, 27–51. Cambridge: Cambridge University Press, 1995.

Koenig, Harold G. *Faith and Mental Health: Religious Resources for Healing*. Philadelphia: Templeton Foundation, 2005.

Lammers, Stephen E., and Allen Verhey, eds. *On Moral Medicine: Theological Perspectives in Medical Ethics*. 2nd ed. Grand Rapids: Eerdmans, 1998.

Lewis, Lisa, and Roger Verdon. "Menninger, Karl." In *The Encyclopedia of Positive Psychology*, 1st ed., edited by Shane J. Lopez, 613–14. Malden, Mass.: Wiley-Blackwell, 2009.

Lightner, David L. *Asylum, Prison, and Poorhouse: The Writings and Reform Work of Dorothea Dix in Illinois*. Carbondale: Southern Illinois University Press, 1999.

Linder, Robert Dean, Daniel G. Reid, Bruce L. Shelley, and Harry S. Stout, eds. *Dictionary of Christianity in America*. Downers Grove, Ill.: InterVarsity, 1990.

Logan, James Samuel. *Good Punishment? Christian Moral Practice and U.S. Imprisonment*. Grand Rapids: Eerdmans, 2008.

Lovelace, Richard F. *The American Pietism of Cotton Mather: Origins of American Evangelicalism*. Grand Rapids: Christian University Press, 1979.

Lowder, Virgil E. "Menninger Relates Religion and Psychiatry." *Christian Century*, April 11, 1951, 474–76.

Luccock, Robert Edward. "Seminary in Retrospect." *Christian Century*, April 26, 1950, 523–25.

Lysaught, M. Therese. "Patient Suffering and the Anointing of the Sick." In Lammers and Verhey, *On Moral Medicine*, 356–64.

MacIntyre, Alasdair C. *After Virtue: A Study in Moral Theory*. Notre Dame, Ind.: University of Notre Dame Press, 1984.

Maisel, Albert Q. "Bedlam 1946: Most U.S. Mental Hospitals Are a Shame and a Disgrace." *Life*, May 6, 1946, 102–18.

Manis, Jerome G., Chester L. Hunt, J. Brawer Milton, and Leonard C. Kercher. "Public and Psychiatric Conceptions of Mental Illness." *Journal of Health and Human Behavior* 6, no. 1 (1965): 48–55.

Marsden, George M. *Religion and American Culture*. San Diego: Harcourt Brace Janovich, 1990.

Marty, Martin E. "The Clergy." In Hatch, *Professions in American History*, 73–91.

———. "Religion and Healing: The Four Expectations." In *Religion and Healing in America*, edited by Linda L. Barnes and Susan Starr Sered, 487–504. New York: Oxford University Press, 2005.

Mason, Robert Lee. *The Clergyman and the Psychiatrist—When to Refer*. Edited by Carol B. Currier and John Russell Curtis. Chicago: Nelson-Hall, 1978.

Mather, Cotton. *The Angel of Bethesda*. Edited by Gordon W. Jones. Barre, Mass.: American Antiquarian Society, 1972.

———. *Diary of Cotton Mather: Volume I, 1681–1708*. Boston: Massachusetts Historical Society Collections, 1911.

———. *Diary of Cotton Mather: Volume II, 1709–1724*. New York: F. Ungar, 1957.

———. *Essays to Do Good; Addressed to All Christians, Whether in Public or Private Capacities*. 2nd ed. London: Williams and Smith, Burtton, Conder, R. Ogle, and C. Taylor, 1808.

May, William F. *The Patient's Ordeal*. Bloomington: Indiana University Press, 1991.

McCall, Donald D. "Anomie My Enemy." *Christian Century*, July 24, 1968, 941–43.

Mencken, F. Carson, Paul Froese, and Lindsay Morrow. "Mental Health and Spirituality." In *The Values and Beliefs of the American Public: Wave III Baylor Religion Survey*, 10–13. Waco, Tex.: Baylor University, 2011.

Menninger, Karl A. "Forward." In *Psychiatry and Religious Faith*, edited by Robert G. Gassert and Bernard H. Hall, xiii–xiv. New York: Viking, 1964.

———. *The Human Mind (1930)*. 1st ed. New York: Knopf, 1930.

———. *The Human Mind (1942)*. 2nd ed. New York: Knopf, 1942.

———. *The Human Mind (1949)*. 3rd ed. New York: Knopf, 1949.

———. *Man against Himself*. New York: Harcourt, Brace, 1938.

———. "The Minister's Consultation Clinic." *Pastoral Psychology* 7, no. 1 (1956): 5.

———. "Psychiatrists Use Dangerous Words." *Saturday Evening Post*, April 25, 1964.

———. "Religio Psychiatri." *Pastoral Psychology* 2, no. 16 (1951): 10–18.

———. *The Selected Correspondence of Karl A. Menninger, 1946–1965*. Edited by Howard J. Faulkner and Virginia D. Pruitt. Columbia: University of Missouri Press, 1995.

————. *The Vital Balance: The Life Process in Mental Health and Illness*. New York: Viking, 1964.

————. *Whatever Became of Sin?* New York: Hawthorn Books, 1973.

Menninger, Roy W. "The Legacy of Menninger." *Bulletin of the Menninger Clinic* 66, no. 4 (2002): 353–61.

Menninger, William Claire. "Psychiatry and Religion: Both Aim at the Re-establishment of a Sense of Relatedness, of Self-dignity, of Self-acceptance in Man." *Pastoral Psychology* 1, no. 1 (1950): 14–16.

Menninger, W. Walter, M.D. "Contributions of Dr. William C. Menninger to Military Psychiatry." *Bulletin of the Menninger Clinic* 68, no. 4 (2004): 277–96.

Meyer, Donald B. *The Positive Thinkers: Popular Religious Psychology from Mary Baker Eddy to Norman Vincent Peale and Ronald Reagan*. Middletown, Conn.: Wesleyan University Press, 1988.

Migliore, Daniel L. *Faith Seeking Understanding: An Introduction to Christian Theology*. Grand Rapids: Eerdmans, 1991.

Miller, Perry. *The New England Mind: From Colony to Province*. Cambridge, Mass.: Harvard University Press, 1953.

————. *The New England Mind: The Seventeenth Century*. Cambridge, Mass.: Harvard University Press, 1954.

Moss, David M. "Karl Menninger: A Centennial Tribute." *Journal of Religion and Health* 32, no. 4 (1993): 253–59.

Myers-Shirk, Susan E. *Helping the Good Shepherd: Pastoral Counselors in a Psychotherapeutic Culture, 1925–1975*. Baltimore: Johns Hopkins University Press, 2009.

Nelson, John Oliver. "Trends toward a Relevant Ministry." *Christian Century*, April 26, 1950, 525–27.

Nelson, J. R. "Bioethics and the Marginalization of Mental Illness." *Journal of the Society of Christian Ethics* 23, no. 2 (2003): 179–97.

Nelson, Susan L. "Facing Evil: Evil's Many Faces." *Interpretation* 57, no. 4 (2003): 398–413.

Neufeld, Vernon H. *If We Can Love: The Mennonite Mental Health Story*. Newton, Kans.: Faith and Life, 1983.

Newman, Elizabeth. *Untamed Hospitality: Welcoming God and Other Strangers*. Grand Rapids: Brazos, 2007.

New York Times. "Rev. Seward Hiltner, 74, Dies; Taught at Princeton Seminary." November 28, 1984.

Niebuhr, H. Richard. *The Kingdom of God in America*. Middletown, Conn.: Wesleyan University Press, 1988.

Noll, Mark A. "The Rise and Long Life of Protestant Enlightenment in America." In *Knowledge and Belief in America: Enlightenment Traditions and Modern Religious Thought*, edited by William M. Shea and Peter A. Huff, 88–124. Cambridge: Cambridge University Press, 1995.

North, Carol, and William M. Clements. "The Psychiatric Diagnosis of Anton Boisen: From Schizophrenia to Bipolar Affective Disorder." In Asquith, *Vision from a Little Known Country*, 213–28.

Nouwen, Henri J. M. "Anton T. Boisen and Theology through Living Human Documents (1968)." In Asquith, *Vision from a Little Known Country*, 157–75.

———. *Reaching Out: The Three Movements of the Spiritual Life*. Garden City, N.Y.: Image Books, 1986.

Numbers, Ronald L. "The Fall and Rise of the American Medical Profession." In Hatch, *Professions in American History*, 51–72.

Numbers, Ronald L., and Darrel W. Amundsen. *Caring and Curing: Health and Medicine in the Western Religious Traditions*. 2nd ed. Baltimore: Johns Hopkins University Press, 1998.

Oden, Amy. *God's Welcome: Hospitality for a Gospel-Hungry World*. Cleveland: Pilgrim, 2008.

Oman, John B. "Church Help for the Mentally Ill." *Christian Century*, January 23, 1952, 100–101.

Orians, George Harrison, ed. *Days of Humiliation: Times of Affliction and Disaster; Nine Sermons for Restoring Favor with an Angry God (1696–1727)*. Gainsville, Fla.: Scholars' Facsimiles & Reprints, 1970.

Phelan, Jo C., Bruce G. Link, Ann Stueve, and Bernice A. Pescosolido. "Public Conceptions of Mental Illness in 1950 and 1996: What Is Mental Illness and Is It to Be Feared?" *Journal of Health and Social Behavior* 41, no. 2 (2000): 188–207.

Pohl, Christine D. *Making Room: Recovering Hospitality as a Christian Tradition*. Grand Rapids: Eerdmans, 1999.

Porterfield, Amanda. *Healing in the History of Christianity*. New York: Oxford University Press, 2005.

Powell, Robert Charles. *Anton T. Boisen, 1876–1965: "Breaking an Opening in the Wall between Religion and Medicine."* AMHC Forum. Buffalo: Association of Mental Health Clergy, 1976.

Presbyterian Life. "Church Club Helps Discharged Mental Patients." December 15, 1959, 31.

Pruden, Edward Hughes. "Nerves of Defense Workers Crack: Psychiatrist Condemns Capital Strain." *Christian Century*, April 1, 1942, 440.

Pruyser, Paul W. "Religio Medici: Karl A. Menninger, Calvinism and the Presbyterian Church." *Journal of Presbyterian History* 59 (1981): 59–72.

Purves, Andrew. *Reconstructing Pastoral Theology: A Christological Foundation*. Louisville, Ky.: Westminster John Knox, 2004.

Reese, Justin G. "Sick Minds Are a Community Problem." *Christian Century*, June 18, 1947, 766–68.

Reinders, Hans S. *Receiving the Gift of Friendship: Profound Disability, Theological Anthropology, and Ethics*. Grand Rapids: Eerdmans, 2008.

Reiss, Benjamin. *Theaters of Madness: Insane Asylums and Nineteenth-Century American Culture*. Chicago: University of Chicago Press, 2008.

Reiss, Oscar. *Medicine in Colonial America*. Lanham, Md.: University Press of America, 2000.

Reynolds, Thomas E. *Vulnerable Communion: A Theology of Disability and Hospitality*. Grand Rapids: Brazos, 2008.

Richardson, Tim. "Menninger through the Years." *Topeka-Capital Journal*. http:// cjonline.com/indepth/menninger/stories/100100_menninger.shtml (accessed February 14, 2012).

Rothman, David J. *Conscience and Convenience: The Asylum and Its Alternatives in Progressive America*. New York: Aldine de Gruyter, 2002.

Rothstein, William G. *American Physicians in the Nineteenth Century: From Sects to Science*. Baltimore: Johns Hopkins University Press, 1985.

Roukema, Richard W. *Counseling for the Soul in Distress: What Every Religious Counselor Should Know about Emotional and Mental Illness*. New York: Haworth Pastoral, 2003.

Rush, Benjamin. *The Autobiography of Benjamin Rush: His "Travels through Life" together with His Commonplace Book for 1789–1813*. Edited by George Washington Corner. Princeton: Princeton University Press for the American Philosophical Society, 1948.

———. Letters from Rush to Board of Managers of Pennsylvania Hospital dated November 11, 1789; April 30, 1798; and September 24, 1810. In "Letters of Benjamin Rush on the Treatment of Insanity at the Pennsylvania Hospital." *American Journal of Insanity* 58, no. 1 (1901): 193–96.

———. *Medical Inquiries and Observations upon the Diseases of the Mind*. 1812. 4th ed., Philadelphia: John Grigg, 1830.

Russell, Letty M. *Just Hospitality: God's Welcome in a World of Difference*. Edited by Kate M. Ott and J. Shannon-Clarkson. Louisville, Ky.: Westminster John Knox, 2009.

Shryock, Richard H. *Medicine in America: Historical Essays*. Baltimore: Johns Hopkins University Press, 1966.

Shuman, Joel James. *The Body of Compassion: Ethics, Medicine, and the Church*. Boulder, Colo.: Westview, 1999.

Silva, Cristobal. *Miraculous Plagues: An Epidemiology of Early New England Narrative*. New York: Oxford University Press, 2011.

Silverman, Kenneth. *The Life and Times of Cotton Mather*. New York: Harper & Row, 1984.

Simpson, Amy. *Troubled Minds: Mental Illness and the Church's Mission*. Downers Grove, Ill.: IVP Books, 2013.

Smith, Ted A., and David D. Daniels III. "History, Practice, and Theological Education." In *For Life Abundant: Practical Theology, Theological Education, and Christian Ministry*, edited by Dorothy C. Bass and Craig R. Dykstra, 214–40. Grand Rapids: Eerdmans, 2008.

Solberg, Winton U. "Science and Religion in Early America: Cotton Mather's 'Christian Philosopher.'" *Church History* 56, no. 1 (1987): 73–92.

Stamm, Ira. "Menninger Has a Distinguished Past but What Is Its Future?" *Topeka-Capital Journal*. http://cjonline.com/indepth/menninger/stories/010602_bus_menninger.shtml (accessed February 14, 2012).

Stevens, Rosemary. *American Medicine and the Public Interest*. Berkeley: University of California Press, 1998.

Stout, Harry S. "The Life and Times of Cotton Mather." *Reformed Journal* 35, no. 8 (1985): 23–25.

Stroup, Herbert H. "Keeping Sane in a Crazy World." *Christian Century*, September 18, 1959, 1338–40.

Surin, Kenneth. *Theology and the Problem of Evil*. Oxford: Blackwell, 1986.

Sutherland, Arthur. *I Was a Stranger: A Christian Theology of Hospitality*. Nashville: Abingdon, 2006.

Swinton, John. *From Bedlam to Shalom: Towards a Practical Theology of Human Nature, Interpersonal Relationships, and Mental Health Care*. New York: P. Lang, 2000.

———. *Raging with Compassion: Pastoral Responses to the Problem of Evil*. Grand Rapids: Eerdmans, 2007.

———. *Resurrecting the Person: Friendship and the Care of People with Mental Health Problems*. Nashville: Abingdon, 2000.

Tanaka, Hideo. "The Scottish Enlightenment and Its Influence on the American Enlightenment." *Kyoto Economic Review* 79, no. 1 (2010): 16–39.

Tanner, Kathryn. "Christian Claims: How My Mind Has Changed." *Christian Century*, February 23, 2010, 40–45.

Taves, Ann. *Fits, Trances, & Visions: Experiencing Religion and Explaining Experience from Wesley to James*. Princeton: Princeton University Press, 1999.

Thorkelson, Willmar L. "Chaplains Serve State Hospitals: Minnesota Launches New Program for Mentally Ill." *Christian Century*, September 20, 1950, 1114–15.

Tiffany, Francis. *Life of Dorothea Lynde Dix*. 1891. 13th ed., Boston: Houghton Mifflin, 1918.

Time. "The Kansas Moralist." August 6, 1973, 2.

———. "Psychiatry and Religion." April 16, 1951, 65–66.

Tomes, Nancy. *A Generous Confidence: Thomas Story Kirkbride and the Art of Asylum-Keeping, 1840–1883*. New York: Cambridge University Press, 1984.

———. "Notes and Documents: The Domesticated Madman; Changing Concepts of Insanity at the Pennsylvania Hospital, 1780–1830." *Pennsylvania Magazine of History and Biography* 106, no. 2 (1982): 271–86.

Trimmer, James Maurice. "C.O.'s Bring Reforms in Mental Hospitals." *Christian Century*, September 22, 1943, 1082.

Upham, Thomas C. *Outlines of Imperfect and Disordered Mental Action*. New York: Harper & Brothers, 1855.

Vacek, Heather. "Opening Hearts and Hands to Those in Need: Mental Illness, Stigma, and the Church." *Hinge: A Journal of Christian Thought for the Moravian Church* 10, no. 1 (2012–2013): 3–13.

Venable, Charles Leslie. "Call for Reform in Institutions: Chicago Ministers Urge Congregations to Work for Improvement in State Hospitals for Mentally Ill." *Christian Century*, June 11, 1947, 748.

———. "Hiltner Stresses Role of Church as Healer." *Christian Century*, November 10, 1943, 1316.

———. "Launch Campaign for Mentally Ill." *Christian Century*, April 23, 1947, 531–32.

———. "Modernize Treatment of Mental Illness." *Christian Century*, August 11, 1943, 926.

Verheyden, Clyde J. "Healing the Whole Man." *Christian Century*, August 6, 1952, 901.

Wallace, Edwin R., and John Gach, eds. *History of Psychiatry and Medical Psychology: With an Epilogue on Psychiatry and the Mind-Body Relation*. New York: Springer, 2008.

Wallerstein, Robert. "Karl A. Menninger, M.D.: A Personal Perspective." *American Imago* 64, no. 2 (2007): 213–28.

Walton, O. M. "Pacifists Protest Beating of Insane: Conscientious Objectors Are Discharged from Ohio Hospital." *Christian Century*, December 8, 1943, 1451–52.

Warner, Margaret Humphreys. "Vindicating the Minister's Medical Role: Cotton Mather's Concept of the *Nishmath-Chajim* and the Spiritualization of Medicine." *Journal of the History of Medicine* 36, no. 3 (1981): 278–95.

Warren, Michael. *At This Time, in This Place: The Spirit Embodied in the Local Assembly*. Harrisburg, Pa.: Trinity International, 1999.

Wigger, John H. *American Saint: Francis Asbury and the Methodists*. New York: Oxford University Press, 2009.

Wilkinson, Harmon. "Conditions in Mental Hospitals." *Christian Century*, April 10, 1946, 465–66.

Williams, Peter W. *America's Religions: Traditions and Cultures*. New York: Macmillan, 1990.

Yong, Amos. *Hospitality and the Other: Pentecost, Christian Practices, and the Neighbor*. Maryknoll, N.Y.: Orbis Books, 2008.

Index

alienists, 68–79, 83, 94–95, 98; *see also* asylum movement
American Eugenics Society, 138
American Medical Association, 68, 105, 128
American Medico-Psychological Association, 218n78
American Psychiatric Association, 121–22, 130, 134–35, 149–50, 154, 157
American Psychoanalytic Foundation, 122, 150
The Angel of Bethesda (Mather), 9 14, 18–19, 23–24, 26
Appeal to Matter of Fact and Common Sense (Fletcher), 32
Arminianism, 62
Association of Medical Superintendents of American Institutions for the Insane, 76, 82, 95, 101, 218n78
Association of Mental Health Clergy, 119
asylum movement: and clergy, 97, 99–100; critique of, 85–86, 94, 101, 103; and institution building, 72–73, 81–83, 86, 96; marginalization of, 104–7, 109; and medical professionalization,

68, 76–79, 83, 94–95, 98; and moral treatment, 18 49; shifts in, 70–71, 78, 81, 146
authority, 202n5; and Boisen, 90–92, 112, 117; of clergy, 14, 16, 24, 62, 72, 91, 114–15, 160, 189n53; and Dix, 56, 63, 84, 87; and Enlightenment empiricism, 31–32, 56; and Mather, 9, 14–16, 29; of medical profession, 13, 16, 29, 35, 105, 108, 123, 160, 189n53; and Menninger, 122, 148; shifts in, 6, 17, 13, 57, 68, 98, 100, 102, 146, 148

back places, 167
Baglivi, Gjuro, 186n24
Bancroft, Aaron, 64–65
baptism, 168, 176, 178
Batchelder, Alice, 93–94, 109, 119
"Bedlam 1946," 130
benevolence societies, 56
Bernard, Claude, 233n114
Bethlehem Hospital, 46, 47, 199n116
biological causes of mental illness, 20, 29–30, 40, 42, 143
biological treatments, 41, 132

265